The Systems Model of Creativity

Mihaly Csikszentmihalyi

The Systems Model of Creativity

The Collected Works of Mihaly
Csikszentmihalyi

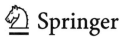 Springer

Mihaly Csikszentmihalyi
Division of Behavioral & Organizational
  Science
Claremont Graduate University
Claremont, CA
USA

This volume contains prepublished material
Name of the set: The Collected Works of Mihaly Csikszentmihalyi
ISBN set: 978-94-017-9083-3

ISBN 978-94-017-9084-0   ISBN 978-94-017-9085-7   (eBook)
DOI 10.1007/978-94-017-9085-7
Springer Dordrecht Heidelberg New York London

Library of Congress Control Number: 2014938476

Printed on acid-free paper

Springer is part of Springer Science+Business Media (www.springer.com)

Contents

Introduction to Set "The Collected Works of Mihaly Csikszentmihalyi"

In looking over these volumes of *Collected Works*, there is no question that a few themes run through the four decades of their writing. For instance, the first report of my studies of creativity appeared in 1964 and, in 2010, *Newsweek* magazine reported on my latest investigations on this topic. Other topics that I have written about, off and on over the past 40 years, are cultural evolution, play, and adolescent development. Each of these themes is vital to the continuing prosperity, if not the survival, of the human race. I hope this rather ambitious collection will embolden other psychologists to take on the big issues of our time, and laypersons to think about how to find more creativity and joy in their lives.

In looking at these articles I cannot help wondering about their origin: How did I end up writing all these words? What convolutions of the brain, what sequence of events and experiences led me to choose these topics, and conjured to keep me involved in them long enough to say something new about them?

I know that asking such questions undermines whatever scientific credibility I might have. After all, science is supposed to be an impersonal endeavor. One's history and subjective experience are in comparison trivial epiphenomena of no consequence to the unfolding of objective truth.

Yet, as a student of human nature, I cannot subscribe to this belief. The sciences—physics and chemistry, and the human sciences even more—are human constructions; even at their most rigorously abstract, their knowledge is a product of *human* minds, expressed in words and symbols most accessible to other human minds. And each mind consists of information coded chemically in the brain, plus the information collected by living in a particular environment at a particular time. Thus, scientific knowledge bears the stamp of the unique combination of genes and memes contained in the minds of those individuals who formulated and transmitted it. Hence I must conclude that whatever I have written over these past 40 years has been filtered through my own unique place in the cosmos, and that therefore a brief acquaintance with the place where I am coming from may help the reader to put the ideas contained in these writings in a more meaningful context.

I remember quite clearly the first time I entertained the possibility of leaving a written record of my attempts to understand human nature. I was about 15-years old, standing across the Termini railroad station in Rome. It was a typical torrid summer day: dust was blowing under the sycamore trees, buses were honking, trolleys were screeching on the rails, crowds were pushing in all directions. I was waiting for a bus to take me away from this maelstrom to the cool serenity of the Palatine hill, where I had been invited by a friend to spend the afternoon in his parents' luxurious apartment. I was poor—my father, who had been briefly appointed Hungarian ambassador to the Italian government, had almost immediately resigned his position in 1948, after a new Communist government had been put in power by the Soviet armies in Budapest, to replace the lawfully elected deputies of the centrist Small-holders' Party. Like many other choices my father made in his life, this had been the right one; on the other hand, he had to pay for his integrity by giving up his job and all we owned back in Hungary. We became stateless refugees in a country that was slowly recovering from the ravages of World War II and hardly in a position to help the stream of homeless refugees from Central and Eastern Europe.

So while waiting at the bus stop, I only barely had the price of the fare in my pocket. Worse than that, I felt very ambivalent about this trip. My friend was a thoughtful, kind boy; nevertheless I dreaded having become, in a matter of months, dependent on his generosity. The previous year, our fathers had been colleagues— his was the envoy of the Spanish government, as mine had been of the Hungarian. Now he continued to live the pampered life of the diplomatic corps, while I quit Junior High School in order to make some money translating and doing odd jobs. My friends and his parents were vaguely aware of my family's situation, and expressed sympathy and concern. When I was visiting, they made sure I ate well, offered me delicacies to take home, and occasionally had their chauffeur take us to watch a soccer game. None of this, however, helped salve my pride. In fact, it made matters even worse; not being able to reciprocate, I felt myself sinking deeper and deeper into a condition of helplessness I abhorred.

In this disconsolate condition, trying to avoid being pushed off the sidewalk by the cheerfully vociferous throngs of people walking towards the Esedra Fountain and the bulk of the Baths of Emperor Diocletian hovering in the background, I held one thing in my hand that was like a talisman linking my carefree past to a future that, while bleak at the moment, I was resolved to make shining again. Improbable as this sounds, it was one of the volumes of Carl Jung's *Complete Works* from the Bollinger series. I had encountered Jung's writing only recently, but was captivated by his vision. "Waiting for the bus, a question suddenly popped into my mind: if he could write about such things, there is no reason why I could not also ...."

After all, my short experience of life had prepared me to ask some of the same questions that Jung was confronting. I had seen just a few years before what seemed like a solid society fall to pieces, a permanent way of life collapse. Both my older half-brothers had been drafted at the last moment to defend Budapest against the advancing Soviets, and both were lost—Karcsi, barely 19-years old, died with all but half a dozen of the 1200 or so students of the Engineering School of the University, trying to hold up an armored division with ancient muskets just issued to them out of an armory; my brother Moricz disappeared without trace in some Russian gulag. Grandfather Otto starved hiding in the basement during the freezing cold of the 1944–1945 winter siege, and aunt Eva, just out of medical school, was blown apart by an artillery shell as she was caring for the wounded on the streets. In other words, it had been a typical mid-century childhood for that part of the world—senseless, brutal, and confusing.

The war was now over, but few seemed to ask the question: How did this happen? How can we prevent it from happening again? Of course there was a lot of blame going around, with the Left pointing its finger at the bourgeoisie for having collaborated with Fascism, and the Right explaining the tragic turn of events by the brutality of the godless Commies; but these arguments could not be the whole story, right? There must be something deeper, something we didn't understand yet, that held the keys to such irrational behavior … Yet most adults seemed to take these events in stride, chalk them up to unfortunate conditions that were unlikely to happen again. In the meantime, let's sweep our sorrows under a rug and try to resume life as if nothing had happened.

This attitude did not make sense to me. I felt that WWII had been a warning sign of a systemic fault in the human condition, one that needed a radical remedy before the Four Horsemen saddled up again. Because none of the grownups seemed interested in taking seriously this radical perspective, I had turned early in my teens to literature, philosophy, and religion, where radical perspectives abounded. Yet, I felt that these approaches to solving the mysteries of human behavior were often disconnected from the realities I experienced in everyday life; too often they relied on simplistic explanations or on mystical revelation, and— true as many of their conclusions might have been—they required leaps of faith that I felt unable, or unwilling to take.

Then, as a result of some really serendipitous circumstances, I happened to read one of Jung's books. I was not even aware that a discipline called "psychology" existed. I thought at first that Jung was a philosopher, or perhaps a historian, or one of those scholars who wrote literary criticism. But whatever he was, I recognized in his writing the passion for going beyond the conventional assumptions about life, a radical re-evaluation of culture, society, and biology that I been looking for but had not yet found.

Waiting for the bus in front of Stazione Termini was the first time it ever occurred to me that I might follow in the footsteps of scholars like Jung, and the other psychologists I had read following his writings. I should add that this epiphany took only a few minutes of that hot afternoon; almost immediately the realities of my position as a destitute high-school dropout took over. The idea was attractive, but shamefully ridiculous. I never went back to it consciously after that day, although at some level the hope must have survived, because 6 years later, when I was making a career for myself in Italy using the linguistic skills I had acquired at home and during our travels, I decided instead to leave for the USA and study psychology.

The decision to become a scholar was rather unusual in our family. On both sides, landowning had been the career of choice. Father's family also included military men and a physician or two. My mothers' ancestors included several judges and provincial administrators as well as physicians. In recent generations, visual artists—both men and women—were superabundant; among nephews and nieces there is a well-known sculptor, a children's book illustrator, a photographer, a textile designer, and the dean of the Hungarian Institute for Industrial Design. But no one, to my knowledge, had ever dabbled much in abstract knowledge.

The one exception was my mother. Although she—like most women of her generation—did not finish high school, Edith was very interested in literature; for instance, she translated Goethe's *Merchen* into Hungarian, and then into Italian. More to the point, throughout her adult life she kept adding to a manuscript she had started at the time she married my father, who had been recently widowed; it was a history of humankind seen from a Christian perspective, as a slow unfolding of knowledge that was to lead to the Kingdom of God. She was deeply influenced in this endeavor by Teilhard de Chardin, a French Jesuit who at one point taught physics to my brother Moricz at the Lycee Chateaubriand in Rome. It was mother who gave me a copy of Chardin's *The Phenomenon of Man*, a book that opened up wondrous vistas to my teenage eyes. My mother's History was a brave endeavor; the onion-skin pages of the manuscript fluttered in the candlelight of World War II, with its optimistic message seemingly grossly inappropriate given the atrocious realities. She laid her copy away in disgust several times, but then took out her battered typewriter again, to add a few more centuries to the progress of goodness on earth.

These childhood experiences—the senseless butchery of WWII, my mother's belief that history had a meaning, the evolutionary vision of Teilhard, the contemporary psychology of Jung—must all have helped shape the writings contained in these volumes. At the same time, the path that led to them was a tortuous one. Because, when I arrived in Chicago in 1956 and took my entrance exams to the University of Illinois, I soon found out that neither Carl Jung, nor (God help!) Teilhard de Chardin were considered serious scholars. Reading them exposed one to ridicule, and citing their work in a student essay earned big question marks from the teacher's red pen.

The period I spent at the University were the final years of the academic hegemony of *Behaviorism* and *Psychoanalysis*, the two currents of thought that had been ruling American psychology for the past two generations. There were useful truths to be found in both these perspectives, but by the late 1950s they already seemed more like historical relics than keys to the future.

What follows is a record of how I tried to combine what I thought were the best insights of the visionary Europeans who had shaped my childhood, with the skeptical empiricism of my new homeland. Even though I have not found definitive answers to the questions that initially motivated my investigations, I can look back on this half century of work with some feeling of accomplishment. I hope that the reader will also agree that the chapters that follow provide fresh light on some of the mysteries of human existence.

Introduction to the Volume

Art and Creativity

Preparing to start a line of research that would lead to a doctoral dissertation, I was in a deep quandary. None of the problems that were considered scientific enough to be researched for a thesis were very interesting to me. The years I had spent working at various jobs after dropping out of high school, had served to buffer me from an unquestioning acceptance of academic wisdom. Without intending to do so, I kept reading what psychologists were teaching from something like a meta-perspective (or perhaps just from a common-sense perspective). Now that I was about to become an academic myself, I could not accept academic orthodoxy uncritically. It was clear that to get a good job as a professor of psychology at a good university I should either study rats in bio-psychology mazes, or study unwary college sophomores being misled in a social psychology lab, or observe small children learning such things as object-constancy in a cognitive develop-mental lab. All worthwhile pursuits if what you wanted to accomplish was a respectable career as a psychologist. But, I felt that being a psychologist was a means to understanding how to live a better life, not an end in itself.

One subject that I thought might help to get me where I wanted to be, and at the same time had some legitimacy in the profession, was the topic of creativity. After all, much—or most—of what makes our lives interesting, meaningful, and worthwhile, is the result of creativity. And, because of the influence of J. P. Guilford, a psychologist from USC who had then become President of the American Psychological Association (or APA), creativity had just become a legitimate topic to study.

The resurgence of scientific interest in creativity is in itself an instructive story about how fads in science are swayed by political and economic forces. During the hegemony of behaviorism (roughly from 1920 to 1950) creativity was something that psychologists had no interest in studying. It was too soft, too subjective, too complicated a notion to be studied within the reigning stimulus–response paradigm that had become the only credible perspective for understanding human behavior. Neither were cognitive psychologists very interested in the topic, because the IQ and its measurement seemed to provide all the information we needed to know about the functioning of the human mind.

Then after the U.S. entered WWII, the Air Force came across an unforeseen problem. At the time, pilots were selected through variety of physical tests and by the conventional measures of IQ. Yet, as the air war escalated and ever more complicated planes were introduced, pilot errors increased resulting in tragic losses of life and equipment. What was puzzling was that high IQ did not prevent unforeseen errors from occurring. A very smart pilot, confronted by a sudden emergency, tended to go "by the book" even when the book had no solution for the problem. Hence the brass in the Air Force decided that in addition to IQ, they should also use some creativity test to screen would-be pilots. Because there were no tests to measure creativity, they turned to Guilford, a professor of psychology at USC who looked at intelligence from a broader perspective than most of his peers, to provide one.

The rest, as they say, is history. Although I know of no data showing that Guilford's tests helped the War effort by decreasing air casualties, there is certainly ample evidence that they made creativity a popular topic among psychologists. Apparently pursuing the study of creativity was in the national interest; there was even good money to be had from the Department of Defense to build laboratories and careers.

Unfortunately, this scenario is not that unusual. Even the IQ tests, originally developed in Paris for testing children applying to private schools, became the most popular psychological tool after the US Army adopted it as a screening test for recruits in World War I. It is like a page from Greek mythology, where Hephestus, the ugly and lame god, became so useful to his peers enchanted by the inventions he forged in his lab under Mount Etna, that Aphrodite—the most desirable goddess on Mt. Olympus—agreed to marry him. Everyone was more or less happy until Ares, the god of war (and therefore the main costumer of Hephestus' inventions), became interested in Aphrodite. She, in turn, could not resist a god in uniform; so while Hephestus kept toiling at his forge, Ares and Aphrodite gamboled in the bed upstairs. Thus do the claims of war often trump the honor of thinkers.

In any case, Guilford made creativity an acceptable topic for a dissertation. To make things easier, a professor in my department at the University of Chicago, Jacob Getzels, had just co-authored a book entitled *Creativity and Intelligence*, in which he and his colleague Philip Jackson reported research where they compared students high in intelligence and high in creativity (as measured by Guilford-type tests), with children equally high in intelligence but *low* on creativity. The first group was in many respects more interesting and more promising than the second, yet the latter was preferred and esteemed much more by teachers.

Getzels had developed a theory of creativity based on the concept of problem-finding. Basing his argument on anecdotal evidence from the lives of creative scientists, he concluded that these individuals differed from less creative peers not so much in the ability to *solve* problems, but in their knack for seeing new problems, and formulating these in ways that then could lead to a solution. One of his favorite sayings was attributed to Albert Einstein to be something to the effect of: a creative scientist is like a detective, but a detective who first must commit the crime that needs to be solved. This explained in part why teachers did not like creative students, no matter how intelligent they were; students are supposed to solve the crimes put before them by their elders, not their own.

With Getzels' support, I was able to immerse myself in the study of creativity. But instead of counting responses to Guilford-type tests, which I thought to be a very pale reflection of creativity, I wanted to study some actual instance of the creative process. I chose artistic creativity for two reasons. First, following in the footsteps of many of my relatives, I had myself painted canvases as a teenager, as well as illustrated magazine articles and movie posters. Familiarity with the process made it likely that I would better understand what other artists were doing and saying. Second, because the development of the creative process is much more transparent and public in the visual arts than in any other field where creativity occurs, one can follow the development of a drawing online, so to speak—the artist starts with a blank surface, and an observer can watch the creation of a work of art from beginning to end, with all the choices, false starts, changes, and new developments that the process entails. In other words, observing artists at work allowed one to study the creative process as it occurs, instead of trusting the recollection of the artist with the inevitable editorial cuts and embellishments that memory provides.

I was able to obtain permission from the School of the Art Institute of Chicago (SAIC), one of the premier art schools of the country, to use office and studio space on their premises, and to test and interview students. This work took over a year, and culminated with a series of intensive observation of fine art students drawing in the studio under semi-experimental conditions.

The data collected at SAIC allowed me to write my doctoral thesis and resulted in a book Getzels and I wrote together a few years later entitled *The Creative Vision*. The first two chapters in the pages that follow are examples of the several articles that appeared in journals during these years. Moreover, all the subsequent writings on the subject were influenced to a lesser or greater degree by this first study.

The idea behind my thesis was basically simple: to find a way to operationalize the "problem-finding" process described in the abstract by Getzels and see how it applied to creativity in art. Just to give one example of the dozen measures: I took still pictures of the drawing of the art students every 3 min (this was before video cameras were widely available). Some students' finished drawings (let's call them type A) were recognizable from the first charcoal strokes—the basic structure did not change from beginning to end. Other students' finished drawings (type B) had no resemblance to how the drawing started. Which of these two kinds of drawings, A or B, do you think were judged by experts to be more original and aesthetically valuable? Contrary to what most people would say, it was the type B drawings that were rated higher.

Interviews conducted with the artists right after they had finished drawing revealed that type A drawings were the result of the artist having a clear idea of what he or she wanted to end up with—an idea inspired by previous knowledge of art: "I wanted to convey the sense of despair that you find in Munch's paintings" or "I wanted to create a startling vanishing-point" or "I wanted to play off the similarities between the smooth surface of this bunch of grapes and the shining casing of this automobile carburetor." Artists who approached the task in this way produced drawings that experts rated less original, interesting, and valuable.

Type B drawings evolved during the process of drawing. The artist typically had a strong emotional response to the objects he chose to draw (the experimenter provided a choice of 30 objects from which the artist could choose as many as he wished to create a still life; after that point, he was told he could ignore the objects, and draw whatever he wanted). But the objects were not chosen because they could well represent art theory or history, as was true for the artists who ended up making Type A work. Instead of their smooth surface, one artist chose to draw a bunch of grapes because an uncle had a vineyard in Michigan where the artist had spent many a nostalgic summer vacations. But once he arranged a still-life to draw, Artist B would let the first strokes suggest what the next ones should be; the drawing developed organically—it was *discovered* rather than *re-presented*. Type-B artists reported in their interviews that by the time the drawing was well advanced, it took on a life of its own: the artist was solving a problem that had no known precedent, a problem that emerged out of the process itself. In other words, they were like Einstein's detective who had to commit his own crime before solving it.

The distinction between problem-finding and problem-solving is further illuminated by one of a series of published exchanges with Herbert Simon, then the only psychologist to have won a Nobel Prize in Economics, for his work on decision making (Daniel Kahneman has now joined him as the second psychologist to be given the Prize). Simon, in his presidential address to the APA, claimed that the computer program he wrote, *when given the right information*, could come up in a few minutes with discoveries in chemistry and physics that took the original discoverer years to make. From the elliptical pattern that the planets follow to the synthesis of urea, Simon's program could make one creative discovery after another in a fraction of the time it took humanity to make. From this, he concluded that creativity was nothing more than fast problem-solving.

Of course, what Simon did was to transform what historically had been a *discovered* problem into a *presented* problem. Tycho Brahe and Friedrich Wöhler had to decide what was the right information necessary to solve planetary motions and the synthesis of urea, respectively; Simon's software was handed the necessary information and the method for reaching the solution. In so doing, anything resembling creativity was leached out of the process. Chapter 5 contains one of the stages of our debate.

But the study of young artists at the SAIC had included much more than problem-finding. In fact, only Chap. 1 deals with it directly. Chapter 2 deals with another recurrent theme in creativity: the personality of the artist. Here the major surprise was that art students majoring in different areas—Fine Arts, Applied Arts, Advertising Art, Art Education—turned out to have very different patterns of values and personality traits. For instance, students with artistic talents and social values ended up majoring in Art Education, but those with high political values chose Advertising Art. Skilled artists who held high theoretical and aesthetic values became Fine Artists. This finding from 1973 is echoed in Chap. 14, published in 2004, where the conceptual framework for understanding the artistic personality is further developed.

Other sub-themes are the influence of the social context on creativity (running through Chaps. 6, 7, 9, and 13) and developmental issues addressing how creativity unfolds from childhood to old age (dealt with in Chaps. 9–11, 15, and 18).

But what probably will be seen as the major contribution to the topic of creativity starts in Chap. 3, and continues throughout Chaps. 4, 8, 10, and 13–15. These chapters develop the conceptual model and theory of what became known as the *Systems Model of Creativity*. Because this model has been widely discussed and occasionally applied by other authors, it may be useful to describe briefly how and why it came about.

By the 1980s, I had had time to digest the results of our studies at the SAIC. The findings did not sit quite well with me. For instance, in a longitudinal follow-up of the former students 18 years after they graduated, it turned out that some of the most promising and gifted young fine artists were employed in real estate, were teaching, or remodeling old houses. One was a thriving plumbing contractor in New Jersey, another designed sweaters in Paris. Although they might have been doing their work quite creatively, the promise of an independent, creative artistic career that had motivated them in the Art School had either never materialized, or had been cut short. Another instance: at SAIC women students had outscored men in the various creativity tests we used, and they had better ratings from art teachers in terms of artistic promise. Eighteen years later, not one of the women artists were known professionally or were exhibiting their work, while at least half a dozen of the men were getting to be established artists.

These findings suggested that if you wanted to know how creative products came about—how new music was composed, novel books were written, or scientific theories elaborated—knowing how "creative" a person might be was not enough. Studying individuals to determine how creative they were was like listening to one hand clapping. Creativity, I concluded, could not be understood unless one took into account the impact a person had in his or her community of peers; its causes could not be understood without taking into account the traditions from which the novelty came, and the contribution society made to the individual's ideas.

I remembered, for instance, when I was about 11-years old and my father took me for the first time to see Giotto's cycle of frescoes on the walls of the Scrovegni Chapel in Padua. For days he spoke in awed tones about the wonderful treat in front of us: we were going to witness, with our own eyes, one of the most significant steps in Western art—the transition from the stiffly anorexic Gothic style of representing the human form, to the more fluid, expressive forms that presaged the great art of the Renaissance. Many years later I did not remember much of our visit, except one conclusion I drew from it: that the man who drew the Walt Disney comics I had loved so much was a much greater artist than Giotto.

This experience reappeared a generation later. Now I had a way to understand it better: creativity was a *social construction*. The mother who taped her child's first finger paintings on the fridge door, the first grade teacher who called some children "creative" if they had a vivid imagination, the advertising copy-writer who came up with a nifty slogan, the scientist who first stumbled into a novel concept—were all called creative because someone believed the products each made were new and worth admiring. When I saw the Scrovegni frescoes I was not impressed because I lacked the art connoisseur's knowledge that provided a context for Giotto's accomplishments. The paintings looked at with fresh eyes, so to speak, were anything but remarkable. The context by which a mother judges her child's daubs is her knowledge that, just a few months before, her child had been a baby incapable of controlling its fingers; but now just look how boldly the colors are smeared across the paper!

The creativity of a work of art emerges against the background of previous art, which constitutes the *domain* of art. Past traditions are the background from which a new work emerges, and judged to be worth preserving in the domain—by including it in museums, collections, art books, and journals. Similarly, a scientific theory or experimental finding emerges against the background of the domain of science, and if considered an advance, will be added to it in its own turn.

But, the attribution of creativity is not a democratic process. When Einstein first published his papers on relativity, it is said that only four physicists in the world understood the importance of his ideas. But because these four were recognized as some of the leading thinkers of the time, their opinion of Einstein quickly trickled down to the second tier of scientists, then to the third; within a decade or so his name was familiar to men on the street. In most human endeavors, the opinion of a small elite determines what's new, what's not; what is valuable and what is not; what belongs to the domain and what should be excluded from it. This elite is what we call the *field*.

The field of basketball, made up of coaches and experts in that game, decides who should be the Most Valuable Player of the NBA each year; the fields of Toyota, Ford, or General Motors decide what new models will be produced next year; the field of pop music—recording studios, producers, and distributors—decide which new songs to release. The only domains that are truly democratic are those in the mass market, where each consumer votes with his or her pocketbook which products will enter the ephemeral domain of products to which they belong.

Of course fields are often "wrong" in the sense that later generations of experts indignantly castigate the choices made by the earlier ones. For instance, now we laugh at the nineteenth-century academic painters who were preferred by the field of art over the Impressionists, Cubists, Expressionists, and so on. How could the experts have been so short-sightedly wrong? How come no one recognized the greatness of Van Gogh while he was still living? The point is, the early experts were not "wrong" and the current experts are not necessarily "right." Walt Disney might still be remembered as a greater artist than Giotto. As our knowledge, life experience, and tastes change, so does our appreciation of previous accomplishments change, like patterns in a kaleidoscope. And less obviously, the same shifting appreciation of the field holds for the sciences: the names of men who were considered great innovators fade from memory, while those of others who were ignored in their lifetimes shine with renewed vigor in following generations.

This is as it should be. If creativity is a social attribution, it makes sense that the attribution should change as society changes. But this message is hard to accept these days, when creativity has become something of a mystical substance, a secular variant of the belief that each of us carries a spark of the divine spirit. The Systems Model is a first step toward a de-mystified, scientific understanding of how certain actions, and the individuals who act them out, end up being considered creative.

In the last analysis, however, important as the Systems Model is, being a psychologist I was most interested in the individuals whose actions lead to the attribution of creativity. What kinds of people achieve a reputation for creativity? What kind of lives do they live? An unexpected opportunity allowed me to provide some answers to these questions. One summer day in the late 1980s, Larry Cremin, then the president of the Spencer Foundation, called me up unexpectedly as I was vacationing in Vail, Colorado, and asked me if I would be interested in studying how creativity unfolds during the lifetime of eminent individuals. If I was, he said, the Spencer Foundation might be interested in funding such a study. I had never met Cremin, but his proposal sounded intriguing, to say the least.

To make a long story short, with the generosity of the Spencer Foundation, I, along with several of my student, was able to conduct long in-depth interviews with 91 individuals who by any measure would be considered creative in their respective domains: historians like John-Hope Franklin and William McNeill; musicians like Oscar Peterson and Ravi Shankar; poets like Hilde Domin and Mark Strand; chemists like Manfred Eigen and Ilya Prigogine; physicists such as Hans Bethe and Subrahmanyan Chandrasekhar; and many others of equal stature in other fields. Twelve of them had earned Nobel Prizes, two of them—Linus Pauling and John Bardeen—twice.

Out of this study we wrote several journal articles and a book, *Creativity: Flow and the Psychology of Discovery and Invention*, which was first published in 1996 and has since been translated into eight languages. The initial study also stimulated many interesting applied studies, ranging from the production of successful new motion pictures to the creative collaboration among space scientists from different national backgrounds in the launching of the probe exploring the moons of Saturn. In the present volume, the study of creative individuals in touched upon in Chaps. 9, 11, 12, 15, 17, and 18.

Finally, in recent years I had the good fortune to establish a collaboration with a young Swedish neuroscientist, Fredrik Ullen, who offered his knowledge and laboratory facilities to do an fMRI study of creativity. Ullen had been recommended by one of the creative scientists I featured in my book—George Klein, who was then the head of the tumor biology lab at the Karolinska Institute in Stockholm. So, Ullen, his student Sarah Bengsten, and I designed an interesting experiment, where professional pianists were asked to improvise a short melody while monitored in a magnetic resonance "tube," and then to repeat their improvisation. The areas of the brain significantly more active while playing in the *improvise* versus the *replicate* conditions were assumed to be implicated in thought processes of a more creative kind.

This study—reported in Chap. 16—is only a first step, but suggests very interesting directions for future research. What I found particularly suggestive is that the area of the brain most specifically active when improvising, the Dorso-Lateral Pre-Frontal Cortex (or DLPFC for short), is also very active when playing poker. Not chess, but poker. It appears to be where decisions are made when one has insufficient information to reach a rational conclusion. I cannot but wonder, do schools ever exercise this part of the brain? Children are taught to solve problems with learned algorithms—rules of spelling, arithmetic; they learn to memorize dates and names. They learn to solve problems by accepted methods. In other words, they learn to solve *presented* problems—but they do not learn how to find *discovered* problems, which requires improvisation. And this, in turn, apparently needs the cooperation of the DLPFC, an area of the brain left dormant in schools.

The 18 chapters in this volume are a representative selection from the best articles on creativity I published in scientific journals. They cover a lot of ground, and they point in several directions. Taken together, I hope the reader will find in them new ideas as well as a comprehensive view of this fascinating domain.

Chapter 1
Discovery-Oriented Behavior and the Originality of Creative Products: A Study with Artists

Mihaly Csikszentmihalyi and Jacob W. Getzels

In order to examine the significance of the "problem-formulation" stage of creative activity, 31 advanced art students were observed in a quasi-naturalistic setting of an art school while carrying out an assignment to produce a still-life drawing. Observations of "discovery-oriented" behavior were recorded for each subject from the time he began organizing the still-life objects until he completed the actual drawing. The finished art work was independently evaluated by an expert panel on three dimensions: overall value, originality, and craftsmanship. A positive relationship was found between discovery-oriented behavior at the problem-formulation stage and the originality (but not the craftsmanship) of the creative product. The study affirms the theoretical and empirical importance of the problem-formulation stage of the creative process and suggests a method for observing and analyzing behavior at this stage.

Despite much recent research on creativity, perhaps the most critical aspect of the problem has eluded systematic inquiry: the process of creative production itself. Although the literature contains numerous self-reports by people engaged in creative tasks (Arnheim 1948; Guitar 1964; Ruitenbeek 1965; Tomas 1964) or interviews with creative individuals regarding their psychological states while at work (Barron 1969; Halasz 1966), and despite the fact that the importance of understanding the creative process rather than merely recording the characteristics of creative people has also long been recognized (Ghiselin 1959; Taylor 1959), the difficulties involved in obtaining reliable observations of such elusive phenomena

---

Requests for reprints should be sent to Mihaly Csikszentmihalyi, Committee on Human Development, University of Chicago, Chicago, Illinois 60637, US.

M. Csikszentmihalyi (✉) · J. W. Getzels
University of Chicago, Chicago, USA
e-mail: Mihaly.Csikszentmihalyi@cgu.edu

M. Csikszentmihalyi, *The Systems Model of Creativity*,
DOI: 10.1007/978-94-017-9085-7_1,
© Springer Science+Business Media Dordrecht 2014

1

have left us essentially without indicators of the relevant variables, to say nothing of empirical data, regarding the *process* of creative production.

The present report, part of a larger study of artistic creativity (Getzels and Csikszentmihalyi 1964, 1965, 1966b), attempts to fill this lack by (a) delineating a theoretically derived set of behavioral variables for the observation and measurement of a creative process in a "real-life" setting and (b) examining the relation of these measures to the quality of the creative product. Although the study was limited to artistic creativity, it seems likely that the concepts and methods should yield useful results in other areas of creative endeavor as well.

Previous work in creativity has suggested the fruitfulness of a conceptual distinction between *discovered problem situations* and *presented problem situations* (Getzels 1964; Getzels and Csikszentmihalyi 1965, 1966a, 1967). Problem situations can be meaningfully distinguished in terms of how much of the problem is clearly given at the start, how much of the method for reaching a solution is already at hand, and how general the agreement is as to what constitutes a good solution. At one end of the continuum there are presented problems, that is, situations where the problem, the method, and the solution are already known, and the problem solver needs only adopt the "correct" procedural steps to arrive at the satisfactory solution. At the other end, there are discovered problems, that is, situations where the problem itself has not yet been formulated but must be identified and the appropriate method for reaching a solution and the nature of the satisfactory solution are unknown.

It would seem that creative work is the outcome of a more or less pure form of the discovered problem-solving process. Outstanding instances of creative achievement involve solutions to problems which were not even formulated as such, but first had to be identified as problems (Kuhn 1962). In the words of Einstein and Infeld (1938):

> The formulation of a problem is often more essential than its solution, which may he merely a matter of mathematical or experimental skill. To raise new questions, new possibilities, to regard old problems from a new angle, requires creative imagination and marks real advance in science [p. 92].

This appears to be the situation in art as well. The importance of discovering the problem in the creative problem-solving process has also been noted by Dewey (1910), Ecker (1963), and Macworth (1965).

If the discovery of problems is central to the creative process, then a crucial dimension of creativity is the disposition of individuals to perceive problems as either discovered or presented. In a preceding interview study, differences between art students were observed in terms of their reported perception of the artistic task. This dispositional variable was tentatively identified as *concern for discovery*, and it was found to be significantly related to the originality of the solutions that the subjects produced (Csikszentmihalyi and Getzels 1970).

The present study was designed to answer the following question: Is discovery-oriented behavior in a real-life situation involving creative production related to the assessed creativity of the product?

The form of creative production observed was the completion of a drawing. The process of producing any work of art implies the same questions that any other problem-solving task does: What is to be done? How is it to be done? When is it completed? These questions can be approached either as discovered or presented. Furthermore, the manifest process of conceiving and executing a graphic work of art can be observed more easily than almost any other processes involving creativity; the steps in the process lend themselves readily to observation and analysis in terms of the discovery model; and the outcome of the process, that is, the finished work of art, can be assessed as to its creative value with reasonable reliability. In view of the theoretical considerations, it was expected that there would be a positive relationship between discovery-oriented behavior and the assessed creativity of the product.

Method

Subjects and Procedure

The sample consisted of 31 male juniors and seniors at one of the foremost art schools in the country. Although the subjects were all in school, some had already won prizes in competition with nonstudent artists, some were exhibiting their work regularly in public and private galleries, and some had won national scholarships; all had survived at least 3 highly competitive years in the art school at considerable financial and personal sacrifice.

Of the data collected in the larger studies (Getzels and Csikszentmihalyi 1964, 1965, 1966b), three items are relevant to the questions raised in this paper. These are (a) an art work from each subject with a variable degree of creativity which could be assessed, (b) an assessment by well-known artist critics of the degree of creativity of the art work, and (c) a set of behavioral measures relating to discovery orientation taken while the subject was working on the artistic product.

Although Categories *a* and *b* above include the dependent variables of the present study and *c* contains the independent variables, for the purpose of greater clarity, it will be more expedient to describe the dependent variables first.

1. *The creative product.* Each of the 31 subjects was asked to produce a drawing in a studio of the art school under initially constant conditions. The conditions were as follows: Twenty-seven objects were placed on a table; among the objects were a small human figure, an antique book, a bunch of grapes, a polished gear shift, a floppy velvet hat, etc. Each subject was asked—1 at a time—to set up on a second table in the same studio a composition that suited him with any of the available objects. He was then to work on a drawing until he felt that it was completed, using a variety of dry media that were also made available. No time limit was given. While the subjects were involved with their task, an observer was present with them in the studio, taking notes and photographs.

Subsequent interviews suggested that the subjects saw the situation as differing very little from the free creative conditions to which they were accustomed.

Twenty-three of the 31 subjects (72 %) said that the difference from their usual free working conditions, if any at all, was minimal. They declared that once they began to work, they proceeded in their customary way. Four of the subjects (14 %) declared that the experimental conditions resembled a typical art school assignment rather than a free creative situation. Only 4 of the subjects (14 %) reported that they felt uncomfortable in the research setting. Given their straightforward responses to other questions of the interview, there is no reason to assume that the process of producing the experimental drawing was seen as essentially different from their way of working either in their own studios or in the studios of the school.

2. *The assessment of the relative creativity of the products.* The 31 drawings produced by the subjects under the conditions outlined above were given to five well-known artists and artist critics for independent rating. The judges were unaware of the subjects' identities. Each judge was asked to make three evaluations: first, on the *craftsmanship* or technical skill of the product (regardless of its originality); second, on its *originality* or imaginativeness (regardless of its craftsmanship); and finally, on its overall *aesthetic value*. (How would you rate these drawings if you were to award prizes in a competitive art show?) The ratings were made on a 1–9-point scale with a "pre-normalized" distribution.

It was expected that the three dimensions of evaluation would overlap considerably, and this, in fact, proved to be the case. The correlation between the combined ratings of the five artist critics on overall aesthetic value and the combined ratings on originality was 0.90 (product-moment correlation); the correlation between overall value and craftsmanship was 0.82, and the correlation between originality and craftsmanship was 0.76. However, as will be seen below, the three dimensions arc sufficiently distinct to yield meaningful insights into the problem of creativity. The agreement among the five judges, that is, the reliability of the ratings on each dimension, was determined by intraclass correlation. The coefficient for overall aesthetic value was 0.29 with a reliability-of-sum coefficient of 0.67; for originality the two coefficients were, respectively, 0.31 and 0.69; for craftsmanship they were 0.22 and 0.58 (Getzels and Csikszentmihalyi 1969). These correlations, although all significant statistically, are obviously not high. The reasons for the lack of closer agreement are discussed in detail elsewhere (Csikszentmithalyi 1965). Part of the unreliability is due to the purposely open instructions given to the judges and some to the deviant ratings of one of the judges, who had a very personal interpretation of what was original and aesthetically valuable. (He equated both with "honesty" and "naivete.") In any case, it must be noted that the combined score based on the live ratings correlated very highly with each of the five individual ratings, and thus it may be considered a representative measure of each artist's definition of the dimension.

3. *The behavioral measures: Discovery orientation.* The process of discovered problem solving could be observed as beginning right after the task was explained to the subjects upon their arrival to the experimental studio. Three sets of behavioral variables were recorded between the time the task was explained and the time that the subjects began to draw. These behaviors were called *discovery at the stage of problem formulation*, since they preceded actual attempts at solution.

The three separate observations were categorized and quantified as follows. (a) *Number of objects manipulated (A1)*: the score on this process variable was a count of how many of the 27 objects were touched by a subject prior to the beginning of drawing. The count was based on the record taken by the observer. (b) *Uniqueness of the objects chosen (A2)*: this score was based only on the objects selected by any given subject and actually transferred by him from the first to the second table. Each object was given a score corresponding to the rank-order frequency with which it had been used by the sample as a whole. Thus, the *book*, the most frequently chosen object, was assigned a score of 1; the *lens*, chosen by the fewest subjects, had a score of 25.5. A subject's score on this variable consisted of the averaged rank score of all the objects he selected. (c) *Discovery-oriented behavior during selection and arrangement (A3)*: this variable was scored as follows. A score of 1 was given if the subject just picked up the objects from the first table and placed them on the second table. A score of 2 was given if the subject was observed holding an object up to his eyes, feeling its weight, texture, etc. A score of 3 was given if the subject experimented with the objects, for instance, by looking through the prism and lens, folding the hat into different shapes, trying to work mechanical parts, etc. A score of 5 was given when actions for both Scores 2 and 3 applied. (d) *Total problem-formulation score (AA)*. Whenever a subject was above the median for the sample on one of the three preceding variables, he was given a score of 1. By adding these scores, the total problem-formulation score was obtained. A constant of 1 was added in order to give a numerical value to subjects who otherwise would have had a score of zero. The total problem-formulation score had, therefore, a range of 1–4.

The next set of three observations was made after the subject began working on his drawing. These variables may therefore be said to represent *discovery at the stage of problem solution*. They were quantified as follows: (a) *Openness of problem structure (B1)*. To score this variable, the sequence of photographs taken at 6-min intervals during the experiment was examined. For each subject, that photograph was scored which for the first time revealed the final structure of the drawing in all its essential elements. The score consisted of the number of minutes which elapsed between the beginning of the experiment and the taking of the given picture, divided by the total time in minutes taken for the drawing as a whole. The score is, therefore, the percentage of the total drawing time elapsed before the final structure of the drawing was essentially completed. (b) *Discovery-oriented behavior while drawing (B2)*. This was scored as follows: The subject received a score of 1 if he just drew without interruption. The subject received a score of 2 if he changed paper or switched from one medium to another. The subject received a score of 3 if he changed the arrangement of objects, substituted, or manipulated the objects. A score of 5 was obtained if both 2 and 3 applied. (c) *Changes in problem structure and content (B3)*. A score of 1 was received if the subject just copied the arrangement. A score of 2 was received if he introduced changes in perspective. A score of 3 was received if he changed the relative magnitude of objects, or left one or more of the objects out. A score of 4 was received if he changed the position of objects on the paper. A score of 5 was received if there was an addition of

Table 1.1 Correlation matrix of six discovery-process variables and two subtotals

Item	Problem formulation				Problem solution			
	A1	A2	A3	AA	B1	B2	B3	BB
Problem formulation								
A1								
A2	0.44**							
A3	0.48***	0.22						
AA	0.64****	0.60****	0.77****					
Problem solution								
B1	0.51***	0.24	0.15	0.25				
B2	0.05	0.14	0.18	0.13	−0.11			
B3	0.30*	0.34*	0.56***	0.48**	0.02	0.44**		
BB	0.26	0.14	0.35*	0.34*	0.34*	0.58***	0.43**	

Note N = 31
* $p < 0.05$
** $p < 0.01$
*** $p < 0.005$
**** $p < 0.0005$

nonexistent objects or major visual elements. A score of 9, if both actions for Scales 4 and 5 applied. (d) *Total problem-solution score (BB)*. Whenever a subject was above the median for the sample on one of the three preceding variables, he was given a score of 1. By adding these scores, the total problem-solution score was obtained. A constant of 1 was added in order to give a numerical value to subjects who otherwise would have a score of zero. The total problem-solution score had, therefore, a range of 1–4.

The reliability of the scoring of the six process variables and the two subtotals was tested by having two raters assess each protocol; the product-moment correlations between the two raters ranged from 0.82 to 0.98; none of the significance levels rose above a percentage of more than 0.0005. It is to be noted that scores on Variables A1, A3, and B2 were based exclusively on the record compiled by the observer. Reliability in recording the observations was not established; however, the variables in question are of such self-evident nature that little or no error in their recording seems to have been possible.

The internal correlations between the six process variables and two subtotals are presented in Table 1.1. It is clear from the pattern that while some of the variables (A1, B3) have a relatively high degree of commonality with the others, the overall overlap is not so large as to make any variable redundant. In other words, it is possible for a subject to engage in what appears to be discovery-oriented behavior at one stage of the problem-solving process without doing so at either an earlier or at a later stage.

There are two main reasons why these six variables were chosen to measure the theoretical construct of discovery orientation. In the first place, they are genuine variables that occur "naturally" whenever artists approach their task. Second, each variable was derived from the model of discovery orientation, as follows. The successful envisagement of a discovered problem would require that (a) a large number of problematic elements be considered before the problem becomes structured (A1); (b) either unusual elements are to be selected as foci of the problem (A2), or (c) a more usual element is selected, but it is thoroughly explored through multiple sensory channels before it becomes a parameter of the problem (A3).

The successful solution of a discovered problem is seen as requiring the following processes: (a) After the problematic elements are selected, the problem begins to be stated, and solutions are attempted. It seems important that the problem solver should not view his problem as having achieved structure too early, lest the problem fail to develop along original lines (B1). (b) As the problem is stated, various forms of solutions are tried out, some of which involve old methods, others involve the discovery of new methods (B2). (c) During the solution of the problem, the problematic elements lose their accepted interpretation —their structure and symbolic content undergo hitherto unforeseen transformations which recombine into a new meaningful whole (B3).

These steps, of course, are not intended to exhaust the requirements for a successfully discovered problem-solving process.

Results

The data in Table 1.2 present the relationship between the amount of discovery-oriented behavior observed during the process of artistic problem solving and the evaluation of the ensuing product. The results follow, in general, the expected direction. More specifically, five of the six behavioral variables were significantly related to the "originality" of the resulting product, four of the six variables were related to its "overall aesthetic value," and two of the six reached significance when correlated with the "craftsmanship" dimension.

The strongest relationship appears between discovery-oriented behavior during the formulation of the problem and the originality of the drawing, as rated by the judges. Of the six variables, the only one that did not support the expectation even in part was the one we have called "openness of problem structure" (B1).

In view of the results reported in Table 1.2, and keeping in mind the fact that the three dimensions of evaluation—overall aesthetic value, originality, and craftsmanship—share a great amount of common variance, one might question the real relationship between the discovery variables and each dimension of evaluation taken individually, shorn of the variance held in common with the others. Table 1.3 shows rather clearly that when the overlapping variance of the three dimensions of evaluation is artificially removed through the statistic of partial correlations, the only significant positive correlations that remain are those between the discovery-process variables (in particular at the stage of problem formulation) and the originality of the product. The high negative correlation ($r = -0.50$) between discovery-oriented behavior at the stage of problem formulation and

Table 1.2 Correlations between discovery-process variables and evaluation of the artistic products by five artist critics

Process variable	Dimension of evaluation		
	Overall aesthetic value (total 5 raters)	Originality (total 5 raters)	Craftsmanship (total 5 raters)
Problem formulation			
A1—Manipulation	0.48****	0.52****	0.16
A2—Unusualness	0.35*	0.42***	0.22
A3—Exploration	0.44***	0.58*****	0.34*
AA—Total	0.40**	0.54****	0.28
Problem solution			
B1—Structure time	0.09	0.08	−0.18
B2—Exploration	0.22	0.37**	0.01
B3—Changes	0.44***	0.61****	0.37**
BB—Total	0.27	0.38**	0.12

Note N = 31
* $p < 0.05$
** $p < 0.025$
*** $p < 0.01$
**** $p < 0.005$
***** $p < 0.0005$

Table 1.3 Second-order partial correlations between the discovery-process-variable totals and the evaluation of the product

Item	Overall aesthetic value (with originality and craftsmanship held constant)	Originality (with overall aesthetic value and craftsmanship held constant)	Craftsmanship (with overall aesthetic value and originality held constant)
Problem formulation total (AA)	−0.50	0.67	−0.24
Problem solution total (BB)	0.01	0.35	−0.25

Note N = 38

the rating of overall aesthetic value is probably due to the near-perfect correlation between the ratings of overall aesthetic value and originality ($r = 0.90$). Once the commonality of the two variables is artificially removed by means of partial correlation, the small residual variability of the rating of overall aesthetic value is negatively related to discovery orientation. The small amount of residual variance may reflect rater error almost entirely, thus producing meaningless correlations. Alternatively, the negative correlation might suggest that in the present cultural climate, originality is a more important criterion of creativity than what was measured by the rating of overall value.

Discussion and Conclusion

The operational measures of discovery orientation introduced in this study appear to be useful tools for the study of creative production. Of special importance is the operationalization of the concept of discovery at the stage of problem formulation, the importance of which has been previously recognized in theory, but has remained inaccessible to empirical observation.

A question raised by the present study is whether the same relationship between discovery orientation and the originality of the product obtains in other fields of creative endeavor, such as mathematics, the sciences, poetics, statesmanship, and so on. While the present study cannot shed light on this issue, the method employed here allows for an empirical answer to it, once the measurement of discovery is appropriately reformulated, so as to be applicable to problem solving in different fields.

Perhaps a word should be added to clarify our view as to the nature of the discovery-process variables. The experimental conditions used in the setting of this study seem to have brought out in the open and made observable a process which normally goes undetected in the artist's awareness whenever he is involved in the production of a work of art. Under ordinary circumstances the artist does not inspect, touch, or manipulate concrete objects before he decides what to paint, but he does consider, weigh, and analyze feelings or sensory material in his awareness. We have assumed for the purposes of this study that the two processes—the manifest and the latent—follow similar laws, and we used the former as an index of the latter. A more complete elaboration of this point has been presented else-where (Csikszentmihalyi (1965); Csikszentmihalyi and Getzels 1970). In any case, surely one should not extrapolate from the observed relationships any implication that touching many objects, choosing unique objects, etc., "causes" originality.

A less basic, but unresolvable, question concerns the universality of the findings in time and space. Would discovery orientation be related to the originality of the painting of artists living a 100 years in the past or in the future? Cultural trends wax and wane with regard to the importance allotted to originality as a component of the creative process. It could perhaps be safely said that in history originality has more often been seen as hindering rather than as fostering great accomplishment.

An awareness of cultural fluctuations in the value attributed to originality helps to point out the strengths and limitations of the concept of discovery. The attitude of discovery orientation in problem solving might not eventuate in a "successful" product except under sociocultural conditions that reward originality. The findings of this study suggest the conclusion that in a cultural milieu which strongly equates originality with overall value, an attitudinal and behavioral approach to problem solving characterized by discovery orientation leads to results which will be considered valuable; and it presents a method by which such orientation can be empirically measured.

References

Arnheim, R. (Ed.). (1948). *Poets at work*. New York: Harcourt, Brace.

Barron, F. (1969). *Creative persons and creative processes*. New York: Holt, Rinehart & Winston.

Csikszentmihalyi, M. (1965). Artistic problems and their solutions (Unpublished doctoral dissertation, University of Chicago).

Csikszentmihalyi, M., & Getzels, J. W. (1970). Concern for discovery: An attitudinal component of creative production. *Journal of Personality, 38*, 91–105.

Dewey, J. (1910). *How we think*. Boston: Heath.

Ecker, D. (1963). The artistic process as qualitative problem solving. *Journal of Aesthetics and Art Criticism, 21*, 233–290.

Einstein, A., & Infeld, L. (1938). *The evolution of physics*. New York: Simon & Schuster.

Getzels, J. W. (1964). Creative thinking, problem-solving, and instruction. In E. R. Hilgard (Ed.), *Theories of learning and instruction. Sixty-third year book of the national society for the study of education*. Pt. 1. Chicago: University of Chicago Press.

Getzels, J. W., & Csikszentmihalyi, M. (1964). *Creative thinking in art students: An exploratory study* (HEW Cooperative Research Rep. No. E-008). Chicago: University of Chicago Press.

Getzels, J. W., & Csikszentmihalyi, M. (1965). *Creative thinking in art students: The process of discovery* (HEW Cooperative Research Rep. No. S-080). Chicago: University of Chicago Press.

Getzels, J. W., & Csikszentmihalyi, M. (1996a). Portrait of the artist as an explorer. *Transaction, 3*, 31–35.

Getzels, J. W., & Csikszentmihalyi, M. (1996b). The study of creativity in future artists: The criterion problem. In O. J. Harvey (Ed.), *Experience, structure, and adaptability*. New York: Springer.

Getzels, J. W., & Csikszentmihalyi, M. (1967). Scientific creativity. *Science Journal, 3*, 80–84.

Getzels, J. W., & Csikszentmihalyi, M. (1969). Aesthetic opinion: An empirical study. *Public Opinion Quarterly, 33*, 34–45.

Ghiselin, B. (1959). The nature of imaginative action. In C. W. Taylor (Ed.), *The third (1959) University of Utah research conference on the identification of creative scientific talent*. Salt Lake City: University of Utah Press.

Guitar, M. A. (1964). *Twenty-two famous painters and illustrators tell how they work*. New York: McKay.

Halasz, L. (1966). Az iroi Tehetseg osszehasonlito vizsgalata. *Psichologiai Tanulmanyok, 9*, 367–382.

Kuhn, T. S. (1962). *The structure of scientific revolutions*. Chicago: University of Chicago Press.

Macworth, N. H. (1965). Originality. *American Psychologist, 20*, 51–66.

Ruitenbeek, H. M. (Ed.). (1965). *The creative imagination*. Chicago: Quadrangle.

Taylor, L. A. (1959). The nature of the creative process. In P. Smith (Ed.), *Creativity: An examination of the creative process*. New York: Hasting House.

Tomas, V. (Ed.). (1964). *Creativity in the arts*. Englewood Cliffs: Prentice-Hall.

Chapter 2
The Personality of Young Artists: An Empirical and Theoretical Exploration

Mihaly Csikszentmihalyi and Jacob W. Getzels

Despite venerable stereotypes and even some recent empirical observations regarding the personality of artists, the following questions remain unanswered in any objective way: (1) Do personality factors differentiate art students from other students of the same age and sex? (2) Is there a relationship between the personality of art students and the values they hold? (3) Are there differences in the personality factors of art students in tha several fields of specialization, e.g. commercial art *v.* fine art? (4) Is there a relationship between the personality factors of art students and their performance in art school? (5) Finally, what is the relationship between the personality factors of successful young artists and eminent scientists, both groups presumably engaged in creative endeavour? The present investigation of a sample of 205 advanced art students applied Cattel's 16 Personality Factor Questionnaire supplemented by the Allport–Vernon–Lindzey Study of Values in an attempt to answer these questions. The findings are placed in a tentative theoretical framework regarding the personality of artists and the expectations of their professional role.

Artists have been viewed with suspicion for at least four centuries, i.e. since the time of the Renaissance historian Vasari, who wrote that the artists he knew all shared an 'element of savagery and madness' (1550, 1959 ed., p. 232). Paradoxically, the disturbing qualities attributed to artists are also believed to fulfil a positive function. As Hauser (1960, p. 325) suggests, these qualities have been widely held a necessary component of creativity.

But does this paradoxical image of the artist have any basis in reality? And if it does, are the 'negative' factors in the artist's personality necessary to the performance of his task *qua* artist, or are they simply accidental by-products of his vocation? These are the two main general questions to be explored empirically and

M. Csikszentmihalyi (✉) · J. W. Getzels
Committee on Human Development, and Departments of Education
and Psychology, University of Chicago, Chicago, IL, USA
e-mail: Mihaly.Csikszentmihalyi@cgu.edu

M. Csikszentmihalyi, *The Systems Model of Creativity*,
DOI: 10.1007/978-94-017-9085-7_2,
© Springer Science+Business Media Dordrecht 2014

theoretically in this paper. In so doing we hope not only to clarify some central issues of creativity, but also to delineate some connections between personality traits and culturally defined requirements for role performance in art.

The psychological literature already contains many studies dealing with the artist's personality; for instance, those by Kris (1952), Roe (1946), Anderson (1959, 1960), Barbon (1969), Cross et al. (1967). Most of this work, however, has focused on professional and often eminent artists who had long since been settled in their careers; and, with the exception of the study by Cross et al., the data tend to consist of depth-psychological material not amenable to comparative or quantifiable analysis.

Ours is an attempt to contribute to the literature by applying normative personality instruments to a sample of young artists who are at the intermediate stage between being students and professionals. Although still in school, a number of them were already selling and exhibiting their work professionally, and winning prizes and commissions in the process. The relative advantage of such a sample (while also having some obvious limitations) is that it allows the study of fledgling artists before their answers on personality tests might have changed as a result of long-term identification with the established artist's way of life; it allows comparisons with other young people of the same sex and educational level; it allows comparisons between more successful and less successful young artists as defined by the training institution, thus contributing to an understanding of the selective factors operating in the *process* of becoming an artist; and finally, it allows comparisons among a large number of young artists who have had relatively similar formal training and exposure to art.

Method

Sample and Procedure

The study was conducted at tho School of tho Art Institute of Chicago, one of the largest and most respected art schools in the country. The data for this report are derived from a larger investigation of students at that institution (Getzels and Csikszentmihalyi 1964, 1966). Available for the present analysis were the protocols of 205 s- and third-year students (94 males, 111 females) on Cattell's 16 Personality Factor Questionnaire (Cattell 1958; Cattell and Stice 1962) which ia the focal instrument of this inquiry, plus 179 completed protocols of the Allport–Vernon–Lindzey Study of Values (1960), as well as school grades and other relevant information collected both through testing and from the school files. The sample completing the 16 PFQ constituted 56 percent of all students registered at the School in the two classes. It did not differ from them on any of the descriptive variables such as age and sex, or any of the other measures such as intelligence or course grades which were available for the two classes as a whole. The instruments were administered and scored according to standard directions given in the Manuals.

Results

The data obtained will be presented in five sections structured around the main empirical questions of this study, namely: Are there personality factors differentiating art students from the relevant age and sex norms? Is there a relationship between personality factors and the values held by art students? Are there internal differentiations in terms of personality factors within the sample of art students depending on future career goals (e.g. commercial art as opposed to fine art)? What is the relationship between personality factors and success in art school? And finally, what is the relationship between the personality profile of successful young artists and eminent scientists, both groups presumably engaged in creative endeavours? In the concluding section of the paper the answers to these questions will be related to yield a model of the interaction of personality variables and social expectations, which it is hoped will begin to describe the dynamics of career choice and activity in this field.

It should be noted that the personality variables used in this study (i.e. the 16 PF factor scores) are not presented as ultimate traits but only as measures of certain motivational trends. Although several recent studies have had difficulty in replicating the factor structures claimed by Cattell (Eysenok and Eysenok 1969; Greif 1970; Schneewind 1970; Sell et al. 1970; Howarth and Browne 1971), a substantial number of other studies find high reliability and behavioural correlates using the 16 PF test; see, for instance, Demangeon 1968; Aberman and Chansky 1970; Roubertoux 1970; O'Dell 1971; Baohtold and Werneb 1971. The situation here is no different from that obtaining with other inventories of the sort. Given the present state of the art, reference to personality characteristics based on factor scores must be read with a note of caution.

Art Students and College Norms

The comparison of the subjects' scores with those of average college students on Cattell's 16 PFQ is presented in Table 2.1. It is readily apparent that both male and female subjects differ significantly from the respective norms on 11 of the 16 factors; on six of the 11 factors both sexes differ jointly and in the same direction.

The factors on which *both* sex groups differ significantly from the norms, and in the same direction, are factors A, F, G, M, Q_1, Q_2. They outline a personality syndrome that could be summarized as follows: young artists, compared to college students of their age and sex, tend to be significantly more socially reserved and cool, aloof in their relations with other people (factor A). They tend to be serious and introspective as opposed to carefree and other-directed (factor F). They are low on 'superego strength', which points to alienation from conventional social and cultural standards (factor G). They are 'unconventional, bohemian, self-

Table 2.1 16 PFQ personality factors: comparison of male and female art student means with general college norms

Personality factors		Art school males (n = 94)	College males (n = 535)	Significance level of t	Art school females (n = 111)	College females (n = 559)	Significance level of t
A	Cyolothymia	7.63	9.79	0.001	8.89	12.08	0.001
B	Intelligence	8.04	7.92	n.s.	8.08	7.57	0.05
C	Ego strength	13.99	15.35	0.01	14.06	14.58	n.s.
D	Dominance	14.17	13.78	n.s.	12.96	10.61	0.001
F	Surgenoy	12.70	16.00	0.001	13.19	16.09	0.001
G	Superego	11.24	12.64	0.01	9.68	13.14	0.001
H	Parmia	11.41	12.99	0.01	12.27	12.20	n.s.
I	Premsia	9.95	8.65	0.01	11.88	11.95	n.s.
L	Protension	10.10	8.76	n.s.	9.45	8.00	0.01
M	Autia	14.34	11.49	0.001	15.65	12.71	0.001
N	Shrewdness	10.46	10.96	n.s.	9.43	10.56	0.01
O	Guilt	11.38	10.14	0.01	11.33	11.24	n.s.
Q_1	Radicalism	10.36	9.65	0.05	10.34	8.74	0.001
Q_2	Self-sufficiency	13.33	9.86	0.001	13.49	9.66	0.001
Q_3	Self-sentiment	9.72	10.08	n.s.	9.38	10.81	0.01
Q_4	Ergio tension	14.02	12.26	0.01	13.86	13.51	n.s.

absorbed, imaginative and creative', with an intensely subjective mental life (factor M). The high score on factor Q_1 indicates an inclination to experiment with problem solutions and a radically questioning attitude towards experience. And finally, the high score on Q_2 points to a trait possessed by persons who, according to the Test Manual, are 'resolute and accustomed to making their own decisions'.

Thus the personality profile of this sample of aspiring artists suggests that as students they tend already to have the characteristics usually associated with 'artistic temperament': they are asocial, introverted, amoral as defined by cultural norms, subjective, questioning and self-contained. The personality scores of second-year students and those of third-year students were almost identical, suggesting—however tenuously, given the small difference in experience between second- and third-year students—that the personality profile of the young artist is most likely not the result of socialization into the professional training institution, but was present prior to entrance into the art school. It is also important to note that five of these six factors which significantly differentiate subjects from their age peers are included among the ten factors cited by Cattell (1963) as characteristic of the ' creative personality'. Another way of analysing the data in Table 2.1 is to apply the weights recommended by Cattell. When the weighted scores are added and converted into sten scores, the means of both male and females correspond to the eighth sten on a normal curve, indicating that by this criterion the mean 'general creativity' of the sample is higher than the 89th percentile of the normative college population.

While the six factors mentioned above might be considered as 'core artistic personality' factors in that they yield large differences for both sex groups, Table 2.1 shows also some strong differences between male and females. For instance, female subjects score significantly higher on Dominance (factor E) than their norms, while male subjects do not differ significantly on this factor from other males. At the same time, male subjects score significantly lower on Parmia (factor H) than the norms, suggesting that they are more shy, withdrawn, less adventurous in an outgoing physical sense than is 'normal' for males of their age and status. Furthermore, male sub-subjects score higher on Premsia (factor I) than the norms, indicating higher sensitivity and more 'effeminacy of feeling' than other college men. Female subjects, on the other hand, do not differ significantly from their norms on factors H and I. This pattern suggests a reversal in culturally defined sex-appropriate personality characteristics among artists. Male artists are more timid, more sensitive, more feminine in feelings than they should be according to social expectations, while female artists are more dominant or masculine than they should be. The patten brings to mind Torrance's (1962) observation that creativity in children dips sharply when heavy demands for 'sex-appropriate behaviour' are placed on them. A boy who is not allowed to express 'feminine' interests, or a girl who has to repress 'masculine' traits, are in effect deprived from using a part of their potential range of feeling and expression. Apparently artists have either been 'improperly' socialized as to sex-related attitudes, or they have learned to transcend the limitations imposed upon their range of admissible feelings.

Personality Factors and Values

A way to test the internal validity of tho findings reported in the section above is to correlate the 16 PFQ factors with the values from the Allport–Vernon–Lindzey Value Scale that have been found to discriminate most between artists and non-artists. Several studies (Deignan 1958; MacKinnon 1964; Getzels and Csikszentmihalyi 1968a, b) indicate that the value structure of artists and art students is characterized by very high Aesthetic Values and very low Economic Values. Table 2.2 presents the correlation between these two values and the 16 personality factors.

The correlation coefficients reported in Table 2.2 tend to support the validity of the personality profile and the significance of the individual personality factors discussed above. For instance, Superego strength (factor G), Shrewdness (N) and Self-sentiment (Q_3) are *positively* correlated with Economic Value but *negatively* with Aesthetic Value for both male and female subjects. Conversely the factors of Sensitivity (I), Imagination (M) and Self-sufficiency (Q_2) are *negatively* correlated with Economic and *positively* with Aesthetic Value.

Considering only those factors that attain significance in at least three of the four possible correlations with the two values, one can say that subjects who have

Table 2.2 Correlations between art students' economic and aesthetic values, and scores on the 16 PFQ personality variables

Personality factors		Economic value		Aesthetic value	
		Males ($n = 86$)	Females ($n = 93$)	Males ($n = 86$)	Females ($n = 93$)
A	Cyclothymia	0.16	0.16	− 0.26[*]	− 0.15
B	Intelligence	− 0.17	− 0.11	0.14	0.16
C	Ego strength	0.21	0.04	− 0.13	− 0.18
E	Dominance	0.07	− 0.06	0.05	0.25[*]
F	Surgency	0.16	0.06	− 0.12	0.05
G	Superego	0.11	0.24[*]	− 0.24[*]	− 0.28[**]
H	Parmia	0.20	0.03	− 0.18	0.11
I	Premsia	− 0.45[***]	− 0.33[**]	0.46[***]	0.27[**]
L	Protension	− 0.12	− 0.09	0.19	0.06
M	Autia	− 0.40[***]	− 0.19	0.42[***]	0.30[**]
N	Shrewdness	0.30[**]	0.36[***]	− 0.25[*]	− 0.26[*]
O	Guilt	− 0.04	0.05	0.14	− 0.03
Q1	Radicalism	− 0.12	− 0.13	0.06	− 0.04
Q2	Self-sufficiency	− 0.25[*]	− 0.36[**]	0.18	0.23[*]
Q3	Self-sentiment	0.22[*]	0.26[*]	− 0.20	− 0.29[**]
Q4	Ergio tension	− 0.14	− 0.06	0.30**	0.19

[*] $P < 0.05$
[**] $P < 0.01$
[***] $P < 0.001$

low Superego strength (G), who tend to be unspoiled rather than worldly-wise (N), who do not model themselves on social expectations (Q_3), also tend to have significantly lower Economic Values and higher Aesthetic Values. Low Economic and high Aesthetic Values are held by subjects who are highly sensitive (I), imaginative (M) and self-sufficient (Q_2).

Personality Differences Among Artists in Different Fields of Specialization

The total sample of art students can be further analysed into four subgroups based on the specific art field in which the student 'majors'. The four curricular specializations available in the School are Fine Arts, Art Education, Advertising Arts, and Industrial Arts. Although the faculty and the administration of the School claim that there is no difference in the entrance qualifications of students who subsequently choose one or the other of these four divisions, and despite the fact that the first two years' curriculum is largely similar for all students, one would still expect personality differences between students specializing in one or the other of these fields. A young person who majors in Fine Arts ought to be even more extreme on the 'core artistic personality' factors than his peer who chooses to concentrate on the applied and educational aspects of art. This expectation is confirmed by the result reported in Table 2.3. The analysis of variance indicates significant differences due to the field of specialization on six factors. With only a few exceptions, the Fine Arts students do in fact tend to be at the appropriate end of the distribution of scores.

Viewing each factor separately, one notes that on Cyclothymia (A), which measures personal warmth and sociability, there are significant F values due to both sex and field of specialization. It is clear that female subjects are more 'sociable' than males. More important are the noteworthy differences due to the field of specialization:

Fine Arts majors of either sex are more cold and aloof than any other group, while the Advertising Arts majors are more 'sociable'. A t test shows that on this factor both male and female fine artists are significantly different from all three other groups.

This pattern recurs with some regularity throughout the factors: the Fine Arts majors also score lowest on adherence to conventional morality (G), while the future Advertising artists score highest (the t test shows significant difference for both sexes); the Fine Arts majors score highest on sensitivity (I) while the Advertising Arts majors are significantly lower on this factor. Again, the Fine Arts majors score highest on the imaginative factor (M); here the Advertising Arts majors are again significantly lower, followed closely by the Industrial Arts majors. The same pattern tends to be repeated for the other two factors on which significant differences result in the analysis of variance, namely Shrewdness (N), and Self-sentiment (Q_3), although the t test shows significant differences only for the female art students.

Students who plan to become full-time fine artists possess to the highest extent four of the six characteristics measured by the 'core artistic personality' factors previously identified. Those students who plan to become commercial artists or advertising illustrators are lowest on these characteristics. In between are the future art teachers and product designers. As far as it goes, the pattern makes good sense. At the largely undifferentiated stage of the common school curriculum, these students already show a separation into vocational groups that corresponds to certain presumably deeply ingrained personality characteristics: aloofness lack of conventionality sensitivity, etc. The next and perhaps more critical question is, are these personality traits related only to choice of vocation, or are they also relevant to success? In other words, is personality related to achievement in art school?

Personality and Success in Art School

The most obvious criterion of success for art students is the grade-point average in art courses (as opposed to courses in art history, humanities, etc.) accumulated during residence at the School. This criterion has also some obvious limitations: there is no assurance, for instance, that the best art students will also become the

Table 2.3 Comparison of art students in different fields of specialization on the 16 PFQ personality factors: analysis of variance, means and F values

Field of specialization	Personality factors															
	n	A	C	E	F	G	H	I	L	M	N	O	Q_1	Q_2	Q_3	Q_4
Male																
FA	35	6.28	13.28	13.54	11.83	10.60	10.23	11.14	10.48	15.26	9.66	11.28	10.74	13.54	9.34	14.16
AE	12	8.50	14.58	13.00	11.17	11.92	11.83	10.50	8.92	14.75	11.00	10.83	11.17	14.67	10.58	12.75
AA	16	9.19	13.44	14.50	15.25	12.62	12.19	8.62	10.87	13.87	10.87	13.00	10.12	12.62	9.31	14.31
IA	23	7.78	15.30	15.00	12.78	11.35	11.48	10.61	9.65	13.74	11.13	10.69	10.00	13.13	10.61	14.39
Female																
FA	44	8.13	14.48	13.48	13.34	8.73	12.23	12.52	10.16	16.66	8.43	11.34	11.16	14.34	8.61	14.41
AE	15	9.67	13.27	11.67	11.40	10.00	11.07	11.80	8.80	15.13	10.00	11.87	10.60	13.27	8.67	13.80
AA	7	10.43	16.28	12.43	12.57	12.00	13.00	10.43	6.14	13.57	12.43	8.28	10.43	11.86	10.86	10.43
IA	27	9.48	13.37	12.55	13.52	10.74	12.44	11.48	9.30	14.52	10.41	11.81	9.67	12.44	10.74	13.85
F value effects																
Sex		13.57***	0.03	4.57	1.01	9.17**	2.21	14.75***	3.52	3.50	3.88	0.00	0.01	0.09	0.97	0.40
Major		5.48c	0.12	1.16	2.61	6.41***	0.38	6.14***	2.23	5.37**	8.68***	0.03	1.85	2.75	4.14**	0.67
Interaction		0.12	2.78	1.24	1.39	0.62	0.51	0.48	3.63*	0.48	1.69	3.13	0.29	1.18	1.73	1.14

* $P < 0.05$
** $P < 0.01$
*** $P < 0.001$

F = Fine arts
AE = Art education
AA = Advertising arts
IA = Industrial arts

best practising artists. However, inasmuch as the grades are given by recognized artist-teachers it is not unreasonable to assume that at this stage in the subjects' development, the art-grade average is as viable a predictor of future performance as one can feasibly obtain. At any rate, for most art students no other criterion is as yet available.

An analysis of the relationship of personality and artistic accomplishment, however, has to be undertaken *within each subgroup* rather than for the total sample. It has previously been found (Getzels and Csikszentmihalyi 1966) that the criterion of success is not related uniformly to other variables within subsamples that differ in terms of sex and field of specialization. A successful young female Advertising Arts major, for instance, tends to have quite different perceptual, cognitive and value attributes from a successful female Fine Arts major or, for that matter, even a male Advertising Arts major. Both on commonsense grounds and in terms of the results reported in the previous section, it can be assumed that Fine Arts majors are probably the most representative art students, those who embody the artistic temperament and goals *par excellence*. It is therefore only with male students in this subgroup that the present analysis will be concerned.

Table 2.4 compares the mean score on the 16 PFQ for male college norms, for male Fine Arts students, and for the 10 male Fine Arts majors in the highest third of the distribution of art course grade-point averages and the 10 Fine Arts majors in the lowest third of the distribution. The first observation is that on all six factors identified as 'core artistic personality' factors without exception the scores of the successful subjects are at the expected extreme relative to the scores of the unsuccessful subjects. The successful subjects are less warm (A), less outgoing (F), less conventional (G), more imaginative (M), more radical (Q_1), and more self-sufficient (Q_2). However, on only one of these six factors (G) does the difference reach a statistically significant level.

In evaluating the magnitude of the differences it should be noted that on all six 'core' factors the whole sample had scored at a significantly different level from the norms, and that Fine Arts majors had further differed from the rest of the art student sample. Thus it is indeed difficult to obtain additional differences within this already so refined and differentiated subgroup. In light of this fact the pattern in Table 2.4 appears to recommend itself to attention despite the lack of more 'significant' differences.

Besides the six 'core' factors, two more attract attention in the table. The first is the factor of Ego strength (C), on which a relatively large, but not significant, difference exists. This suggests that too strong an ego is not an advantage for artistic achievement in the school. The largest difference between the two subgroups is found in the factor measuring Self-sentiment (Q_3), a difference significant at the 0·005 level. Cattell defines Self-sentiment as 'conforming to socially accepted behaviour' as well as 'self-control', 'foresight' and 'exacting will-power'. One might interpret this to mean that the subjects who achieve success in school tend to hold an image of themselves which is not dependent on other people's expectations or approval; their self-concept is autonomous, their

Table 2.4 Mean personality scores (16 PFQ) for college norms, male fine arts students, and high and low achieving male fine arts students

Personality factors		Male college norms ($n = 535$)	Low achieving male fine arts students ($n = 10$)	Male fine arts students ($n = 35$)	High achieving male fine arts students ($n = 10$)	Direction of difference on 'Core' factors for high and low achieving students
A	Cyclothymia	9.8	6.7	6.7	5.3	Expected
C	Ego strength	15.4	14.3	13.3	11.3	–
E	Dominance	13.8	13.4	13.5	13.3	–
F	Surgency	16.0	12.3	11.8	10.4	Expected
G	Superego	12.6	11.8	10.6	8.8	Expected
H	Parmia	13.0	9.5	10.2	9.3	–
I	Premsia	8.7	11.7	11.1	12.1	–
L	Protension	9.8	11.3	10.5	10.8	–
M	Autia	11.5	15.4	15.3	16.0	Expected
N	Shrewdness	11.0	9.7	9.7	9.6	–
O	Guilt	10.1	11.9	11.3	11.4	–
Q_1	Radicalism	9.7	9.7	10.7	10.7	Expected
Q_2	Self-sufficiency	9.9	13.0	13.5	13.6	Expected
Q_3	Self-sentiment	10.1	10.3	9.3	7.2	–
Q_4	Ergio tension	12.3	14.8	14.5	14.5	–

'Cora artistic personality' factors are given in italics

self-respect independent of outside judgement. The similarity between this factor and the other in which the difference attains significance (factor G) should not escape notice (Fig. 2.1).

Finally, when the 'composite creativity score' is obtained from the 16 PFQ according to the weights suggested by Cattell (1963), it is found that the 10 'high' subjects have a mean creativity score equivalent to sten 10 on a normal curve (higher than that of 99 percent of the normal college population), while the 10 'low' subjects place at sten 8. Thus even within such an already highly selected sample (the whole male Fine Arts group's mean score was at sten 9), personality differences, however small, are apparently related to differences in artistic success.

Comparison of the Personality of Successful Young Artists with that of Eminent Researchers

The results have shown that a specific personality configuration tends to distinguish art students in general from college students, future fine artists from art students in general, and the successful from the unsuccessful young fine artist. The configuration includes the six 'core personality' factors, namely low Cyclothymia, Surgency, Superego strength, high Autia, Radicalism and Self-sufficiency. To

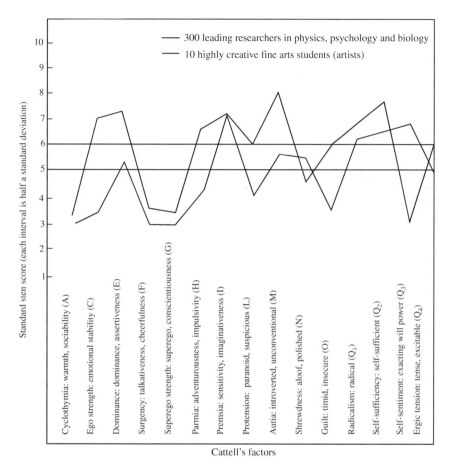

Fig. 2.1 Comparison of the personality profile (16 PFQ) of highly creative fine arts students and of leading researchers in science

these one might add, at least for male fine artists, high Premsia and low Self-sentiment; finally, to round out the picture, one should remember that high Aesthetic Values and low Economic Values are also always present in the pattern.

This configuration is essentially the same that Cross et al. (1967) found in practising artists, and is in several significant ways similar to that of leading researchers in physics, psychology and biology. In fact, when the personality profile of the 10 successful subjects in Table 2.4 is compared with that of Creative scientists studied by Cattell and Drevdahl (1955), it is seen that both Fine Arts students and scientists score very low on factors A, F and G, and relatively high on factors I, Q_1 and Q_2.

Both successful art students and successful scientists tend to be aloof, non-gregarious, unconcerned with moral standards, sensitive, radical and self-sufficient. On five of the six 'core artistic personality' factors art students and scientists score alike, suggesting that these factors are relevant to creativity in general, not just to an artistic vocation. On the other hand, relative to successful scientists, successful art students have much lower ego strength (C)—the difference in means is of the order of two standard deviations—are less adventurous (H), more suspicious (L), more subjective (M), more insecure (O), and significantly lower on self-sentiment (Q_3).

Discussion

Despite the fact that an association between certain personality characteristics (as measured by the 16 PF factor scores) and an artistic vocation—even more, a *successful* artistic vocation, at least during the art school stage—seems clearly established, the nature of the association is still in question.

A distinction might help to clarify the various connections that are logically possible between personality and artistic activity. The personality configuration found in this study could be a necessary aptitudinal factor which is intrinsic to the task requirements of 'artistic' activity. In other words, a person who is outgoing, conforming, gregarious, objective, etc., might simply not engage in the kind of behaviour that is necessary to produce art. There are certain intrinsic requirements for most occupations that pre-select the type of person intending to perform within their given limits. For instance, a career in classical music not only excludes people who are tone-deaf, but also those whose personality characteristics make them unwilling to concentrate, who lack self-discipline, or dislike sedentary activities. The professional behaviour of a salesman requires a personality that is gregarious, extraverted and not likely to become deeply concerned about casual encounters. Personality characteristics that are so to speak built into the function of the task we shall call *task requirements.*

But it is also possible that the personality configuration that has emerged in this study has nothing to do with the functional, intrinsic, substantive characteristics needed to do artistic work. Its presence might reflect only social-structural or extrinsic *context requirements.* That is, it could be that a person who is outgoing, conforming, gregarious, etc., will avoid becoming an artist not because he is incapable of performing the activities required to produce art, but because he cannot accept the conditions of the artistic role, which at the time includes poverty, ostracism, loneliness, and so on. It is possible to distinguish logically at least four reasons why artists will have a particular personality configuration: (1) it is a task requirement for any Creative work; (2) it is a task requirement for any work in art; (3) it is a context requirement for any Creative person; (4) it is a context requirement for any artist. Which one of these four reasons seems most cogent, given the present findings? The easiest and safest answer is that all four are involved in producing the reported pattern of associations. Yet despite the difficulty involved in extricating antecedent–consequent relations, it is possible to try locating with more precision the conditions that account for an artist's personality system.

The data plus common sense suggest that high Sensitivity (I) and Self-sufficiency (Q_2) might be task requirements for producing any creative work. A person who is insensitive and lacks confidence in his own powers can hardly be engaged in the arduous challenge to existing norms that a Creative effort requires. Of course a person possessing these traits necessary for creative production might not necessarily be successful in his efforts; in fact, under certain frequent social conditions, he might be actively ostracized. In several historical periods creativity was not considered a positive value. In the splendid Egyptian civilization, for instance, hundreds of years passed during which innovation and originality—at least in art —were actively discouraged (Gombrich 1966, pp. 40–41). Europe in the Middle Ages, the Byzantine civilization, and perhaps the Soviet Union in the past half-century, were not so much incapable of artistic creativity as disinterested in it. The accepted art style was all of a piece with the rest of the culture and the social system, and any 'creative' artist was seen as a disruptive element to be contained and isolated. The successful artist in such a society was not the type of person we would call creative. Despite the fact that creativity as we understand it is not always conducive to recognition, we might say that *creative work can be accomplished only by people with high sensitivity and self-sufficiency.* This description matches the profile of both our artists and creative scientific researches (Cattell and Drevdahl 1955, 1956; Cattell and Butcher 1968, pp. 298, 349; Cattell and Eber 1970).

But there are other personality factors on which both the young artists and the scientists score similarly. These are factors A and F, the first implying coldness and aloofness, the second a reserved and taciturn disposition (Cattell and Butcher 1968, pp. 298, 349). Are these *task requirements* for creative production? While this question cannot be answered definitely, these two traits seem to be more *context requirements* for a creative worker in our days rather than being intrinsically necessary for creativity activity. It is possible that under certain socio-cultural conditions, when 'creativity' is neither discouraged as it was in ancient Egypt, nor popularized and vulgarized as it is in our day, the creative individual need not withdraw from interaction with other people to preserve his unique vision. From what we know of artists of the past, it would seem that in early Renaissance Florence the great creative geniuses were working in an unselfconscious manner, cheerfully integrated within the social matrix of their peers. But a few generations later, when the milieu of Renaissance culture had become aggressively innovative and originality-seeking, the genius who wanted to be true to his vision had to isolate himself and withdraw from the limelight (Vasari 1550). *Withdrawal and seclusiveness seem to be necessary for any creative person, whether artist or scientist, only under certain socio-cultural conditions.*

There are, finally, the personality factors that appear to be specific to artists as opposed to creative scientists. These include low emotional stability or Ego strength (C), low conformity to norms (G), high subjectivity and imagination (M), and low Self-sentiment (Q_3). Of these, a low G and a high M seem to be *task requirements* for carrying on artistic activities. It could be argued that low Ego strength is prevalent only when art is conceived of as dealing with unconscious contents, as in historical periods of a romantic persuasion. It is questionable whether artists would tend to have weak egos in periods of classical art, or in what Sorokin (1963) has called 'ideational' phases of culture. Similarly, low Self-sentiment need only be a characteristic of the artist's personality in historical periods when he experiences his goals and values to be incongruent with those of the rest of society.

In summary, on the basis of the findings one might advance the hypothesis that high Sensitivity (I) and Self-sufficiency (Q_2) are *task requirements* for all individuals who are to perform creatively; while high Autia (M) and low Superego (G) are *task requirements* for artists only. Low Cyclothymia (A) and low Surgency (F) seem to be *context requirements* for creative people who want to preserve their autonomy under conditions when creativity is either repressed or over-popularized. Finally, low Ego strength (C) and low Self-sentiment (Q_3) are *context requirements* that are operative only when artists live under adverse cultural conditions. Creative people will also exhibit more of the characteristic traits of the opposite sex than is usually considered 'normal' by the definition of a given culture. This can be explained in terms of a *task requirement* for artists to use a full range of cognitive and emotional responses regardless of sex-linked socio-cultural expectations.

Admittedly the issues raised in the last section are speculative in nature, and they are offered only as hypotheses open to falsification, in the hope that future work will be able to sort out the correct inferences from the faulty ones. One suggestion for further methodological research is also in order. Whatever personality inventory is to be used, the results should be submitted to independent item factoring. Although we have no reason to doubt the applicability of the Cattell factors based on prior item groupings, it would be useful to see whether artists do in fact respond within the expected factorial structures. In any case, the results of this study indicate that the present factors of the 16 PF do meaningfully differentiate between various gradations of artistic vocation and success.

Finally, while it is important to know more about what personality traits characterize the creative person, and the creative artist in particular, it is also important to know more about the interaction of the personality traits of such an individual with the pattern of role expectations that impinge on him in his social environment.

References

Aberman, H. M., & Chansky, N. (1970). Factor analysis of two personality tests with differing conceptual frameworks. *Psychological Reports, 27*, 476–480.

Allfort, G. W., Vernon, P. E., & Lindzey, G. (1960). *Manual: A study of values*. Boston: Houghton Mifflin.

Anderson, H. H. (1959). Creativity in perspective. In: H. H. Anderson (Ed.) *Creativity and its cultivation*. New York: Harper.

Anderson, H. H. (1960). The nature of creativity. *Studies in Art Education, 1*, 10–17.

Baohtold, L. M., & Werneb, E. E. (1971). Personality profiles of women psychologists over three generations. *Dev Psycol, 5*, 273–278.

Barbon, F. (1969). *Creative persons and creative processes*. New York: Holt, Rinehart & Winston.

Cattell, R. B. (1958). *Objective-analytic test battery*. Champaign: Institute for Personality and Ability Testing.

Cattell, R. B. (1963). *IPAT information bulletin no. 10*. Champaign: Institute for Personality and Ability Testing.

Cattell, R. B. & Butcher, H. J. (1968). *The prediction of achievement and creativity*. Indianapolis: Bobbs-Merrill.

Cattell, R. B., & Drevdahl, J. E. (1955). A comparison of the personality profile (16 PF) of eminent researchers with that of eminent teachers and administrators, and of the general population. *British Journal of Psychology, 46*, 248–261.

Cattell, R. B., & Eber, H. W. (1970). *Handbook for the sixteen personality factor questionnaire*. Champaign: Institute for Personality and Ability Testing.

Cattell, R. B., & Stice, G. F. (1962). *Handbook for the sixteen personality factor questionnaire*. Champaign: Institute for Personality and Ability Testing.

Cross, P. G., Cattell, R. B., & Butcher, H. J. (1967). The personality pattern of creative artists. *British Journal of Educational Psychology, 37*, 292–299.

Deignan, F. J. (1958). Note on the values of art students. *Psychological Reports, 4*, 566.

Demangeon, M. (1968). A propos d'une tentative de validation do l'échello d'anxiété de Cattell sur un échantillon d'étudiants français. *BINOP, 24*, 309–323.

Drevdahl, J. E. (1956). Factors of importance to creativity. *Journal of Clinical Psychology, 12*, 21–26.

Eysenok, H. J., & Eysenok, S. B. G. (1969). *Personality structure and measurement*. San Diego: Knapp.

Getzels, J. W. & Csikszentmihalyi, M. (1964). Creative thinking in art students: an exploratory study. University of Chicago, Chicago, U.S. Office of Education (HEW) Cooperative Research Project Report E-008.

Getzels, J. W., & Csikszentmihalyi, M. (1966). The study of creativity in future artists: The criterion problem. In O. J. Harvey (Ed.), *Experience, structure, and adaptability*. New York: Springer.

Getzels, J. W., & Csikszentmihalyi, M. (1968a). The value-orientations of art students as determinants of artistic specialization and creative performance. *Studies in Art Education, 10*, 5–16.

Getzels, J. W., & Csikszentmihalyi, M. (1968b). On the roles, values, and performance of future artists: A conceptual and empirical exploration. *The Sociological Quarterly, 9*, 516–530.

Gombrich, E. G. (1966). *The story of art*. New York: Phaidon.

Greif, S. (1970). Untersuchungen zur deutschen Übersetzung des 16 PF Fragebogens. *Psychologie Beitraege, 12*, 186–213.

Hauser, A. (1960). *The social history of art* (Vol. 2). New York: Vintage Books.

Howarth, E., & Browne, J. A. (1971). Investigation of personality factors in a Canadian context. I. Marker structure in personality questionnaire items. *Canadian Journal of Behavioural Science, 3*, 161–173.

Kris, E. (1952). *Psychoanalytic explorations in art*. New York: International Universities Press.

MacKinnon, D. W. (1964). The creativity of architects. In: O. W. Taylor (Ed.) Widening horizons in creativity. New York: Wiley.

O'Dell, J. W. (1971). Method for detecting random answers on personality questionnaires. *Journal of Applied Psychology, 55*, 380–383.

Roe, A. (1946). The personality of artists. *Educational and Psychological Measurement, 6*, 401–408.

Roubertoux, P. (1970). Personality variables and interest in art. *Journal of Personality and Social Psychology, 16*, 665–668.

Schneewind, K. A. (1970). Wie universell Sind Cattella objektive Persönlichkeitefaktoren. *Diagnostica, 16*, 94–97.

Sell, S. B., Demaree, B. G., & Will, D. P. (1970). Dimensions of personality. I. Conjoint factor structure of Guilford and Cattell trait markers. *Multivariate Behavioral Research, 5*, 391–422.

Sorokin, P. (1963). *Modern historical and social philosophies*. New York: Dover.

Torranoe, E. P. (1962). *Guiding creative talent*. Englewood Cliffs: Prentice-Hall.

Vasari, G. (1550). Lives of the most eminent painters, sculptors, and architects. New York: Random House (1959).

Chapter 3
Culture, Time, and the Development of Talent

Mihaly Csikszentmihalyi and Rick E. Robinson

The literature on giftedness gives the impression that most authors *conceive* of talent (*talent, giftedness* and *prodigious performance* will be used interchangeably) as a stable trait that belongs to a person. Although some writers have warned us not "to view giftedness as an absolute concept—something that exists in and of itself, without relation to anything else" (Renzulli 1980, p. 4), most people consider giftedness as an objective fact, something you either have or don't have, like green eyes or a mole on the nose. Our 20 years of research with mature artists and other creative individuals suggests a different view, which might be summarized as follows:

1. Talent cannot be observed except against the background of well-specified cultural expectations. Hence, it cannot be a personal trait or attribute but rather is a relationship between culturally defined opportunities for action and personal skills or capacities to act.
2. Talent cannot be a stable trait because individual capacity for action changes over the life-span, and cultural demands for performance change both over the life-span and over time within each domain of performance. Thus, it cannot be assumed that a 5-year-old prodigy will be considered outstanding as a teenager or adult. (Artificially restricted definitions of talent based purely on test performance, such as an IQ score, are a partial exception to this rule.)

These two points may seem to have only obscure, ivory-tower academic interest. But their implications have a rather substantial bearing on what we think giftedness is, how we measure it, and what predictions we think are warranted by our measurements. The reminder of this chapter will attempt to explicate these

---

M. Csikszentmihalyi, *The Systems Model of Creativity*,
DOI: 10.1007/978-94-017-9085-7_3,
© Springer Science+Business Media Dordrecht 2014

implications as suggested by our longitudinal studies of gifted individuals struggling to develop their talents in the real world.

The researches referred to in this article were supported by the Spencer Foundation (longitudinal study of artists) and by an SSRC grant to study gifted mathematics students.

The Sociocultural Constitution of Giftedness

Investigators in the field of giftedness occasionally remark that, whereas there are young prodigies in music, chess, foreign languages, sports, or mathematics, there are no child prodigies in the realms of morality, altruism, politics—or even art and poetry. This fact is interpreted to mean that children are able to develop precocious skills in music, math, and the like, but not in morality.

An entirely different interpretation is also possible. We do not see early talent in morality, not because children lack the appropriate skills, but because what we mean by morality has never been as clearly articulated as, say what we mean by mathematics. Without a clear definition, we have no criteria for recognizing in young children the behaviors that might develop into outstanding moral ability. It is not simply that we are lacking the right test or scale, but that, when dealing with domains that have not been fully and consensually defined by society, we do not even have a good grasp of what it is we are looking for. More than 20 years ago, in their exploration of creativity, Getzels and Jackson (1962) suggested that "psychosocial excellence" was as important a skill as outstanding intellectual ability was, and they began to investigate the characteristics of highly moral teenagers. But when, last year, Howard Gruber, of the Committee on Giftedness of the Social Science Research Council, organized a symposium on moral giftedness at Yale University, it was as if every participant had to rethink and redefine the concept of morality from ground zero. Instead of fostering a greater consensus, the intervening twenty years seem to have served only to increase confusion about the nature of morality.

Musical or mathematical talent can be easily recognized, because Western culture long ago developed a fairly clear and unanimous agreement as to what these domains are. Equally important, for every well-defined domain there is a well-elaborated set of criteria that permits specification of what constitutes excellence at any of a number of points in the life-span. Thus, accuracy and excellence in those domains is easy to assess. Those trained in the field have the means to recognize superior performance at once. Consequently, an outstanding performance can label the performer as having a "gift", which can then be reinforced and nurtured through a series of increasingly demanding challenges that the medium (music, mathematics, swimming, etc.) presents. Domains that are less clearly defined also lack the articulated series of challenges and criteria for evaluation. Therefore, it becomes exceedingly difficult to identify the precursors of excellence and those who may possess them. Furthermore, those who do possess potentials in such domains are given none of the systematic support necessary to refine and develop potentials into abilities commensurate with the needs of society and demands of the domain.

The Reification of Giftedness

The quintessence of a talent that has been quantified in light of its societal definition is the one measured by the IQ score. The IQ was developed as a measure of performance in Western academic institutions, and for the sake of the argument, its effectiveness in such settings might be granted. But it is important to realize that intelligence as defined by the IQ did not exist before Binet invented it. Therefore, the whole argument about the relative contributions of nature and nurture to intelligence is meaningless. Intelligence refers to patterns of thought evolved by culture and recognized by society. It cannot exist outside its social context. Of course, like all human behavior, it is mediated by the biochemical processes of the nervous system. But to locate intelligence within the brain is to reify a phenomenon that manifests itself only in interaction. The IQ refers to a peculiar process adapted to its peculiar environment—the Western academic bureaucracy—just as skill in chess is a mental process adapted to the particular setting of the chess game. A superior IQ or a high chess ranking indicate the ability to function exceptionally well within the rules of the appropriate social system. It takes a bit of magical thinking to believe that these abilities have any value beyond the school or the tournament. Outside their social context, they retain only the attraction of whatever stands out because of its scarcity—much like a rare postage stamp or an unusual stone.

The precise measurement of the IQ makes it possible for scholars and educators to ask such questions as: What proportion of the population is truly gifted? Is it 3 or 5 %? There are two meanings such questions can have, what we might call a *naturalistic* meaning and an *attributional* meaning (Brannigan 1981). The naturalistic assumption is that giftedness is a natural fact, and therefore the number of gifted children can be counted, as one might count white herons or panda bears. If this is the sense in which people are asking the question, the question is meaningless. The attributional assumption recognizes that giftedness is not an objective fact but a result jointly constituted by social expectations and individual abilities. From this perspective it is obvious that the question "What proportion of the population is gifted?" means "What proportion of the population have we agreed to call gifted?"

In other words, no objective criterion "out there" will ever reveal how many gifted children there are. The collectivity as a whole must make up its mind where to draw the line. One can argue that any child who can move, see, speak, and think is gifted—after all, how rare such skills are in the empty vastness of the galaxies! And if we reflect on what small proportion of these gifts are developed in the schools or used by the culture, we realize what an enormous task it is to help unfold the basic giftedness of our normal children. On the other hand, one might argue that giftedness is more properly reserved as a title for those boys and girls who show truly exceptional performance in some important domain—the "prodigies" whose skills are perhaps one in a million, or one in 10 million. And there is nothing wrong in claiming that the gifted constitute 5 % of the population either, as long as we admit that this figure is not the result of any scientific deduction, but the outcome of a purely pragmatic consensus.

Then there are vast areas of human action in which precise quantifications, or even comparisons, are either difficult or impossible. Variations in ability certainly exist in these areas, but they have not been conceptualized in terms amenable to quantification. It is easy to find out in what percentile one ranks in terms of the IQ scale. It is easy to ascertain that someone is the 14th best tennis player in the world, or someone else the 6th ranked mathematician in his age group, But who is the best mother? Or the 5th most honest politician?

The fact that we can detect talent in chess but not in moral behavior does not mean that chess is more important than morality. Nor does it mean that it is a superior talent. It simply means that, being a rational activity conceived by humans, anything that happens in chess can be completely encompassed by the mind, and ability in it can be accurately measured—whereas morality will evade quantification until the culture evolves a general enough consensus about its nature.

It is in fact equally plausible to advance an opposite claim: that the activities in which prodigious performance can be easily detected are by definition relatively trivial. What makes giftedness so exciting in these domains is not the value of the performance but its clearly measurable extraordinariness. Precocious talent in these fields shares with the feats chronicled in *The Guinness Book of World Records* an appeal to our propensity to respond to the improbable—be it freak or genius.

It is more likely that neither of these claims is completely the case. Still, it is important to keep in mind that precision in measurement is not tantamount to significance or value. The IQ score, the GRE test, or mathematical ranking may be reliable and exact, but precision says nothing about the individual or social value of what is being measured. What remains to be elucidated through the study of the constitution of domains are the socio-cultural factors, as well as factors intrinsic to the domains, that determine the degree to which any given domain is clearly defined and talent within it correspondingly quantifiable. But how valuable the domains themselves are must be assessed in light of a general theory of social priorities.

Variations Within the Domains

The cultural expectations that make the expression of talent possible differ not only from one domain to another, as between poetry and physics, but also, within the same one over time. For instance, it was much easier to recognize artistic talent in the Renaissance than it is in the present, because at that time a child who could draw lifelike pictures had something important to contribute to the art of the time. Giotto's gift was supposedly recognized by the Pope's envoy who was riding by the pasture where the young shepherd was sketching his lambs using a flat rock and a bit of charcoal. Most of the artists whose lives Vasari describes were noted at an early age for their skill at reproducing likeness. By contrast, during the height of abstract expressionism in the 1950s and 1960s, drawing lifelike pictures no longer constituted a valuable talent. Spontaneity and emotionality were considered the key elements in the production of good art. Young people who had these qualities were thought to have talent by the gatekeepers of the domain—the art teachers, gallery owners, curators, critics, and collectors. Then, during the following decades, painting returned to much more controlled styles, such a hard-edge and photo-realism. The qualities that had identified promising abstract expressionists were no longer in demand.

Children with graphic talents for rendering natural forms, or for evoking emotions through their drawing, certainly still exist. Indeed, such children art is encouraged as a charming expression of spontaneity and innocence by parents, by progressive educators, and by producers of UNICEF Christmas cards. But these talents are no longer considered relevant to mature artistic performance by the gatekeepers of the domain—if anything, they are believed to be detrimental. We see, then, that as the nature of the domain changes over time, the selection criteria for young talent vary accordingly. Because' of the Interactive and socioculturally constituted nature of talent, as its social definition changes, so does its manifestation—children who in a previous era" would have been thought gifted no longer stand out, and others who would not have been noticed now appear to have talent.

How Many Talents?

The sociocultural constitution of giftedness also provides a relevant perspective on the debate as to whether talent is a unitary gift or whether there are multiple "talents". It has been recognized for a long time that the reduction of giftedness to a unitary dimension is completely arbitrary. Some writers have also taken the next step by admitting that the number of distinct talents we wish to recognize (like the level at which we wish to set the threshold of giftedness) is purely a matter of convention and convenience. There being no "natural" talents, their number and kind depend entirely on distinctions we are willing to make. For example, Paul Torrance wrote as follows:

> It is quite clear that there is a variety of kinds of giftedness that should be cultivated and are not ordinarily cultivated without special efforts. It is clear that if we establish a level on some single measure of giftedness, we eliminate many extremely gifted individuals on other measure of giftedness. It is also clear that intelligence may increase or decrease, at least in terms of available methods of assessing it, depending on a variety of physical and psychological factors both within the individual and within his environment (Torrance 1965, p. 49).

Recently, Feldman (1980) has focused our attention on the existence of different *domains* in which giftedness manifests itself, and has pointed out that, whereas some domains seem to be universal, others are more dependent on the culture or on a restricted subset of performances within it. Howard Gardner's (1983) latest book describes *multiple intelligences,* each potentially resulting in one of seven relatively independent basic talents. Which of these "raw intelligences", if any, a child develops depends on differences in neurological organisation that make the child more sensitive to a particular range of stimuli and better able to function within it at a superior level.

These departures from previous orthodoxy point to the direction in which the field is likely to be moving in the future. Yet even these progressive concepts appear to be rooted in a somewhat naturalistic view of giftedness because they conceive of domains as being either more or less dependent on culture. But from an attributional perspective, every domain of thought is entirely constituted by culture, and at the same time entirely dependent on individual physiology. To think of thought as an "interaction" is misleading because it suggests that the two components act separately, that thinking is a combination of discrete biological and cultural factors (Freedman 1980). In actuality, every act of thought, every symbolic connection, is shaped simultaneously by endogenous biological patterns and by exogenous cultural patterns. It is, of course, possible to alter the content of, or the process of, thought by modifying either template separately. But when a child's thinking is changed through the cultural template, the resulting thought is no more dependent on culture than it was before. The biological processes that make thought possible are just as essential as they ever were. And vice versa: Culture shapes even the most universal, the most basic, conceptual domains.

Perhaps a thought experiment will help clarify these points. Let us suppose that somewhere in the world a new game is invented and given the name of *mo*. (Johann Huizinga, the Dutch cultural historian, has argued that most of the hallowed human institutions—such as Science, religion, warfare, the law, poetry— were originally games and only later became serious and binding; thus, the example is not altogether trivial.) To play *mo* well, one must recognize fine spatial and color distinctions, one must be very agile, and one must have a high tolerance for alcohol. With time, the game of *mo* becomes my popular among the cultural elite, and good players are in great demand. But few people possess all the skills necessary to excel in the game, so extensive searches for *mo* prodigies are instituted. The question is, will they find them? As the reader will probably agree, it is logically certain that young *mo* geniuses will indeed be found. It could not be otherwise: Because people differ in spatial perception, agility, and tolerance for alcohol, it follows that there must be a small number of individuals who will be relatively outstanding in all the three skills. This concludes the thought experiment. Now comes the interpretation of its results: Should we conclude that talent in *mo* was by physiological factors? Certainly, because all the component skills depend on demonstrably neurological processes. Or should we say that talent in *mo* is culturally constituted? Certainly, because the combination of physiological skills was meaningless before the game was invented.

It would be too facile to resolve this paradox by saying that talent in *mo* is the result of an interaction between individual skills and cultural rules. It is more a question of codevelopment in which latent potentials are shaped by expectations that in turn were made possible by the existence of biological potentials. It is idle to try separating these two components in the genesis of talent.

Implications of the Sociocultural Model

These considerations suggest that to reify talent as some kind of preformed gift that exists within the child is a mistake. The homuncular view of giftedness does not fit the facts. It is not that the child's talent reveals itself and it recognized by society. It is closer to the truth to say that the possibility to reveal talent is provided by the cultural environment, and that it is this possibility that the "talented" child recognizes.

The clearest practical implication of this perspective is that ideas about identifying gifted children need to be reformulated. Early identification and accurate prediction (the acid test of any identification paradigm) have been the goal toward which much giftedness research has been working. Yet that entire endeavor is predicated on an assumption of giftedness as a stable, intra-individual trait. Recognizing that giftedness is socioculturally constituted means it would be premature to dismiss as infertile the domains where precocity is not now evident (such as morality). Further, we must realize that, as the domain changes through history or across the life-span in response to shifting sociocultural demands, what constitutes an expression of giftedness will also change. Delisle and Renzulli's (1980) "revolving door" model of programming is one approach that already takes this notion into account during the school years.

In addition, a skillful marriage of this attributional perspective with the concepts advanced by Feldman (1980) and Gardner (1983) suggests profitable new directions to explore. On the one hand, we need to know more about multiple intelligences or the potential skills that children possess but that go unrecognized and undeveloped because we are blind to their existence. On the other hand, we must know more about the organization of the domains in which talent manifests itself, because it is what we expect of a chess player, pianist, artist, mathematician, or *mo* player that defines what will constitute talent.

And, what is perhaps most important, we might ask ourselves what it would take to *create* talent in domains that are important to our survival, such as nurturance, wisdom, or frugality. Perhaps all it would take is agreement on the criteria of performance, and then—as if by magic—talent will reveal itself.

The Temporal Constitution of Giftedness

Because the great majority of research in the field of giftedness consists of cross-sectional studies of children, it is easy to fall into the habit of thinking that the "gifted child" is a permanent entity. Such children may grow and develop, may even lose their gift, but basically it is assumed that gifted children studied at 5 and 10 years of age will retain their relative superiority over time, unaffected by qualitative transformations.

Even longitudinal studies (Terman 1925; Oden 1968) seem to assume that the passage of time is simply something akin to friction in mechanics, a variable that slowly decreases the predictive power of an early diagnosis of talent. Even when it is recognized that developmental stages in the human life-span introduce qualitative transformations, as in the recent article by Mönks and Ferguson (1983), the authors describe the gifted teenager as a static entity moving through the vicissitudes of adolescence, rather than as a person who may change ways of thinking, wishing, and acting beyond recognition—and hence who may also cease to be gifted by the original diagnostic criterion.

The point is that, if we agree talent depends on social attributions rather than on a naturalistic trait locked in the child's physiology, then it follows that talent should be thought of not as a stable characteristic but as a dynamic quality dependent on changes within the individual and within the environment.

Below, we examine four developmental vectors that express this dynamic: the psychosocial, the cognitive-developmental, the domain, and the field. Although we explicate each separately, it should be borne in mind that movement along each is concurrent with movement along the rest, and that all four are complexly interdependent.

Giftedness Through the Life-Span

A child of 10, born with an exceptional sensitivity to sounds, might enjoy developing his "talent" in music under the guidance of his parents and teachers. In the preadolescent years, as some developmental psychologists have observed, the main challenge confronting a child is to find out whether he can act with competence, whether he can master increasingly complex tasks (Erikson 1963; Havighurst 1951). So for the preteen boy, practicing the piano happens to coincide with a possible resolution of this central developmental task. He can throw all his energies into playing music.

After puberty, our little pianist turns into a person with new impulses, new desires, and with a different conception of self related to different experiences and social expectations. He is, to all intents and purposes, an entirely different organization of psychic energy. If we are to follow the Eriksonian map of psychosocial development, we would say that the need to establish his identity becomes the boy's main concern. According to Havighurst, the boy will be mostly concerned to establish his autonomy from the family. In either case it is easy to see that for the teenage boy to play the piano might now conflict with his developmental task: He might feel that he cannot find his identity or establish his autonomy as long as he continues to devote all his energies to what his parents expect of him. Yet, without constant practice, he cannot fulfill his promise. A great number of talented youngsters presumably succumb to the reorganization of psychic energy ushered in at adolescence.

Similar changes in priority await the growing boy a few years later. The issue of intimacy, of developing close and stable relations with another person is the salient task for most people in late adolescence. It is a task that is both a challenge and a new opportunity. Those who respond to it may find their old goals reshuffled once more. Practicing the piano may become meaningless compared with a date.

Another reorganization of motives awaits the growing man when he begins to establish a family of his own. We might, with Erikson, call this the crisis of generativity. It involves choices about where to allocate one's psychic energy in terms of replicating one's identity over time. The basic choice is whether to put the most effort into replicating one's *genes* or one's *memes* that is, whether to raise offspring or to pass on ideas; whether to transmit the information contained within one's biological structure or that contained within one's memory. The Romans used the saying, *libri aut liberi* "books or children" to indicate the dilemma. Of course, there are many examples, headed by that redoubtable patriarch J. S. Bach, of men and women who left both children and works of genius to an appreciative posterity. But by and large it is true that many adults who have succeeded in keeping their talent intact up to their twenties feel they must choose between *libri* and *liberi*. In our studies, we found that promising artists who decide to continue in fine arts as adults tend to marry less often and have fewer children than their colleagues who opt out of their domain of giftedness to pursue more secure careers. This is especially true of women, for whom the competition between bearing (and rearing) children and dedication to art is more acute than for men. Many artists who have placed their talent on a back burner admit that family responsibilities had to take precedence; just as many other confess they simply had to give up marriage and children because their talent exerted an uncompromising attraction.

Although these conflicts have long been recognized, it has been generally assumed that real genius perseveres despite all the upheavals of the life cycle. "Talent will out" is the common opinion; those who are distracted from its Relentless unfolding are obviously the weak and the less gifted. But, of course, we do not know if this is indeed the case. Perhaps it is the most talented people, the ones most sensitive, to the possibilities of existence, who drop out of the single-minded pursuit necessary to maintain excellence in a domain of giftedness. In a trivially circular sense it is true, by definition, that the most talented are those who persevere. We do not know, however, whether this is also true in an empirical sense—nor is there a way we can see how this proposition could be tested.

Identity, intimacy, generativity: In our culture, these are themes that offer the typical person a chance to restructure his or her self around new goals. They are themes that tend to emerge in a sequence, at predictable times along the life cycle, at the confluence of maturational changes and social expectations. How do they affect the development of the once gifted youngster? Under what conditions will talent emerge untouched from the crisis, and when will it be transformed beyond recognition or abandoned?

Of course, there are also myriad unpredictable events and accidents, some private, some historical, that will affect the development of talent. An illness, the death of a parent, an economic depression, or a sudden epiphany might either reaffirm the young person in his or her goal or change the direction of life forever. At this point, there is no way to take the impact of these random events into account. But the universal regularities of the life cycle, with the dynamic inter-action of its psychosocial phases, presents a set of predictable conditions that can be related to the unfolding of talent. In fact, unless such relations are established, it is difficult to see how an early diagnosis of giftedness can have any prognostic value.

Giftedness and Cognitive Development

Superimposed on the sequence of changes in goal structure at different stages of life are transition points between cognitive stages. The development of thought, as Piaget has shown, does not consist of a simple quantitative increase in the content of knowledge or the ability to reason. It proceeds, rather, by discontinuous reorgani-zations in the way we think. As Carter and Ormrod (1982) have shown, gifted children (or at least children with IQs above 130) pass through the same sequence of transformation in thinking strategies as normal children do, but faster; at age 13, the average gifted child thinks in terms of formal operations, whereas the average normal child 2 years later still combining concrete and formal operations in his thought.

The qualitative transitions in thought processes introduce another source of unpredictability in the development of giftedness. Passing from sensorimotor learning to concrete operations, or from concrete to abstract thought, it appears that the growing child might lose the edge of superiority he or she had at the previous stage. Excellence at the concrete-operational stages in no way guarantees excellence at the stage of formal operations.

Bamberger (1982), for example, interprets the large dropout rate of talented musicians in adolescence as due to an inability on their part to continue to excel after the transition to formal thought. A child prodigy is music need not operate at the abstract level; superior sensorimotor skills can mark him or her as a genius. But by adolescence, teachers and the critical public begin to expect from the budding genius a sensitivity to the formal relationships in the music he or she plays. According to Bamberger, many brilliant performers must face the realization that the superior skills that served so well at the previous stage do not necessarily allow them to meet the new set of expectations. Presumably, the opposite pattern obtains as well. "Late blooming" may occur when a child who is not particularly good at the sensorimotor or concrete-operational level enters the stage of formal thinking and finds himself at home there.

The complexities of interdependence among the different lines of development begin to be apparent when we note that the main stage in the reorganization of personal goals—that of identity formation and search for autonomy—overlaps in time with the period during which most young people grapple with the transition from concrete- to formal-operational thought. Clearly, then, this is a phase of life in which genius might either vanish a shine with a renewed light. Of course, there might be transitions in cognitive development other than the ones included in the Piagetian canon, and hence other predictable turning points in the trajectory of talent. As cognitive psychology continues its explorations, its finding will have to be constantly integrated with our understanding of what happens to giftedness through the life-span.

Another way to look at time-related changes in the requirements for though is by adopting the *presented problem-solving* versus the *discovered problem-finding* model of the creative process. This model highlights the fact that when we measure superior performance in children with the IQ or will practically any other test, we are measuring ability to solve problems that an presented. However, superior adult performance in a creative domain inquires the ability to formulate new problems on one's own. The skill needed to solve problems appears to be of an entirely different order from the one necessary to discover problems; hence, predictions based on the former may have little bearing on later outcomes (Getzels 1964). Anyone teaching graduate students suspects, for example, that the indicators of problem-solving ability such as GPA, SAT, and GRE scores, performance on tests and the like are all rather poor at predicting which student will be able to propose an original dissertation. Dropouts from doctoral programs are often brilliant problem-solvers who all through their academic careers were rewarded for their cognitive skills; confronted for the first time with the tasks of formulating a problem of their own, however, they become paralyzed—while candidates far less promising on traditional measures succeed in discovering a worthwhile thesis.

Among artists, for example, it is clear that the ability to find problems is more essential for success than the ability to solve them (Getzels and Csikszentmihalyi 1976). In our current follow-up study, IQ tests and problem-solving ability measures taken 20 years ago bear no relationship, or a slightly negative one, to current artistic recognition. However, the tendency to approach unstructured tasks with a discovery orientation, and the ability to formulate new problems where none were posed, are still good predictors of success 20 years later.

At this point, we know next to nothing about why and how a child may get stuck at the stage of concrete operations, or never be able to formulate a novel problem. Unless we learn more, a cross-sectional assessment of talent in childhood will remain a useless indicator of achievements to come.

Changing Requirements of the Domain

The stages of cognitive development-discussed above presumably. apply to everyone—at least for people growing up in the rationalistic environment of Western culture. But in addition to such more or less "universal" sequences, each domain in which talent can be shown has its own sequences of expected levels of performance, and some of these may require reorganizations of skills that will suddenly inhibit the further development of talent or spur it to new heights.

In mathematics, for instance, the introduction of geometry as a subject at about the first year in high school opens up new opportunities and calls for spatial skills that are apparently based on structures of the brain different from the ones previous computational skills had relied on (Franco and Sperry 1977). This shift in challenges can overwhelm some formerly talented youngsters and allow others to shine for the first time. In general, however, it is probably the case that a change in cognitive demands at a new stage in the domain is more likely to dampen outstanding performance than to enhance it, for the simple reason that the youngsters who were not performing at the top in a previous stage are usually no longer in contention for "gifted" status by the time that status and its attendant support change in ways that might benefit them. In highly competitive domains, such as music, math, or sports, the way down is always much broader than the way up; year by year, it becomes more difficult to catch up, and dropping out becomes increasingly easy.

For psychosocial and cognitive development, theorists such as Erikson, Havighurst, and Piaget have provided models of sequences of development that are valuable heuristics for understanding the order and organization of those vectors. For the domain, which at first may seem more arbitrary the coherently ordered, a model familiar to most researchers in giftedness amplifies a general order across domains: Bloom's *Taxonomy of Educational Objectives* (Bloom et al. 1956). Given that the taxonomy was derived through the analysis of responses to thousands of different tests and test items, it focusing it on domains rather than on individual abilities is a justifiable and possibly more appropriate use of the taxonomy.

Looking at domains in terms of the taxonomy makes it possible to speech transition points where talent is likely to falter or to bloom (with apologies for the pun). Individuals who distinguish themselves by their rapid acquisition and comprehension of knowledge, and facile application of that knowledge to real problems (the first three major levels of the taxonomy) may belie this talent when it comes to analyzing, synthesizing, and evaluating (the three highest levels). Conversely, an individual who has mastered the three lower levels at a more conventional pace, thus never being identified as "gifted" may find in the higher levels the perfect medium for expressing exceptional ability. Werner von Braun, who developed the principles of rocket propulsion failed ninth-grade algebra. Yet, we must assume that he eventually mastered the basics of that domain, even if with less than flying colors, before he was able to achieve his masterful solution to the problem and put humanity a the path to the moon and stars. Albert Einstein, as a teenager, failed the admission exams in science at the Zurich Polytechnic.

A distinction similar to the one that involves Bloon's taxonomy has been drawn by Susanne Langer in her discussion of genius and talent. Langer considers talent to be technical mastery and genius to be "the power of conception". Bloon's taxonomy is clearly a further specification of these general definitions. Langer illustrates the implications of this distinction quite clearly when she writes:

> Precocity [in talent] is commonly taken for a sign of genius; and every year the correct stage, the radio, the screen, and sometimes even the picture gallery hail as an doubted genius some truly amazing child, whose talent overcomes the difficulties technique as a deer takes the pasture bars, and sometimes that child grows up to the art world afire... but far more often its adult life proves to be that of a good professional artist without special distinction.... But it is a mistake to think genius incomplete from the beginning.... Genius, indeed, sometimes appears only with maturity, as in Van Gogh, whose early pictures are undistinguished, and grows at deepens from work to work, like Beethoven's, Shakespeare's, or Cézanne's, long after technical mastery has reached its height (Langer 1953, pp. 408–409).

Although it is obvious that technical knowledge will vary from domain to domain, it is less obvious, but probably true, that the higher-order operations—analysis, synthesis, and evaluation—will also vary significantly across domains. Thus, the abilities that facilitate these operations in, say, music, have no relation to the same operations in physical chemistry. This is, of course, implied in Gardner's concept of multiple intelligences.

Descending once more from the ivory tower, we might point out a practical implication of the distinctions drawn in this section. It has been shown that more rapid cognitive development and technical mastery is one dimension that differentiates "gifted" from "normal" children. This may be termed the quantitative differential. We have also argued that giftedness may manifest itself after certain levels are mastered at a conventional rate on both of these sectors. This type of differentiation is not a matter of rate but of changes in process—a qualitative differential. Quantitative versus qualitative is the basis of the "enrichment" versus "acceleration" debate in curriculum design for the gifted. By considering qualitative and quantitative progression as attributes of the same dimensions, it becomes clear that programming is not a matter of "either/or". Rather, the gifted child builds one upon the other, and programming should be a matter of providing both and modulating their emphasis as the individual develops and changes. The implications for identification should be abundantly clear.

For instance, children placed in a gifted program by virtue of their rapid progress through the early levels of domains may not measure up to the requirements when the quantitative differential ceases to be the primary means of distinguishing the more from the less able. Conversely, as Delisle and Renzulli (1980) have pointed out, the "pool" of potential participants must be kept large and open, so that those who do not distinguish themselves along purely quantitative lines have the opportunity to foster and develop the more qualitative aspects of their abilities when progress through the domain brings them to the point of efficient mastery so as to utilize fully their superior skills at the higher levels. Finally, when higher-order qualitative processes become prerequisites of further progress within a domain, further opportunities arise for assessing the newly emerging skills of students both in and out of the program. Specific domains may differ in terms of when critical shifts in demands for performance occur. If both the domain and the individual involved to it undergo significant changes at these points—as we argue they must—it makes sense for the program and its identification apparatus to undergo a similar reorganization.

Significant work might be done to identify which domains have common abilities necessary for mastery of different levels. As the levels of the taxonomy are worked through for each new domain, the relationship of mastery a one domain to mastery in another also could be ascertained. There are clear parallels between transitions in this hierarchy and those in the other dimensions of our model. An obviously interesting one is the connection between concrete operations, presented problem solving, and the lowest order of a domain and that of the transition to higher orders, formal operations, and discovered problem solving.

Finally, it should be apparent from the earlier discussion that some domain are much more stable than others. These tend to be the ones that are clear defined and thus more amenable to precise measurement. What constitutes a great performance in running has not changed since the first Olympic games almost 3 millennia ago, and the criteria in math, music, or chess are almost as hallowed. In a *closed* domain, constructed by humans according to rational principles, requirements are likely to remain stable because the symbolic system is largely autonomous and self-contained—it need not respond changes in the rest of the culture. Western music or math evolve in term of their own intrinsic logic, to a large extent regardless of what happens elsewhere. There is no clear link between the transition to non-Euclidean geometry, or to 12-tone music, and any changes outside the domain of math of music. These transitions were the outcome of dissatisfaction with symbolic formulations within the specific fields and owed very little to social, politics or technological events or to progress in other symbolic media.

To put it another way, we can draw upon Saussure's (1959) distinction between *langue,* the abstract; synchronic semiotic system of language, at *parole,* or the concrete everyday speech of language users. *Langue* is a closed system with its own rules and internal logic; speech, although rooted in language, is a more open system, more responsive to sociocultural influences. Music is an analogous symbolic system. Popular music may shift in response to historical change, but the semiotics of music remain a relatively closed system that sets the parameters within which the popular variations occur. Criteria of excellence in closed domains will tend to be consistent over time.

By contrast, the plastic arts are relatively more open systems without the set language and rules that music is ultimately based on. Open domain interact more with whatever happens outside their own province. The boundaries are more permeable. Art and poetry are relatively less autonomous than music and math; to be effective, they must stay in touch with what is happening in the rest of the world. The poetry of Rupert Brooke idealizing war lost much of its point after he was killed in a conflict that revealed in sordid meaninglessness, whereas Picasso's *Guernica* owes its success in great part to the fact that it expresses the revulsion we have come to feel in the face of war. Criteria of excellence in open domains are bound to change more often and more drastically than in closed domains, because their parameter are less predictable.

Shifting Requirements of the Field

If by "domain" we mean a culturally structured pattern of opportunities for action, requiring a distinctive set of sensorimotor and cognitive skills—in short, a symbolic system such as music, mathematics, or athletics—we may designate by "field" the social organization of a domain. A field includes all the statuses pertinent to the domain; it specifies the habitual patterns of behavior—or roles—expected from persons who occupy the various statuses. The field of art includes the statuses and attendant roles of art student, teacher, museum visitor, collector, critic, speculator, historian, as well as that of the creative artist.

We like to believe that the gifted are immune to societal pressure—that the jargon of status and role is not relevant in their case. But it takes only the briefest glimpse at the struggles gifted people must undergo in real life to realize how deep the effects of social expectations are on the development of their talent. And to the extent that these expectations change at different stages of the progress within a field, some previously gifted persons will not be able to continue in the role, whereas others might flourish.

A good example involves the transition between the status of art student to that of an independent fine artist. In our culture (at least in the 1960s, when our study was conducted), many young people who were good at drawing entered art school because they were attracted to the artist's role: the bohemian life-style of the solitary, independent, unconventional genius without material concerns. Fine-arts students who internalized this role were rewarded in art school. They received better grades and stood higher in the opinion of their teachers. Many possibly talented young artists dropped out of the field at this stage because they felt uncomfortable in the expected role.

As the young artist began to move out of his student status and tried to establish himself as a practicing artist, an entirely new set of role requirements, often diametrically opposed to the previous ones, came into effect. To be recognized as an artist in our present culture, a young person has to turn from being a withdrawn, introspective loner into becoming a gregarious self-promoter who can attract the attention of the gatekeepers of the field and who can negotiate advantageous terms with gallery owners and collectors. To make it as an artist, he must learn to banter with businessmen, flatter dowagers, and impress foundations. Many talented young persons succumb to these unexpected challenges that strain the adaptive capacity of even the most flexible among them (Getzels and Csikszentmilialyi 1976, pp. 184–208). Of lcourse, in other societies, at different times, the artists' status will require other behaviors, other compromises. In contemporary socialist countries, for example, the artist's role is much less individualistic and unconventional from the very beginning; hence, the later adaptation to the requirements of a collectivistic bureaucracy are less discontinuous.

Similar adjustments are required in other fields. For instance, when a young singer or instrumentalist becomes good enough to enter auditions and competitions, an entirely new set of demands enters the picture, and even the most promising musical talent may be cut short by the pressures of public performance. Later on, one might have to learn to politic and to ingratiate oneself with those who control good singing parts or prizes at competition and the gifted musician may discover he has no gifts for that.

The demand for mathematical talent in society influences the way it is taught in school. The resultant competitive pressures can take a heavy toll ever among the best students. In our current study of gifted high school mathematicians, girls especially express a distaste for the weekly contests that students against each other to determine their relative standing as "mathletes". Typically, if a girl displaces a boy from one of the highest ranks, the other boys will sympathize with their demoted colleague and ostracize the successful girl. But also, many of the boys who are good at math and enjoy working at it are unable to cope with the requirements surrounding their status. Later on, of course, the demands will change again—first in college, then in graduate school, then in the professional roles. The competition remains, although in a less obvious form; many new considerations will also enter the picture. For instance, the number of scholarships available in college the state of the job market, will deter some talented persons or attract other to the field.

The implications of these shifts for the identification of talent are that occur must take into account carefully the role requirements of the next status before making predictions on the basis of success in a previous one. For instance success in school is a rather poor predictor of success in many of the real world settings in which gifted people usually perform. This for at least two reasons: first, because the academic incentive system is typically extrinsical motivated (e.g., grades), whereas genuine creative performance relies a intrinsic motivation and may be hindered by extrinsic rewards (Amabile 1983). Hence talented children who perform well in the school system often become lost after graduation when the extrinsic reward structure can no longer guide their performance. Second, academic institutions emphasize and reveal problem solving, whereas talented performance after school depends heavy on problem finding (Getzels and Csikszentmihalyi 1976). Therefore, we might conclude that a child who is exceptionally well adapted to the social system of the school and excels therein is *ipso facto* less likely to be well adapted to the requirements of a creative role, especially in fields like art, literature, and basic sciences, where extrinsic rewards might be arbitrary and problem finding is at a premium.

The Crossing Paths of Development

Figure 3.1 summarizes what we have said so far about the temporal construction of giftedness. The lowest of the four steplike lines represents the major psychosocial transitions in the life cycle. Erikson's eight stages were used in this illustration, but the number of transitions depends on how fine an analysis is required. For example, Mönks and Ferguson (1983) consider as many as six "transformations in behavioral patterns" during adolescence: attachment friendship, sexuality, achievement, autonomy, and identity.

The second line from the bottom illustrates major changes in cognitive development. Here the traditional Piagetian transitions are indicated, the problem solving–problem finding dimension is alluded to, although as yet there is no evidence about the chronology of that transition. Here again of course, more refined distinctions in the developmental sequence are possible.

Whereas the two lower lines refer to sequences common to most people in our culture, the two upper lines will vary by domain and by field. In this illustration, the domain of the figurative arts was used as an example. Transition points along these two lines are even more approximate than on the lower ones; they are based on experience rather than rigorous data. To identify clearly the stages at which domains require restructuring of performance is one of the challenges for gifted-ness research. If we want to be able to give informed help to the gifted and to assist their development, it seems we ought to identify such transitions and understand their dynamics. For example, we compare a gifted child at around age 5 (line A in Fig. 3.1) and then in his late teens (line B), it is clear that the youngster will be in different developmental stages on all four time lines. And if we chose the same two time points for a different youngster with different abilities in a different domain, the cross sections would be different yet again. The challenges will be qualitatively different and so will the resources one needs to draw on. The traits that make the child gifted at A may not be of much use to the young person at B. If the assumption of giftedness as a stable "trait" is maintained the parent, teacher, or counselor who knows what help A needs to maintain his gifts may well be far off the mark when it comes to helping B.

In the study of gifted high school mathematicians mentioned in the previous section, we met an intriguing problem. When teachers were asked to rate students on "performance as compared to what you see as their potential almost all of the freshmen were rated at or near their potential, where seniors were rated bimodally —half at or near, half "far below". Is this due to sheer difference in ability? It does not seem to be so: The students who live up to their potential are no different on a number of standardized measures of mathematical ability from the students who are not using their talents. Is it due to the *Sturm und Drang* of adolescence? Possibly; the achieving students see getting into a good college as the central current problem of their lives. The underachievers tend to say things such as "figuring out where and where I'm going", or "trying to make peace with mother and at least start talking to my father before I leave for college". Is it due to changing interests as new domains are opened up? Possibly; although they are talking the same courses, achievers spend over twice as much time thinking about mathematics as the nonachievers do. Is the difference due to increasing difficult demands within the domain of mathematics? Again, possibly; trigonometry and calculus are certainly more demanding in an absolute sense, and seniors perceive math work as more challenging than do freshmen. Finally, we must consider the possibility that the whole concept of living up to one's potential is an artifact of the teacher's differential perception of freshmen versus seniors. Teachers have a set of

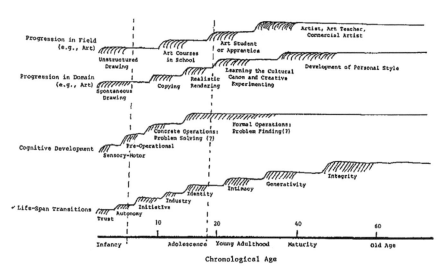

Fig. 3.1 Example of time lines in the development of talents. A measurement of talent taken at point *A* in the life cycle will reflect a very different combination of processes than a measure taken at point *B*

preconceptions as to what constitutes the "proper" progression through a high-powered math program. Students who adapt to these expectations, who fulfill their "proper" role, may be seen as the achievers, whereas those who calculate and integrate to the tune of a different drummer are rated as nonachievers. It is also true that teachers cannot tell whether a freshman does or does not live up to his or her potential; for freshmen, aptitude and achievement are synonymous. Only later in high school is it possible not to live up to one's potential.

Our intuition at this point, though, is that no one of these possibilities gives the full answer for every student. Rather, the relative contribution of each dimension may differ greatly in explaining why each youth did or did not use his or her gift. Of course, only a longitudinal study could answer the questions completely.

To maintain her or his talent over the life-span, a person has to integrate more and more complex experiences in consciousness and behavior. A child prodigy who fails to grow along the four vectors of complexification becomes an increasingly pathetic example of unfulfilled promise. At what age does the unfolding of giftedness stop? There does not seem to be a definite end to its growth. Verdi, who was considered to have talent early in life, composed *Falstaff* when he was nearly 80 years old, and the joy and beauty in that work is like nothing he had ever written before.

Those working with children who are able to perform at exceptional levels in some domain are understandably eager to recognize and to encourage what truly seems to be a precious gift—a rare and enviable possession. It is a natural reaction that we share. But valuing exceptional performance should not lead to blind worship or specious pleading. It is not necessary to subscribe to the naturalistic fallacy, to a position that reifies a process constituted jointly by cultural expectations and by individual abilities.

By reifying giftedness as "scientific fact", one might gain short-term respectability and financial support. But we shall certainly sacrifice long-term growth in understanding. For talent is not the expression of a personal trait but the fulfillment of a cultural potential; it is not just a cognitive process but the focusing of the whole of consciousness on a task; it is not a gift one has to hold on to forever, because changes in the growing person's priorities, and changes in the demands of the domain and of the field, often turn gold into ashes and ashes into gold. To pretend otherwise only serves to obscure reality and prevents a conceptual grasp of the phenomenon.

The directions for research suggested in this chapter may seem circuitous and difficult to follow. They include assuming a perspective alien to those trained in a purely cognitive approach. Yet it is liberating to realize that giftedness is a much more flexible potential than the naturalistic approach asserts it to be, and that in the last resort it is up to us to decide what talents are and how much giftedness there shall be.

References

Amabile, T. M. (1983). *The social psychology of creativity*. New York: Springer.

Bamberger, J. (1982). Growing up prodigies: The midlife crisis. *New Directions for Child Development, 17*, 61–78.

Bloom, B. S., Englchart, M. D., Furst, E. D., Hill, W. H., & Graghwohl, D. R. (1956). *Taxonomy of educational objectives: Handbook. I. Cognitive domain*. Makay: New York.

Brannigan, A. (1981). *The social basis of scientific discoveries*. Cambridge: Cambridge University Press.

Carter, K. R., & Ormrod, J. E. (1982). Acquisition of formal operations by intellectually gifted children. *Gifted Child Quarterly, 26*(3), 110–115.

Delisle, J. R., & Renzulli, J. S. (1980). The revolving door identification and programming model: Correlates of creative production. *Gifted Child Quarterly, 26*(2), 89–95.

Erikson, E. H. (1963). *Childhood and society* (2nd ed.). New York: Norton.

Feldman, D. H. (1980). *Beyond universals in cognitive development*. Norwood: Ablex.

Franco, L., & Sperry, R. W. (1977). Hemisphere localization for cognitive processing of geometry. *Neuropsychologia, 15*, 107–114.

Freedman, D. G. (1980). The social and the biological: A necessary unity. *Zygon, 15*(2), 117–131.

Gardner, H. (1983). *Frames of mind*. New York: Basic Books.

Getzels, J. W. (1964). Creative thinking, problem solving, and instruction. In E. R. Hilgard (Ed.), *Theories of learning and instruction. The sixty-third yearbook of the national society of the study of education, Part 1* (pp. 240–267). Chicago: University of Chicago Press.

Getzels, J. W., & Cskiszentmilialyi, M. (1976). *The creative vision: A longitudinal study of problem finding in art*. New York: Wiley.

Getzels, J. W., & Jackson, P. W. (1962). *Creativity and intelligence: Explorations with gifted students*. New York: Wiley.

Havighurst, R. J. (1951). *Developmental tasks and education*. New York: Longhmans.

Langer, S. K. (1953). *Feeling and form: A theory of art*. New York: Seribner.

Mönks, F. J., & Ferguson, T. J. (1983). Gifted adolescents: An analysis of their psychosocial development. *Journal of Youth and Adolescence, 12*(1), 1–18.

Oden, M. (1968). The fulfillment of promise: 40-years follow-up of the Terman gifted group. *Genetic Psychology Monographs, 77,* 3–93.
Renzulli, J. S. (1980). Will the gifted child movement be alive and well in 1990? *Gifted Child Quarterly, 24*(1), 3–9.
de Saussure, F. (1959). *Course in general linguistics.* New York: Philosophical Library.
Terman, L. M. (1925). *Genetic studies of genius: Mental and physical traits of a thousand gifted children* (Vol. 1). Stanford: Stanford University Press.
Torrance, E. P. (1965). *Gifted children in the classroom.* New York: MacMillan. (Quoted in Barge, V. S. & Renzulli, J. S. (Eds.). (1975) *Psychology and education of the gifted* (2nd ed., pp. 48–55). New York: Wiley.)

Chapter 4
Society, Culture, and Person: A Systems View of Creativity

Mihaly Csikszentmihalyi

The Constitution of Creativity

It is customary to date the renewal of interest in creativity among psychologists to Guillord's presidential address to the APA more than 30 years ago (Guilford 1950). Ever since that date, an increasing tide of publications on the subject has been appearing in our journals. Many of these books and articles have tried to answer what has been thought to be the most fundamental question: *What* is creativity? But no one has raised the simple question that should precede attempts at defining, measuring, or enhancing, namely: *Where* is creativity?

On hearing this question, most people would answer "Why, in the creative person's head, of course". Others might demur at such a subjective location and say that creativity is in the thought, object, or action produced by the person. At any rate, all of the definitions of creativity of which I am aware assume that the phenomenon exists, as a concrete process open to investigation, either inside the person or in the works produced.

After studying creativity on and off for almost a quarter of a century, I have come to the reluctant conclusion that this is not the case. We cannot study creativity by isolating individuals and their works from the social and historical milieu in which their actions are carried out. This is because what we call creative is never the result of individual action alone; it is the product of three main shaping forces: a set of social institutions, or *field,* that selects from the variations produced by individuals those that are worth preserving; a stable cultural *domain* that will preserve and transmit the selected new ideas or forms to the following generations; and finally the *individual,* who brings about some change in the domain, a change that the field, will consider to be creative.

So the question "Where is creativity?" cannot be answered solely with reference to the person and the person's work. Creativity is a phenomenon that results

Reproduced with permission from Conception of Giftedness (Eds. R.J. Sternberg and J. E. Davisdon), pages 325−339, New York, USA. Copyright © 1988, Cambridge University Press.

M. Csikszentmihalyi, *The Systems Model of Creativity*,
DOI: 10.1007/978-94-017-9085-7_4,
© Springer Science+Business Media Dordrecht 2014

from interaction between these three systems, Without a culturally defined domain of action in which innovation is possible, the person cannot even get started. And without a group of peers to evaluate and confirm the adaptiveness of the innovation, it is impossible to differentiate what is creative from what is simply statistically improbable or bizarre.

Three colleagues from three different generations have been especially helpful in developing the ideas in this chapter. J.W. Getzels, who inspired me to the study of creativity, has always been a source of fresh insights and strong values. Howard Gardner, as simulating and generous a colleague as one might wish for, sharpened the thoughts in this chapter through the numerous conversations we have had over the years. And so did Rick Robinson, who is standing out now on the long journey of scholarship.

The importance of this distinction is shown by the muddle that people who ignore it are prone to get into. For instance, Herbert Simon (1985), in his 1985 address to the APA, made the claim that his computer program BACON could replicate the solutions of some of the most creative problems in science—such as the derivation of Kepler's and Newton's laws—and therefore it should be considered to have the attribute of "creativity" (Csikszentmihalyi 1986), His conclusion would follow if one were to accept the premise, clearly articulated by Simon, that if an object or idea A is undistinguishable from another object or idea B, and if we agree that B is creative, then it follows that A must be creative too. This argument might work in the domain of logic, but it does not apply in the empirical world, where creativity exists only in specific social and historical contexts.

To see the weakness in Simon's argument, we need only to consider the case of a forger who can exactly reproduce some painting that we have agreed to recognize as creative—one originally painted by, let us say, Rembrandt. The two canvases, the original and the forgery, are completely indistinguishable. Does it follow from this identity between the two products that Rembrandt and the forger are equally creative, or that the, two paintings are equally creative? If we say yes, then there is no more point in talking about creativity.

My argument, of course, is that the two paintings may be of equal technical skill, of the same aesthetic value, but they cannot be considered to be equal in creativity. Rembrandt's work is creative because he introduced some variations in the domain of painting at a certain point in history, when those variations were novel, and when they were instrumental in revising and enlarging the symbolic domain of the visual arts. The very same variations a few years later were no longer creative, because then they simply reproduced existing forms. The same argument applies to BACON and to any other procedure that replicates a creative achievement.

It is impossible to tell whether or not an object or idea is creative by simply looking at it. Without a historical context, one lacks the reference points necessary to determine if the product is in fact an adaptive innovation. An unusual African mask might seem the product of creative genius, until we realize that the same mask has been carved exactly the same way for centuries, A complex mathematical equation that purports to explain teleportation might impress the layman, but be recognized as pure gibberish by the mathematically trained.

I realized only recently, after writing for over two decades about creativity, that I had never "seen" it. Of course, like most people, I have been exposed to many objects and ideas that we call creative. Some of these might have been arresting, or interesting, or impressive, but I cannot say that I ever thought of them as "creative". Their creativity is something that I came to accept later, if at all, after comparing the object or idea with others of its kind, but mostly because I had been told by experts that these things were creative.

When I was a young child, we lived for a while in Venice, a few steps from St. Mark's Square, in a spot where the density of original works of art is one of the highest in the world. Later we moved to Florence, and every morning I walked past Brunelleschi's elegant Foundling Hospital with its priceless round Della Robbia ceramics. As a teenager I lived on the Gianicolo Hill in Rome, overlooking Michelangelo's great dome. During this time, my father, a redoubtable amateur art historian made sure to point out to me the flowering of Renaissance creativity that surrounded us, I believed him, but I must confess that those masterpieces by and large made no impression on me. Some of them did produce an uncanny sense of serenity; others conveyed a great sense of power, or an undefinable excitement. But creativity? The great breakthroughs of Western art all looked equally old and decrepit to me; to think of them as innovations seemed a silly convention. I am afraid that in those years I would have gladly exchanged Giotto's frescoes in the Scrovegni Chapel for some Donald Duck comics illustrated by Walt Disney.

One might ask what this proves—only that I was ignorant and that it requires a certain amount of sophistication to recognize genuine creativity. I grant my ignorance, but I beg to raise what I think is an important point: Where does the information that gives us the ability to make sophisticated judgments come from? The information does not seem to be in the object itself. If we think about it, the reason we believe that Leonardo or Einstein was creative is that we have read that that is the case, we have been told it is true; our opinions about who is creative and why ultimately are based on faith. We have faith in the domains of art and science, and we trust the judgment of the field, that is, of the artistic and scientific establishments.

There is nothing wrong with this, because it is an inevitable situation. But by recognizing it, we must also accept some of its consequences, namely, that any attribution of creativity must be relative, grounded only in social agreement. And from this it also follows that social agreement is one of the constitutive aspects of creativity, without which the phenomenon would not exist.

It is easiest to see this process in art, where the selection criteria of the field change rather erratically. Kermode (1985) tells how Botticelli was for centuries considered to be a coarse painter, and the women he painted "sickly" and "clumsy". Only in the mid-nineteenth century did some critics begin to reevaluate his work and see in it creative anticipations of modern sensibility. To what extent was creativity contained in Botticelli's canvases, and to what extent did it emerge from the interpretive efforts of critics like Ruskin? One might argue that Botticelli's creativity was constituted by Ruskin's interpretations, that without the latter the former would not exist, and hence that Ruskin and the other critics and viewers who have since looked closely at Botticelli's work are just as indispensable to Botticelli's creativity as was the painter himself.

Similar situations abound in the history of art. In his lifetime, Rembrandt was thought to be a less important painter than Jan Lievens, who was also working at the same time in Amsterdam. How many people know of Lievens now? The powerful canvases of Francisco de Zurbaran were eagerly sought after in the royal court of Madrid until around 1645, when Murillo began to show his more graceful and lively paintings; after a few years Zurbaran was forgotten, and later died in poverty (Borghero 1986). To understand creativity, it seems necessary to know how the attributions of creativity are made. By what process does Rembrandt emerge as more creative than Lievens?

The notoriously fickle realm of the arts is by no means the only one in which social processes determine what is and what is not to be considered creative. As Kuhn (1970, 1974) has noted, the same forces are at work in the hard sciences. In the domains of physics and chemistry, in the domain of mathematics, originality is attributed by social processes that are relative and fallible and that sometimes are reversed by posterity.

Augustine Brannigan (1981) has reviewed several instances of scientific discoveries in which retrospective reinterpretation was at least as important as the original contribution had been. For example, he makes an interesting case to the effect that our view of Mendel's contribution to genetics is generally quite wrong. The impression we have is that Mendel made a series of epochal experiments in the genetic transmission of traits in the 1860s, but that his creativity was not recognized by the scientific community until about 40 years later. This view, according to Brannigan, is radically mistaken in a subtle but essential respect. He argues that Mendel's experiments were not and could not have been contributions to genetics at the time they were made. Their implications for the theory of variation and natural selection were discovered only in 1900 by William Bateson and other evolutionists looking for a mechanism that explained discontinuous inheritance. Within their theoretical framework, Mendel's work suddenly acquired an importance that it had lacked before, even in the mind of Mendel himself. So where was Mendel's creativity? In his mind, in his experiments, or in the use his results were put to by later scientists? The answer, it seems to me, must be that it is to be found in all three. Just as the interpretations of Ruskin and other critics are inseparable from Botticelli's creativity, so the interpretations of Bateson and his fellows are constitutive parts of Mendel's creativity.

Brannigan forces us to see how even ostensibly simple facts, such as what is or is not a "discovery", are really the results of social processes of negotiation and legitimation. Most people would agree, for instance, that Columbus discovered America. But what does "discovery" mean in this context? Certainly it does not mean that he was the first man to set foot on the shores of the Western Hemisphere. Nor did it mean that Columbus knew that he had found a new continent previously unknown to Europeans; until the end he was convinced he had landed in Asia.

It means, as Brannigan shows, that he was the man for whom the field that could legitimize such things (which in his case included the Spanish crown, its royal commission, and various scholars and cartographers) was willing to make a claim of discovery. Not until Vespucci recognized that the so-called West Indies were part of an entirely different continent did Columbus's almost superhuman efforts get retrospectively revised as a "discovery". And if in the fullness of time it turns out that it was Erik the Red who really discovered America, that "discovery" will be as much a result of scholarship and politics as a result of Erik's travels.

A Dynamic Model of the Creative Process

One way to represent the set of relationships that constitute creativity is through the "map" provided in Fig. 4.1. It is important to realize that the relationships shown in the figure are dynamic links of circular causality. In other words, each of the three main systems—person, field, and domain—affects the others and is affected by them in turn, One might say that the three systems represent three "moments" of the same creative process.

The starting point on this map is purely arbitrary, One might start from the "person", because we are used to thinking in these terms—that the idea begins, like the lighted bulb in the cartoon blurb, within the head of the creative individual. But, of course, the information that will go into the idea existed long before the creative person arrived on the scene. It had been stored in the symbol system of the culture, in the customary practices, the language, the specific notation of the "domain." A person who has no access to this information will not be able to make a creative contribution, no matter how able or skilled the person otherwise is. One needs to know music to write a creative symphony. It is difficult to become recognized as a creative Mandarin chef without knowing quite a bit about Chinese cooking.

A corollary of this relationship is that depending on the structure of the domain, it might be either relatively easy or more difficult for a person to innovate. The more precise the notation system, the easier it is to detect change and hence to evaluate whether or not the person has made an original contribution. Other things being equal, it should be easier to establish creativity in mathematics, music, or physics than, say, philosophy, the visual arts, or biology.

But returning to the system "person", we see that its contribution to the creative process is to produce some variation in the information inherited from the culture.

The source of the variation might be an inherited or learned cognitive flexibility, a more dogged motivation, or some rare event in the life of the person. Of course, this is the aspect of the process that almost all psychologists interested in creativity have been studying—unfortunately, this usually is the only aspect studied. And by itself, the process of generating variation will not reveal what creativity is about. The reason is that focusing on the individual out of context does not allow the observer to evaluate the variation produced. It has been said that

Fig. 4.1 The focus of
creativity. This "map" shows
the interrelations of the three
systems that jointly determine
the occurrence of a creative
idea, object, or action. The
individual takes some
information provided by the
culture and transforms it, and
if the change is deemed
valuable by society, it will be
included in the domain, thus
providing a new starting point
for the next generation of
persons. The actions of all
three systems are necessary
for creativity to occur

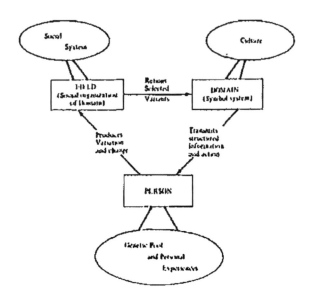

99 % of all new ideas are garbage, regardless of the domain or the status of the
thinker. To sift out the good ideas from the bad, another system is needed.

It is the task of the "field" to select promising variations and to incorporate
them into the domain. The easiest way to define a field is to say that it includes all
those persons who can affect the structure of a domain. Thus, the field of art
includes the following: art teachers and art historians, because they pass on the
specialized symbolic information to the next generation; art critics, who help
establish the reputation of individual artists; collectors, who make it possible for
artists and works of art to survive; gallery owners and museum curators, who
preserve and act as midwives to the production of art; and, finally, the peer group
of artists whose interaction defines styles and revolutions of taste.

Thus, the field of art, like any other field, is made up of a network of inter-
locking roles. Some of them have a better chance than others of incorporating a
selected variation into the domain. The people who fill these privileged roles act as
"gatekeepers" to the domain. For instance, in a field like nuclear physics, the
conviction of a thousand high school physics teachers that a new idea is pure
genius probably would not be enough to get the new idea into the journals and
textbooks that define the domain, whereas the same conviction held by half a
dozen Nobel Prize winners might do it. During the Renaissance, the attention of a
pope, or his mistress, was enough to select out the work of a young artist and slate
it for preservation; once preserved, the work becomes part of the canon and will
filter through, as one item of information in the domain, so that following generations of artists can be inspired to imitate it or reject it.

It goes without saying that fields will differ in the stringency of their selective
mechanisms, the sensitivity of their gatekeepers, and the dynamics of their inner
organization. The fields of botany and genetics in the USSR had only one

gatekeeper for almost a generation, and his criteria of selection were based more on ideology than biology (Lecourt 1977; Medvedev 1971). Critics complain that the fate of American art is decided by only ten thousand inhabitants of Manhattan, but compared with most of the past stages of Western civilization, during which a few princes and bishops held the keys of artistic survival, this is a huge field.

It also follows that a field with fuzzy selection criteri, or one with gatekeepers who are not highly respected, will have great difficulty in establishing the creativity of a new idea. Similarly, but for opposite reasons, a new idea will face difficulties in being recognized as creative if the field is defensive, rigid, or embedded in a social system that discourages novelty. For instance, the aridity of Soviet genetics in the thirties was not, strictly speaking, a fault of the scientists who made up the field, but of the peculiar agenda of the broader social system of which the field was a part.

Every field is embedded in a specific social system. The resources of the larger society help to support tile recognition of new ideas. The flowering of new ideas in Athens in the fifth century BC, or in fifteenth-century Florence, nineteenth-century Paris, or twentieth-century Vienna and New York, was due in large part to the fact that these centers at those times were in the position to pay attention to an unusually great number of new ideas. What does it take for a community to be able to do so? To a certain extent the materialist explanation applies: Disposable wealth is one of the conditions that makes the selection of novelty possible. In addition, it takes disposable attention—people who in addition to being wealthy have the time to take an interest in the domain (Csikszentmihalyi 1978, 1979). A hundred years ago, every aspiring artist in Europe dreamed of being in Paris, where the field of art had the greatest financial clout, as well as being numerically the largest and most sophisticated. It is sobering to remember that even the great Leonardo, that most protean of all known creators, timed his moves to the tides of his patrons' fortunes. As soon as Sforza started spending lavishly, he left Florence for the ducal court in Milan; when the pope became more solvent than the duke, he moved to Rome; he went back and forth between the two Italian courts, but when the finances of King Francis I began to outshine those of both, he packed up for France.

Occasionally, great creative reformulations appear to take place outside of all constituted fields. Gardner (1986) makes this case for Freud: Essentially, he invented psychoanalysis, and at the time he did so there was no social organization specifically qualified to support or suppress his ideas. In a certain sense, the founders of all great systems are in the same position: Galileo may be said to have started the field of experimental physics, and at the time of the Wright brothers there was no field of aeronautics. What happens in such cases is that a subset of people from related fields recognize the validity of the new variation and become identified with the emerging field. In the case of Galileo, it was mathematicians, astronomers, and philosophers who were attracted to his ideas; in the case of the Wright brothers, it was automobile and bicycle mechanics; Freud's first followers were other medical men.

But the model suggests that without people in neighboring fields who become attracted to the new idea, the creative process will be aborted, If no qualified persons are willing to invest their energy in preserving the variation, it will not become one of the "memes" that future generations will know about. In a setting with not enough mechanics interested in flying, the Wrights' efforts would eventually have been forgotten, and aeronautics would not have developed.

The Element of Time in the Constitution of Creativity

In looking again at the complex dynamics represented in Fig. 4.1, it should be clear that time plays an important role in the creative process. It is here that the folk view of the creative idea as a bolt of lightning is least realistic. First of all, an important breakthrough usually follows a long period of gestation in the domain. The atomic theory of matter existed, in embryonic form, 25 centuries before it was given its first satisfactory shape. Medical advances, engineering triumphs, and artistic revolutions typically exist for a long time as unclearly formulated possibilities. During this period of gestation, new converts to the field become inbued by its "problematics". Occasionally there seems to be a discovery that truly comes from nowhere: Roentgen's discovery of radiation and Fleming's discovery of penicillin usually are held to be accidental. But they appear to be accidents only if we abstract the creative person from the context. The behavior of electric current in a cathode tube and the effects of various substances on bacterial cultures were problems that existed in Roentgen's and Fleming's respective domains; we might perhaps even say that they provided an implicit tension, a demand for resolution that exerted an invisible pull on workers in the field. If Roentgen and Fleming had not been sensitive to these potentialities in their work, no amount of lucky accidents would have produced a discovery.

It is not only in the transition from the domain to the person but also in the move from the person to the field, and from the field back to the domain, that time is involved. The only way to establish whether or not something is creative is through comparison, evaluation, and interpretation. Sometimes, as we have seen, the field reverses its judgment: Botticelli moves to the forefront, and Lievens fades into the background; Mendel is hailed a genius, and Lysenko is revealed a fake.

And once the field makes up its collective mind—at least temporarily—it takes a while for the new idea to be included into the canon of the domain. Given current technology and the highly rationalized organization of most fields, this time lag is shorter than at some times in the past. But it has been estimated that it still takes an average of 7 years for a bona fide new discovery to make its first appearance in the textbooks of most domains. This process is faster or slower depending on the structure of the domain and of the field.

I know a particle physicist of great renown who likes to tell a story about an advanced seminar he has taught in Munich, where one of the students once interrupted his blackboard demonstration and jotted down a formulation of the equation different from the formulation he had been developing. The student's version appeared to be more elegant and suggestive than the professor's had been. The story goes that in a matter of weeks, every theoretical physicist in Germany knew of the event, and within a month, physicists on the West Coast of the United States were toying with the new equation. Eventually the student got himself a Nobel Prize.

Such a denouement would be impossible in most other disciplines. It could never happen, for instance, in psychology. Imagine a student, even if he had the most brilliant mind in the world, being able to impress his peers, his teachers, and the community of psychologists by something he said in a seminar! Not even the best known psychologist could achieve such a result. Perhaps in very limited, very specialized subfields it is possible to earn instant recognition for a creative idea, but the lack of common conceptual commitment, the fragmentation of the domain, guarantees that the recognition will remain for a long time parochial.

There is another sense in which time is implicated in the systems model developed in Fig. 4.1. The arrows pointing from person to field to domain. Actually describe an ascending spiral, because every new bit of information added to the domain will become the input for the next generation of persons. Thus, the model represents a cycle in the process of cultural evolution. As the terms suggest, *variation, selection,* and *transmission* are the three main phases of the cycle, and these are also the main phases of every evolutionary sequence (Campbell 1965, 1976). We might conclude that creativity is one of the aspects of evolution. But contrary to biological evolution, in which information relevant to phenotypic behavior is changed chemically in the genes, cultural evolution involves changes in information coded extrasomatically. Dawkins (1976) coined the term "meme" to refer to a "unit of imitation" that was transmitted from one generation to the next, A meme could be a tool like a stone ax, a formula for smelting copper, the Pythagorean theorem, the first bar of Beethoven's Fifth Symphony, the concept of democracy, the smile of the Mona Lisa—in short, any structured information that could be remembered that was worth passing on through time. Using Dawkins's term, we would say that a domain is a system of related memes that change through time, and what changes them is the process of creativity (Csikszentmihaiyi and Massimini 1985).

The Generative Force of the Field

In Fig. 4.1, the arrows go in a clockwise direction from domain to person to field, and then again to the domain—at a later point in time. This sequence, although it accurately represents the main trends, does not exhaust all the possibilities. A field —or the society that harbors it—may stimulate directly the emergence of new ideas in people who otherwise would never have taken up work in a particular domain.

The case of Brunelleschi is a good example. He was clearly one of the most creative individuals of the Renaissance, whose impact on the future of architecture is indisputable. Yet by all accounts he never would have became an artist and architect if he had been born a generation earlier, when the community of Florence was less interested in sponsoring art. Brunelleschi was the son of an upper-class professional, a notary with good political connections, and he went through the best educational training the city had to offer. Everyone expected him to follow a career in the liberal professions. Yet at the age of 23, in 1398, Brunelleschi joined the goldsmiths' guild and started practicing the plastic arts. It was a startling choice for a scion of the oligarchy (Heydenreich 1974, p. 31), but as the demand for good artists became more intense, more of his peers followed Brunelleschi's example.

Florence in the first 25 years of the fifteenth century illustrates well how the field can stimulate the emergence of creativity. There is general agreement that during those few years some of the most enduringly original works of art were produced in what was a relatively small community. An approach to creativity that focused on the person would have to explain what happened in Florence by postulating a sudden and temporary increase in the originality of individual artists, presumably based on genetic drift or some environmental change that increased originality. But the more likely explanation is that individual potentialities remained constant, and the changes that produced the Renaissance took place in the social system, the field of art, and, to a lesser extent, the culture and the domain.

By the dawn of the fifteenth century, Florence had been the foremost financial center of Europe for almost two centuries, and one of its main manufacturing centers. By judiciously lending money to various kings and princes in England, Germany, and France, at least a dozen families in Florence (the Mozzi, Peruzzi, Bardi, Spini, Scali, Pulci, Abbati, Falconeri, Alfani, Alberti, Chiarenti, Cerchi, Buonsignori, Franceni, Rimberti, not to mention the latecomers Strozzi and Medici) had become the leading capitalists in the Western world. There were several dozen wealthy merchant families, and hundreds profited from the making of wool and silken textiles and from working metals. In the words of one historian, "the other great requirement of art, patronage, sprang from the same financial source" (Cheyney 1936, p. 273).

The social situation was not one that would appeal to our democratic sensibilities. According to one sociologist, the Florentine worker was "completely deprived of all civil rights... capital [ruled] more ruthlessly and less troubled by moral scruples than ever before or after in the history of Western Europe" (Hauser 1951, p. 20). Nor were foreign affairs in better shape; during those years, Florence was engaged in constant life-and-death struggles against Milan and Naples (Hartt 1979). Yet rising production led to increased home consumption, and by a fortuitous chain of events, such as the discovery of long-buried Roman buildings and sculpture, and the influence of new ideas from the Middle East, the consumption of the wealthy Florentines was channeled into the patronage of works of art.

It might help to understand the genesis of creativity if we review briefly the events of those crucial 25 years of Florence. Most art historians agree on what were the greatest accomplishments of that period. Any list would include, at the very least, the following: the making of the north doors of the Baptistery by

Ghiberti (1402–1424); the statues of St. Mark (1411) and St. George (1415) that Donatello placed in the chapel of Orsanmichele; the statue of St. Philip (1414) by Nanni di Banco in the same location; Brunelleschi's start on the Foundling hospital (1419), the cathedral cupola (1420), and the Sacristy of San Lorenzo (1421); the frescoes of the Adoration of the Magi by Gentile da Fabriano (1420–1423); and those Masaccio painted in the Brancacci Chapel (1424–1427). These three works of architecture, three sculptures, and two sets of paintings are generally held to be the most notable achievements of the early Renaissance in Florence (Hartt 1979; Heydenreich 1974).

Now, in each of these eight cases, the impetus for doing the work came either from a rich individual who wanted to celebrate the name of his family (the works of Masaccio and Gentile da Fabriano and Brunelleschi's sacristy were commissioned, respectively, by the bankers Brancacci, Strozzi, and Medici for their churches) or from one of the political or guild unions (Ghiberti's doors were commissioned by the merchants' guild; the Signoria asked for and paid for the statues of Donatello and Nanni; the silk weavers' guild got the Foundling Hospital built; and the wool guild supervised the building of the dome).

The building of this famous dome gives a glimpse of how the community directed artistic production. The executive power was in the hands of a 12-man committee, the Operai del Duomo, who were selected from various corporations, with a preponderance of wool merchants and manufactures. The function of this committee was to organize competitions, select the best entries, commission the winning artists, supervise the work in progress; and pay for the finished product. In the case of the cupola, general plans had been drawn up as far back as 1367, but despite several competitions, no architect had been able to satisfy the stringent requirements of the Operai. It is well known that during this period a large proportion of the populace took part in the selection process: suggestions, letters, and criticism flowed steadily from citizens to the Operai, expressing their ideas of how the dome of the cathedral should be built. Finally, more than 70 years after the first plans, Brunelleschi and Ghiberti were entrusted with the great task.

The "Gates of Paradise" that Ghiberti finally built for the Baptistery went through a similar close scrutiny. The Calimala, or merchants' guild, appointed a jury of 34 experts to review the entries, Before the contest, the jury consulted some of the leading scholars of Italy about what the subject matter of each of the 28 panels of the doors should be. Of the several dozen artists who prepared sketches for the commission, six were chosen for the final list. They were given 1 year to prepare a bronze relief that would serve as the test entry, and during this period their production costs and living expenses were covered by the Calimala (Hauser 1951, p. 39). The test consisted in making a panel illustrating the sacrifice of Isaac. After the year had passed, Ghiberti, who in 1402 was only 23 years old and almost unknown, was judged to have done best. For the next 50 years he worked first on the north, then on the east doors, with the continuing financial and critical backing of the guild (Heydenreich 1974, p. 129).

It was this tremendous involvement of the entire community in the creative process that made the Renaissance possible. And it was not a random event, but a calculated, conscious policy on the part or those who had wealth and power. The goal of the Florentines was to make their city into a new Athens (Hauser, 1951, p. 23). In terms of our model, an unusually large proportion of the social system became part of the art "field", ready to recognize, and indeed to stimulate, new ideas,

"In this environment", wrote Heydenreich (1974, p. 13), "the patron begins to assume a very important role: in practice, artistic productions arise in large measure from his collaboration". Hauser's position is even more extreme: "[In] the art of the early Renaissance ... the starting point of production is to be found mostly not in the creative urge, the subjective self-expression and spontaneous inspiration of the artist, but in the task set by the customer" (Hauser 1951, p. 41).

Implications of the Model

At this point, some readers used to the person-centered perspective on creativity might begin to feel that the argument I am developing is a betrayal of psychology in favor of historical or sociological approaches. This is surely not my intention. It seems to me that an understanding of the complex context in which people operate must eventually enrich our understanding of who the individual is and what the individual does. But to do so we need to abandon the Ptolemaic view of creativity, in which the person is at the center of everything, for a more Copernican model in which the person is part of a system of mutual influences and information.

The Domain Level

A long agenda of questions can be generated from this approach, questions that usually are ignored in creativity research yet might hold the key to many important findings.

In terms of the domain, the basic question is "What are the various ways in which information can be stored and transmitted, and how does the structuring of information affect creativity?" We need to develop concepts and measures to evaluate the structuring of information, so as to discover which symbol systems are better able to store creative ideas, and to transmit them over time. The work of Feldman (1980) was a pioneering attempt in this direction, and so is the direction of research pursued by Project Zero at Harvard (Perkins 1981). The newly emerging fields of cognitive science and artificial intelligence (Gardner 1985) also will have much to contribute to answering such questions.

We also need to understand better how access to information is differentially open to various categories of individuals. Basically, this amounts to the question "flow can we make past creativity available to the most people, so as to facilitate future creativity?"

The other side of the coin is the question "How can we motivate people to become involved in a particular domain?" The issue here is not how to provide extrinsic motivation like money and recognition, which more properly belong to the concerns of the field, but rather how to ensure intrinsic motivation, which hinges on the inherent attractiveness with which the information is presented. For no matter how original one might be, if one is bored by the domain, it will be difficult for one to become interested enough in it to make a creative contribution. The ability to attract and sustain interest rests in part on how well the domain is internally organized. How motivation and personality more generally are implicated in creativity has been extensively studied (Amabite 1983; Csikszentmihalyi 1986; Csikszentmihalyi and Getzels 1973; Roe 1946), but we still know very little, about the specific motivational values of different ways of patterning information.

The Person

Because most studies of creativity focus on individual processes, this is the phase of the creative cycle that needs the least attention, being the best known. The main conceptual question here is "How do some individuals get to produce a greater amount of variation in the domain than others?" The answer to this question is going to involve motivational and affective variables as well as cognitive ones. It is likely that some children are born with more sensitivity to certain ranges of stimulation—to light as opposed to movement, or to sound—and therefore might be more advantaged in dealing with the nemes to which they are more sensitive (Gardner 1983). The ways in which various information-processing strategies are used by creative children are being actively investigated (Bamberger 1986; Siegler and Shrager 1984; Sternberg 1984). It is also likely that early experiences (Walters and Gardner 1986) and demographic variables such as sibling position, social class, or religious upbringing will have their effects. The importance of "problem finding" as an approach to creative tasks has been documented longitudinally with artists (Csikszentmihalyi and Getzels 1971, 1988).

Careful studies of truly creative individuals that take into account all the facets of the complex interactions among person, field, and domain are especially needed and in scarce supply. Some examples of attempts in this direction are Gruber's study (1981) of Darwin, Getzels and Csikszentmihalyi's longitudinal study (1976) of young artists, and Feldman's continuing investigations (1986) of prodigiously gifted children.

The Field

It is probably true that less is known about the effects of the social system on creativity than about the other two phases of the cycle. The theoretical issue here is

"What forms of organization facilitate the selection of new variants and their inclusion in the domain?" Bloom (1985) has documented the extensive support system, including devoted parents and committed teachers, that gifted children need in order to master the skills required by a domain. Getzels and Csikszentmihalyi (1968) and Csikszentmihalyi et al. (1984) have shown how social roles interact with artists' personalities to determine success in the field. Simonton (1978, 1984) has conducted extensive studies of the relationship between features of the social system and the frequency of creative behavior.

A start in the right direction has certainly been made. Psychologists studying creativity have begun to realize the relevance of related approaches. The history of science, the history of ideas, cognitive science, artificial intelligence, and organizational sociology are no longer out of bounds for those who wish to get a strong grip on the issues. But all these promising studies—and the many others there was no room to mention—are thus far unrelated to each other, as if these distinct aspects of the creative process could be understood in isolation from each other. Perhaps even more than new research, what we need now is an effort to synthesize the various approaches of the past into an integrated theory. Of course, all this poaching in neighboring territory places an added burden of scholarship on the psychologist. The systems approach demands that we become versed in the skills of more than one discipline. The returns in knowledge, however, are well worth the effort.

References

Amabite, T. (1983). *The social psychology of creativity*. New York: Springer.
Bamberger, J. (1986). Cognitive issues in ihe development of musically gifted children. In: R. J. Stemberg, & J. E. Davidson (Eds.), *Conceptions of giftedness* (pp. 388–416). Cambridge: Cambridge University Press.
Bloom, B. (1985). *Developing talent in young children*. New York: Bailantine.
Borghero, G. (1986). *Thyssen-Bornemisza collection. Catalogue raisonne*. Milano: Edizioni Electa.
Brannigan, A. (1981). *The social basis of scientific discoveries*. Cambridge: Cambridge University Press.
Campbell, D. T. (1965). Variation and selective retention in socio-cultural evolution. In: H. R. Borringer, G. I. Blankston, & R. W. Monk (Eds.), *Social change in developing areas* (pp. 9–42). Cambridge: Schenkman.
Campbell, D. T. (1976). Evolutionary epistemology. In P. A. Schlipp (Ed.), *The library of living philosophers* (pp. 413–463). La Salle: Open Court.
Cheyney, E. P. (1936). *The dawn of a new era: 1250–1453*. New York: Harper & Bros.
Csikszentmihalyi, M. (1978). Attention and the holistic approach to behavior. In K. S. Pope & J. L. Singer (Eds.), *The stream of consciousness* (pp. 335–358). New York: Plenum.
Csikszentmihalyi, M. (1979). Art and problem finding. Paper presented at the 87th annual convention of the APA, New York.
Csikszentmihalyi M (1986) Motivation and creativity: Towards a synthesis of structural and energistic approaches to cognition. New ideas in psychology (in press).

Csikszentmihalyi, M., & Getzels, J. W. (1971). Discovery-oriented behavior and the originality of creative products. *Journal of Personality and Social Psychology, 19*(1), 47–52.

Csikszentmihalyi, M., & Getzels, J. W. (1973). The personality of young artists: An empirical and theoretical exploration. *British Journal of Psychology, 64*(1), 91–104.

Csiksientmihalyi, M. & Getzels, J. W. (1988). Creativity and problem finding in art. In F. H. Farley, & R. W. Neperud (Eds.) *The foundations of aesthetics, art, and art education.* New York: Praeger.

Csiksientmihalyi, M., Gelzels, J. W. & Kahn, S. (1984). *Talent and achievement: A longitudinal study with artists.* Chicago: University of Chicago (Unpublished manuscript).

Csikszentmihaiyi, M., & Massimini, R. (1985). On the psychological selection of bio-cultural information. *New Ideas in Psychology, 3*(2), 115–138.

Dawkins, R. (1976). *The selfish game.* New York: Oxford University Press.

Feldman, D. (1980). *Beyond universals in cognitive development.* Norwood: Ablex.

Feldman, D. (1986). *Nature's gambit.* New York: Basic Books.

Gardner, H. (1983). *Frames of mind.* New York: Basic Books.

Gardner, H. (1985). *The mind's new science.* New York: Basic Books.

Gardner, H. (1986). Freud in three frames. *Daedalus, 115*, 105–134.

Getzels, J. W., & Csikszentmihalyi, M. (1968). On the rules, values, and performance of future artists: A conceptual and empirical exploration. *Sociological Quarterly, 9*, 516–530.

Getzels, J. W., & Csikszentmihalyi, M. (1976). *The creative vision.* New York: Wiley.

Gruber, H. (1981). *Darwin on man.* Chicago: University of Chicago Press.

Guilford, J. P. (1950). Creativity. *American Psychologist, 5*(9), 444–454.

Hartt, F. (1979). *History of Italian renaissance art.* Englewood Cliffs: Prentice-Hall.

Hauser, A. (1951). *The social history of art* (Vol. 2). New York: Vinlage.

Heydenreich, L. H. (1974). *Il primo Rinaseimento.* Milano: Rizzoli.

Kermode, P. (1985). *Forms of attention.* Chicago: University of Chicago Press.

Kuhn, T. S. (1970). *The structure of scientific revolutions* (2nd ed.). Chicago: University of Chicago Press.

Kuhn, T. S. (1974). Second thoughts on paradigms. In F. Suppe (Ed.) *The structure of scientific theories.* Urbana: University of Illinois Press.

Lecourt, D. (1977). *Proletarian science.* London: New Left Books.

Medvedev, Z. (1971). *The rise and fail of Dr. Lysenko.* Garden City: Doubleday.

Perkins, D. (1981). *The mind's best work.* Cambridge: Harvard University Press.

Roe, A. (1946). The personality of artists. *Education and Personality Measure, 6*, 401–408.

Siegler, R. S. & Shrager, J. (1984). A model of strategic choice. In: C. Sophian (Ed.) *Origins of cognitive skills.* Hilisdale: Lawrence Erlbaum.

Simon, H. A. (1985). *Psychology of scientific discovery.* Paper presented at the 93rd Annual APA Meeting, Los Angeles, CA.

Simonton, D. K. (1978). History and the eminent person. *Gifted Child Quarterly, 22*, 187–195.

Simonton, D. K. (1984). *Genius, creativity, and leadership.* Cambridge: Harvard University Press.

Sternberg, R. J. (1984). Toward a triarchic theory of human intelligence. *Behavioral and Brain Sciences, 7*(2), 269–316.

Wallers, J. & Gardner, H. (1986). The crystallizing experience. In: R. Stemberg, & J. Davidson (Eds.), *Conceptions of giftedness* (pp. 306–331). Cambridge: Cambridge University Press.

Chapter 5
Solving a Problem is Not Finding a New One: A Reply to Herbert Simon

Mihaly Csikszentmihalyi

It seems curiously unreasonable that Professor Simon should accuse me of "glorifying unreason" for pointing out that scientific creativity involves processes that are not reducible to rational problem solving heuristics. Since when is stating facts tantamount to glorification? What I argued is that computer models of the creative process do not include affect, motivation, and curiosity, and hence could not be said to replicate what goes on in the mind of a person confronting a problem creatively. Computers simulate some of the rational dimensions of cognition, leaving out the rest.

To point out the variety of dimensions of human thought in no sense implies a "glorification" of non-rational elements. Ignoring them, however, leads to an unrealistic feeling of security about what we do and do not understand. I am afraid that we shall need the Lord's help more if we "get on with the task" as Professor Simon would have us do, without realizing its potentially misleading nature.

But perhaps I underestimated the inclusiveness of BACON's rationality. Perhaps elements of affect and motivation are already built into its programs. I am getting this impression from Professor Simon's description of the heuristics Hans Krebs is said to have employed: (a) *"use whatever comparative advantage* you have...;" (b) *"attack* a problem..." and in the case of Fleming: (c) "keep alert for phenomena...that *violate* your expectations..." (I added the italics to highlight the

Reproduced with permission from the Journal New Ideas in Psychology, volume 6, issue 2, pp. 183-186, 1988, Mihaly Csikszentmihalyi, with permission from Elsevier. Copyright © 1988, Elsevier

Author's reply to H. A. Simon (1988) Creativity and motivation, Vol. 6, No. 2, pp. 177–181.

M. Csikszentmihalyi (✉)
Department of Behavioral Sciences and Education, University of Chicago,
Green Hall, 5848 South University Avenue, Chicago, IL 60637, USA
e-mail: Mihaly.Csikszentmihalyi@cgu.edu

M. Csikszentmihalyi, *The Systems Model of Creativity*,
DOI: 10.1007/978-94-017-9085-7_5,
© Springer Science+Business Media Dordrecht 2014

rhetoric). To the extent that dimensions like competitiveness, aggressiveness, and a sense of being violated by disconfirming data are included in the computer's experience, then I must acknowledge that it does begin, indeed, to simulate the cognitive processes involved in creativity. But if these elements are in fact included, in what sense are they "rational?"

Reason—whether it is defined as sound judgment, good sense, or the ability to reach conclusions from given premises—must take into account a hierarchy of goals. Among these goals the survival of the individual, his or her social context, and the environment on which they depend must always be reckoned as primary. Therefore to work on a bomb that could destroy the planet would not be reasonable, no matter how rational the scientific steps that went into its making. To attack problems with the tools of rationality, simply because they are presented to us, and without considering the reasons for doing so is not reasonable, whether done by man or machine. This vital distinction the artificial intelligentsia is yet to incorporate into its heuristics.

To duplicate the conditions of creativity in real life, the computer must further be able to override its programs and to choose among ill-defined concerns some that it can formulate as problems amenable to solution. Furthermore, it must have the option of refusing to run any of the problems it is presented with—it should be able to pull its plug if it feels like it. Until these features are built into the program we shall never know, for instance, why Fleming took the trouble of inspecting leftover Petrie dishes while thousands of other investigators, presumably just as well versed in problem solving heuristics, did not.

Professor Simon ignores the possibility mentioned in my article that problem solving and problem finding might require opposite, or at least orthogonal cognitive strategies (and by "cognitive" I mean not just rational, but emotional and motivational as well). Hard evidence on this question is still rather scant. But we all know how many brilliant students enter graduate school, with 17 years of training in problem solution under their belt, and how few of them are ever able to isolate an important new problem, or even an interesting one, for their thesis. As long as we convince ourselves that creativity is nothing but rational problem solving, it is difficult to see how this situation will ever get better.

Professor Simon wonders why I ever supposed that anyone doubted the importance of motivation and sustained attention in creativity. The reason is that I could not find in the computer's heuristics any analogue to the motivational and attentional decisions that a person must constantly confront, decisions that will determine whether he or she will persevere in the task long enough to make a creative contribution. In real life, as I pointed out, even a Leonardo or a Newton must work with an information processing apparatus that is much slower than a computer, and he cannot afford the luxury of devoting all his mind to a problem.

For instance, in his response, Professor Simon writes: "With a new academic appointment, Krebs was faced with the task of designing a research program... that was the problem he had to solve." Is this supposed to mean that any academician coming up for tenure will formulate and solve a creative problem? Wouldn't it be nice if that were true. The unanswered question is whether the motivational and attentional patterns involved in creativity are different from those used in problem solving. If Kreb's motivation was nothing but what Simon implies it was, that is the *extrinsic* goal of developing a research program for his lab in view of a job promotion, then his motivation might eventually be simulated by BACON, But it seems that creative people are also motivated by the *intrinsic* rewards of working in the domain of their choice. Do these two reasons for trying to formulate and solve problems give different results as far as creativity is concerned? We won't know the answer as long as motivational issues—of both the extrinsic and the intrinsic kind—are not modeled by the computer, and as long as we assume a priori that creativity is nothing but the application of "normal" problem solving heuristics.

In this context it is revealing that Professor Simon chides me for not quoting the work of my colleague Bloom, "which studies the formative years of creative musical performers, scientists, and athletes in six different fields." I have the highest admiration for Bloom's work, but I don't think, and from what I know neither does he, that his study deals with "creative" individuals, He uses the term *talent* to describe his sample. Generally people tend to distinguish between talent and creativity. The first refers to an innate ability to perform at high levels within a domain such as music or mathematics, without, however, any implication that the performance will be novel or creative. But I can see how someone who has already prejudged the question in favor of equating creativity with problem solving would tend to blur this distinction.

In my paper, I did not mean to claim that creativity is nothing but problem finding. By writing that "The unique property of scientific discovery is problem finding, not problem solving," I asserted that the difference between a more and a less creative outcome does not lie in the ability to solve the problem, but in the capacity to formulate it in an original way. Of course, problem solving must also be involved, Therefore I welcome Professor Simon's demonstrations that much problem solving occurs in the creative process. But unfortunately our positions are not reciprocal; he maintains that creativity is nothing but "problem solving of a normal kind," by extending its definition to cover the discovery of new problems, Whether this is an example of the Fallacy of the Definite Article or not, the reader should decide.

In fact, Professor Simon's answer evades all the basic issues raised by my article. Leaving aside for the moment the crucial questions about affect and motivation, and concentrating solely on the cognitive aspects, there are two points on which BACON bears no relationship to actual creative thinkers: (a) it only finds regularities in data that have been pre-selected because the programmers *already know that the data display regularities;* and (b) it finds regularities only because the ability to describe regularities *was given to BACON directly by the programmers.*

If a reasonably bright high school student was given the same information as BACON, eventually he or she would also be able to simulate the great discoveries of creative scientists. But no one would call the student "creative" on that account. No matter how fast BACON is, as long as all it does is apply borrowed heuristics to a defined set of data, it will never simulate anything creative. It might begin to approach creativity when it can develop its own heuristics, when it is able to perform structural mapping between entirely different domains of data, when it learns to prioritize problems in terms of interest and importance. So far, we seem to be still rather far removed from this creative scenario.

There is one point in Professor Simon's critique that is well taken and where the ambiguity in my writing could understandably have been confusing. It concerns the "serious historical mistakes" about Copernicus and Kepler—that the greatness of their contributions was their "unstated intuitions" about the integration of the various branches of knowledge, rather than the particular solutions they brought to their problems. As the last sentence of the errant paragraph suggested, I had meant to say that the reason Copernicus and Kepler were able to achieve their revolutionary breakthroughs was that they believed in, and tried to express, that unity of knowledge many scholars since Aristotle and Democritus might have accepted, but were unable to formulate.

What we call creativity is a historical, evolutionary process carried out by biological organisms struggling in a social and cultural context. It makes no sense to strip it of all its dimensions except one, and call the simulation of what is left by the same name as the original. Creativity is not a "natural" phenomenon that can be simulated outside its socio-temporal context. Whether an outcome will be creative or not does not depend on the process itself, but on the judgment of whoever has the power to legitimize new discoveries. Hence the notorious difficulties in agreeing as to what is or is not a creative contribution. Perhaps we can learn more about creativity by studying social attribution processes than we can by studying solution heuristics.

Despite how it may seem, I am a great admirer of Professor Simon's work. In the long run—if there is going to be one—I expect that computer programs such as the ones Professor Simon pioneered may in fact replicate the kind of processes we call "creative." But that will only happen if those programs succeed in building into their heuristics the kind of constraints I have been talking about. As long as they only model rational problem solving, they may be better than we are, but they won't be like us.

Chapter 6
Shifting the Focus from Individual to Organizational Creativity

Mihaly Csikszentmihalyi and Keith Sawyer

An organization may be internally creative, through the implementation of cost-saving technologies or new accounting procedures or the development of new technology R&D. However, the biggest impact on profitability and market share most often derives from external creativity, navel responses to new legislation or radical market shifts. Creativity at the internal level is no guarantee of business success at the external level, but it is a prerequisite. The danger is that internal creativity can become isolated, feeding on itself in an incestuous fashion.

Attempts to increase innovation in organizations have been based largely on the belief that by increasing individual creativity, and by identifying and removing fetters to individual creativity, organizations can increase their ability to respond to changes in the external environment. Many creativity researchers and consultants typically have treated creativity as an individual trait and have underestimated its social and organizational components. For instance, a 1993 *Technology Review* article surveyed a wide range of creativity consultants, almost all of whom focused on techniques to foster individual creativity. In contrast, we believe that organizational creativity, which emphasizes social and group creative processes, will be a key factor in corporate success in the future, particularly in industries with complex, changing business environments. After all, innovation is a trait of entire organizations, not of individuals, because it is the full organization that must invest in the development, manufacturing, and marketing of a new product. Although employees' creative insights are necessary, they are a relatively minor factor in the overall innovativeness of the organization. There is no lack of good ideas, the problem is creating a system to manage the research and development.

Reprinted from M. Csikszentmihalyi; K. Sawyer, 1995, Shifting the Focus from Individual to Organizational Society in C.M. Ford and D.A. Gioia (Eds.), Creative Actions in Organizations, pages 167.172 Thousand Oaks, CA: SAGE, Copyright © 1995.

M. Csikszentmihalyi (✉) · K. Sawyer
University of Chicago, Claremont, CA, USA
e-mail: Mihaly.Csikszentmihalyi@cgu.edu

M. Csikszentmihalyi, *The Systems Model of Creativity*,
DOI: 10.1007/978-94-017-9085-7_6,
© Springer Science+Business Media Dordrecht 2014

A Systems Approach

In the early part of this century, Henri Poincaré described his own process of creative mathematical thought in terms of three stages: "this appearance of sudden illumination [is] a manifest sign of long, unconscious prior work... [this unconscious work] is possible, and of a certainty it is only fruitful if it is, on the one hand preceded, and on the other hand followed, by a period of conscious work" (Poincaré 1913, p. 389). Expanding on this notion, psychologist Hadamard (1945) proposed a four-stage model of creative insight. In this model preparation is followed by an incubation stage during which the subconscious repeatedly attempts new combinations of mental elements until one becomes stable and coherent enough to emerge into consciousness, resulting in illumination, the subjective experience of insight; the final stage is verification, or the conscious evaluation and elaboration of the insight.

Our own research confirms the basic outline of the four-stage model. Insights often occur during "idle time" when a person is removed from the tight schedule and time demands of the usual office routine. Of course, idle time would not be productive without the periods of hard work that precede it, it would never lead to practical effect without development and refinement following the insight. Although such stage models are generally accurate, they must be expanded to address how social and contextual factors influence the creative process. When asked to describe a moment of insight, creative people often mention interpersonal contacts, strategic or political considerations, and a knowledge of what questions were "interesting" as defined by others in their sphere of activity. Although the insight often occurs in isolation, it is surrounded and contextualized within an ongoing experience that is fundamentally social, and it would be meaningless out of that context.

The systems view developed by Csikszentmihalyi (1988, 1990) proposed that creativity must be defined with respect to a system that includes individual, social, and cultural factors that influence the creative process and help to constitute a creative outcome. These influences are separated into the "field" (the group of gatekeepers who are entitled to select a novel idea or product for consideration) and the "domain" (the symbolic system of rules and procedures that define permissible action within its boundaries). Examples of domains are the "generally accepted accounting practices" invoked in every annual report or the production processes in place in a factory. Domains are presented to organization members as "given knowledge," the basic factors of the profession. In practice, however, most creativity involves identifying those points at which the domain can be changed for the better, without excessive cost. A novice treats the domain as unchangeable, an expert or virtuoso not only realizes what can or should be changed, but also how difficult such change will be. In the systems view, the creative process involves the generation of a novel creative product, the selection of the product by others in the field, and the retention of selected products that the field adds to the domain.

The "cycle of entrepreneurship" provides a good example of the application of the systems view to business—for instance: A researcher or executive independently develops a novel solution to a market need. The corporation's management, acting as the field, concludes that this novel, creative product is not suited to the domain of their business. The stymied individual then creates a new field and domain, in the form of a start-up corporation. This pattern has resulted in two methods of appropriating the entrepreneur's drive and initiative, either by becoming an investor in the Straight-up (there by joining the new field) or initiating new corporate policy designed to encourage "intrapreneurship" (changing the field's selection process to be more receptive to innovation).

Bringing it to Business

The view of creativity as a system process has strong Implications for organizations. The "field" represents the other employees in the organization, and the "domain" represents the accepted body of practices, often inscribed in formal documentation. Just as physics and literature are different domains, accounting and operations also are different domains. These are examples of horizontally different domains. Similarly, product lines and market segments are vertically distinct domains. Businesses are usually organized either functionally, with fields (organizational units) corresponding to horizontal domains, or in market units, with fields corresponding to vertical domains.

In addition to these domains and fields, corporations must act within an external environment with its own domains and fields, such as market competition and government legislation. Today's increasingly activist consumers form yet another "field" that affects the organization's success. To integrate these multiple, intersecting forces, both within and without the organization, we propose a model that accounts for several levels at which "creativity" might be defined for an organization. In addition to the vertical and horizontal distinctions, both external and internal dimensions must be accounted for. These are distinct domains and fields both inside and outside the organisation.

External forces acting on creativity include such domains of activity as market forces (number of products, cohesiveness of product lines, geographical diversity) and government legislation (regulatory constraints). These external forces also include external fields such as consumers (needs, degree of market segmentation), competitors (number of competitors, market share, brand royalty), politicians, and suppliers (permanent relationships, degree of independence, second-source availability). Internal forces acting on creativity include such domains as technology (limitations, pace of new developments), organizational structure, finance, and product lines. Internal fields include the staff (receptiveness to novelty, degree of rigidity), the corporate culture/informal organization, the individual's location within the organization, major stockholders, and the board.

The relative complexity of this model, incorporating both internal and external systems, and vertical and horizontal levels, can help explain why "creativity" is so difficult to define creativity can occur within any one of these domains—and can be detailed by any one of these fields. Creativity means different things in different industries; an innovation in financial services may have very little in common with a manufacturing process innovation. Furthermore, creativity means different things in different organizational functions; a marketing innovation may have very different characteristics than a technical or accounting innovation. An organization may be internally creative, through the implementation of cost-saving technologies or new accounting procedures or the development of new technology in R&D. The biggest impact on profitability and market share, however, most often derives from external creativity, novel responses to new legislation or radical market shifts.

Creativity at the internal level is no guarantee of business success at the external level, but it is a prerequisite. The danger is that internal creativity can become isolated, feeding on itself in an incestuous fashion. The challenge for organizations is to create corporate cultures that direct internal creativity toward external creativity resulting in increased market share and customer satisfaction. For example, internal R&D creativity that results in a product innovation must be linked with the more mundane creativity of implementation for the organization to become externally successful—a commonly noted failing of American business.

Lessons from Our Research

These ideas can be combined with findings from our research to generate several observations that are directly relevant to creativity in organizations. To recapitulate and integrate some of these findings:

1. The creative process is heavily dependent on social interaction, which takes the form of face-to-face encounters and of immersion in the symbolic system of one or more domains.
2. The most significant insights (e.g., those that lead to innovative new products or uses for new technology) are often characterized by a synthesis of information from multiple domains, which can be as far apart as chemistry is from social norms, or as close as neighboring branches of mathematics.
3. To achieve such a synthesis, there most be: (a) thorough knowledge of one or more domains; (b) thorough immersion in a field that practices the domain; (c) attention on a problematic area of the domain; (d) idle time for incubation that allows insights to emerge; (e) ability to recognize an insight as one that helps resolve the problematic situation; (f) evaluation and elaboration of the insight in ways that are valuable to the field or domain.
4. The most important individual characteristics are strong interest, curiosity, or intrinsic motivation that drive a person or group to commit attention to a

problematic area in a domain, and beyond generally accepted boundaries of knowledge.

5. It is essential not to fill schedules with goal-directed, conscious, rational problem solving, so as to allow for the serendipitous combination of ideas.

6. It is important to provide opportunities for testing insights, to develop their consequences.

Implications for Understanding Organizational Creativity

Our perspective generates several implications. First, that individuals are not the proper level of analysis. Creativity is a systems-level phenomenon defined internally by the corporate culture and externally by the business environment. Second, the multileveled systems view of the corporation suggests a difficulty in translating internal creativity into external creativity, Executives should analyze their organization's multiple domains and fields and attempt to understand how the various internal and external fields are related. Third, because so many key insights result from the combination of more than one domain, organizations should encourage cross-domain fertilization by establishing liaisons among different units. Fourth, creativity takes time; it will not emerge overnight. The more significant the creative insight, the longer the period likely to be required for preparation and incubation. Fifth, some rewards should be in the form of formal "idle time." Promising employees should be assigned to spend time in the library or the lab for a day every week or month, to refresh their patterns of thought. They also should be encouraged to take their allotted vacations and not work too many weekends.

Finally, the systems model of creativity implies that there must be a commitment from the top of the organization. Innovation is often opposed by entrenched political interests. Only strong support from top management will make it possible to overcome the inertia of the status quo.

References

Csikszentmihalyi, M. (1988). Society, culture, and person: A systems view of creativity. In R. J. Sternberg (Ed.), *The nature of creativity: Contemporary psychological perspectives* (pp. 325–339). New York: Cambridge University Press.

Csikszentmihalyi, M. (1990). The domain of creativity. In M. A. Runco & R. S. Albert (Eds.), *Theories of creativity* (pp. 190–212). Newbury Park: Sage.

Hadamard, J. (1945). *An essay on the psychology of invention in the mathematical field.* New York: Dover; Princeton: Princeton University Press.

Poincaré, H. (1913). *The foundations of science.* Garrison: Science Press.

Chapter 7
Creative Insight: The Social Dimension of a Solitary Moment

Mihaly Csikszentmihalyi and Keith Sawyer

There appears to be a general tendency, in all cultures and historical periods, to differentiate between mental processes that are routine, shallow, and trivial on the one hand, and those that are unusual, profound, and important on the other. In the English, language, the word that best denotes the second type of mental process is *insight*, derived from the Old Dutch for "seeing inside." We classify as insightful ideas that seem to get to the core of an issue and people who are prone to have such ideas. Like other words referring to mental processes that are relatively rare and valued—such as wisdom or intuition—insight is likely to have been selected and preserved in the vocabulary because of its adaptive significance (Csikszentmihalyi and Rathunde 1990). In other words, a culture that in principle cannot differentiate between more profound and more superficial aspects of an issue because it lacks the concept of insight is likely to have more trouble coping with its material and ideational environment.

An insight is typically said to occur when an individual is exposed to some new information that results in a new way of looking at a known problem or phenomenon in such a way that its essential features are grasped. The term *insight* often is accompanied by a modifier (e.g., *fresh insight, new insight*, or *powerful insight*). Usually we think of some cause that results in insight: For example, "researchers yield new insights on Japan," or "this new metaphor provides fresh and powerful insights." Insight seems to involve (1) an existing state of mind or set of mental structures relevant to the topic and (2) a moment of realization, consequent to new information or a sudden new way of looking at old information, resulting in (3) a quick restructuring of the mental model, which is subjectively perceived as providing a new understanding. These criteria imply that it is impossible to have an insight about a topic unless the person experiencing the insight *has* had some prior exposure to the issue.

M. Csikszentmihalyi, *The Systems Model of Creativity*,
DOI: 10.1007/978-94-017-9085-7_7,
© Springer Science+Business Media Dordrecht 2014

Although the term *insight* can he used to describe moments that we all seem to have from time to time, in this chapter we propose that insight is best studied through mental processes that result in creative products. Whereas examples of insight in everyday life tend to be elusive and debatable, they are both more public and more convincing when they occur to scientists whose work results in Nobel prizes or to artists and writers who enhance our lives with their creative endeavors. In what follows, we discuss the phenomenon of creative insight as reported in a series of interviews with creative individuals from various fields. The moment of insight emerges, in these interviews, as a central aspect of creativity. We suggest that what we learn about insight in the context of the creative process will help us understand insight more generally.

General Observations About Creative Insight

Recent studies of scientific creativity (Simonton 1988a; Gruber and Davis 1988) and artistic creativity (Getzels and Csikszentmihalyi 1976; Martindale 1990) have focused on mental processes or models of the creative process, following in the cognitivist tradition of psychology established in the early sixties. Counter to this dominant mode, a few researchers have attempted to understand the social and cultural influences and environments in which creativity is manifested (Campbell 1960; Csikszentmihalyi 1988, 1990a; Harrington 1990; John-Steiner 1992; Woodman and Schoenfeldt 1989). As John-Steiner (1992) points out, these two approaches—the first intrapsychic, the second interpersonal—have not yet been successfully integrated. In this chapter, we hope to begin such an integration by showing the relationship between insight, clearly an intrapsychic process, and the social milieu in which it occurs.

Most studies of creative insight have been conducted by psychologists and therefore tend to focus on the cognitive processes during and leading up to the moment of insight- The tendency has been to assume that this moment occurs when the person is alone; hence, insight has been studied mainly as a cognitive process that occurs in isolation. As the peak experience in creative lives, the moment of insight has fascinated creative individuals and their biographers alike. Consequently, many creativity researchers have focused on the moment of creative insight and attempted to analyze it as a purely intrapsychic cognitive process.

In this chapter we will present a different perspective, by expanding out from this moment in time and embedding it within the other relevant stages of the creative process. When we look at the complete "life span" of a creative insight in our subjects' experience, the moment of insight appears as but one short flash in a complex, time-consuming, fundamentally social process. It is true that the individuals we interviewed generally report their insights as occurring in solitary moments: during a walk, while taking a shower, or while lying in bed just after waking. However, these reports usually are embedded within a more complex narrative, a story that describes the effort preceding and following the insight, and the overall sense of these complete narratives stresses the salience of social, interactional factors. It seems that the solitary nature of the moment of insight may have blinded us to the social dimension of the entire creative process.

When we reviewed our interviews, we discovered a common narrative structure in descriptions of creative insight. (For other collections of personal narratives of moments of insight, see Shrady 1972 and Ghiselin 1952) Respondents described moments of creative insight as being contextualized within a four-stage process. The first stage consists of the hard work and research preceding the moment of insight; the second stage is a period of idle time alone; the third stage is the moment of insight itself; and the fourth stage is the hard work and elaboration required to develop and bring the idea to fruition. Most of these eminent people paraphrased the saying: "Creativity is 99 % perspiration and 1 % inspiration."

The periods of hard work that precede and follow a creative insight are fundamentally social, deeply rooted in interaction with colleagues and in the individual's internalized understanding of the culturally constituted domain. The balance of hard work and idle time can also be viewed as a balance between social interaction and individual isolation. The social interaction within which the creative insight is nestled is coincident with this "99 % perspiration." Thus, the traditional models of creativity, which involve stages and which focus on psychological processes, inadequately represent this social, interactional aspect of the process of creative insight.

Multistage Models of Creative Insight

In the early part of this century, Poincaré (1913, p. 389) described his own process of creative mathematical thought using three stages: "This appearance of sudden illumination [is] a manifest sign of long, unconscious prior work.... [This unconscious work] is possible, and of a certainty it is only fruitful, if it is on the one hand preceded and on the other hand followed by a period of conscious work." Hadamard (1949) proposed a four-stage model of creative insight in which *preparation* is followed by an *incubation* stage, during which the subconscious repeatedly attempts new combinations of mental elements until one becomes stable and coherent enough to emerge into consciousness. This results in *illumination*, the subjective experience of insight. The final stage is *verification*, or conscious evaluation of the insight.

Following these early formulations, many contemporary approaches have been based on two- or three-stage models of creative insight. The two-stage models refer to a first stage of *ideation,* a time-consuming, perhaps subconscious, generation of new ideas or combinations, and a second stage, in which certain privileged *combinations emerge into consciousness* (Epstein 1990; Milgram 1990). This second stage is subjectively perceived as the moment of insight. The three-stage models (Feldman 1988; Langley and Jones 1988; Ohlsson 1984; Perkins 1988; Simon 1977; Simonton 1988a) include these two stages but suggest a third and final stage of *evaluation* or *elaboration*, in which the creative insight is developed consciously, with the active use of external sources and prior knowledge, into a communicable symbolic product, whether an artwork or a scientific publication. (See Runco 1990 for a more thorough review of three-stage models.)

Campbell (1960) often is cited as the inspiration for contemporary three-stage models of creativity. He used the evolutionary paradigm to explain the growth of knowledge in general, developing what he called an "evolutionary epistemology," of which creativity is a special case. In his scheme, changes in "ways of knowing" start with (1) a variation stage, during which a large number of novel responses are generated, followed by (2) a selection stage, in which the best-adapted variations are chosen from all the options, and finally (3) a retention stage, during which the selected variants are added to the pool of responses for transmission to the next generation.

Simonton (1988a) developed a theory of scientific creativity based on Campbell's framework. (Perkins 1988 and Martindale 1990 also base their three-stage models on Campbell's evolutionary metaphor.) For Simonton, the variation stage involved the chance permutations of mental elements. He defined these mental elements as "the fundamental units that can be manipulated in some manner" by the creative process (Simonton 1988b). Some of these chance permutations will be more stable than others, and these configurations will emerge into consciousness, resulting in an experience of insight. At this point, Simonton's theory states, the individual must engage in conscious work to transform the chance configuration into a communication configuration, a symbolic form of the insight that allows communication of the insight, such as a journal article or painting.

Although there are subtle variations in the definitions of these stages of creative insight among different researchers, we propose the following unifying framework: The first stage, preparation, which is stimulated by external pressures or by intrinsic motivation, involves focused conscious work, such as studying or analyzing data. These rational thought processes provide the raw material on which the subconscious can begin working. The second stage, which can last a very short time or go on for years, is the stage of incubation. The theorists previously cited disagree about just what occurs in the subconscious; Hadamard (1949) argued that active, guided processing is taking place, whereas most current researchers believe that chance combinations of thought processes below the threshold of awareness provide an adequate explanation (Langley and Jones 1988; Simonton 1988a, b). The third stage, *insight*, occurs when the subconscious combines or selects an idea which, for reasons that remain poorly understood, emerges into consciousness, resulting in an "Aha!" experience. This insight will be useless unless it is *evaluated* by the conscious mind and *elaborated* for presentation to others. Some researchers have used concepts such as implicit theories of creativity or metacognition to characterize how individuals engage in this fourth evaluative phase (Runco 1990; Sternberg 1988).

Social Process Models of Creativity

Stage models such as those just reviewed, have been widely used by psychologists as frameworks for analyzing creativity. These models have focused on psychological stages of the individual's creative process, without attempting to represent social influences. How does the individual integrate his or her insights with an ongoing domain of scientific or artistic activity? To what extent is the preparation stage dependent on the symbolic domain or on the social group within which the individual works? Creative individuals rarely work in a vacuum, isolated from the social systems that constitute their domain of activity. The evaluation and elaboration stage also implies a social dimension: How can an insight be evaluated unless the individual makes use of an internalized model of the domain (e.g., by using the formal mathematical procedures endorsed by the culture) and without an intimate familiarity with experts in the field who help select and define what is worthwhile? How can an idea be elaborated if not within the context of a specific domain of endeavor and with an awareness of the social processes required to communicate the idea through the field?

In our interviews, we found that creative individuals had a strong subjective awareness of external social or discipline influences at each creative stage. When asked to describe a moment of creative insight, they typically provided extended narratives that described not just a single moment but a complex, multi-stage process, with frequent discussions of interpersonal contact, strategic or political considerations, and awareness of the paradigm, of what questions were interesting as defined by the discipline. This was particularly salient in the preparation stage and in the evaluation and elaboration stage. Although the moment of creative insight usually occurs in isolation, it is surrounded and contextualized within an ongoing experience that is fundamentally social, and the insight would be, meaningless out of that context. Therefore, to better understand, the interviews, we needed to incorporate perspectives that explored the ways that social factors influenced the stages of the creative process. We turned to social process models of creativity, recently proposed by several researchers, in an attempt to incorporate social system influences on the creative process.

Harrington (1990) argued for an ecological approach to creativity and compared the influence of the biological ecosystem on the organism to the influence of social environments on the creative individual. Using this metaphor, creativity is described as a psychosocial process that places demands on both individuals and their social contexts, or ecosystems. Extending the ecological metaphor, Harrington discussed the importance of "organism-environment fit" in the creative process and how creative individuals can he active shapers of their environments.

The interactionist model of creativity derived from the symbolic interactionist school within sociology. Woodman and Schoenfeldt (1989) developed this approach to explain how individual differences in creativity might be derived from exogenous factors. The interactionist model explored the combination and interrelation of psychological and environmental factors in human behavior. Woodman and Schoenfeldt proposed the primary components of contextual influences (culture and group, task constraints), social influences (social facilitation, rewards and punishments, role modeling), cognitive style (ideational fluency, problem-solving style), personality traits (autonomy, intuition), and antecedent conditions (past history, socialization, biographical variables). However, their presentation did not attempt to characterize the processes of creativity suggested by stage models.

The systems view developed by Csikszentmihalyi (1988, 1990a) proposed that creativity could not be operationalized at the psychological level alone. Like the ecological and the interactionist models, Csikszentmihalyi argued that individual creativity must be defined with respect to a system that includes not only the individual but also social and cultural factors which influence the creative process and help to constitute creativity. He separated these influences into the *field*, the group of gatekeepers who are entitled to select a novel idea or product for inclusion in the domain, and the domain, consisting of the symbolic system of rules and procedures that define permissible behavior within its boundaries (hence the domain of baseball, chess, or algebra or, more narrowly, a Kuhnian paradigm). The creative process involves the generation of a novel creative product by the individual, the evaluation of the product by the field, and the retention of selected products by addition to the domain. Thus, the creative process involves a recurring circle from person to field to domain and back to the person, paralleling the evolutionary pattern of variation (person), selection (field), and retention (domain).

An Interpsychic Model of Creative Insight

The majority of our interviews included descriptions of the creative process that were consistent with the stage models. However, we noticed that these stagelike narrative descriptions tended to group into two distinct types not formerly discussed in the literature. These types varied in terms of the length of time involved in the overall creative process. Some individuals described working for several years on a problem before the flash of insight hit, whereas others spoke of working for a few hours in the morning and having the insight in the afternoon. Most creative individuals experience both types of creative process. For example, Darwin's journey on the *Beagle* involved a daily ritual of observing the natural environment, taking notes, and reflecting on similarities and differences among animals and plants. Each day's work resulted in new observations about these relationships. However, the culmination of these many small insights into the theory of natural selection was a lengthy process, taking years if one includes not only the journey but the knowledge acquired by Darwin before hoarding the ship. In our interviews, this variation in time scale applies not only to preparation but also to the phase of evaluation and elaboration; In some cases, the evaluation occurred in a matter of minutes, whereas in others it took months or even longer to elaborate or confirm the insight.

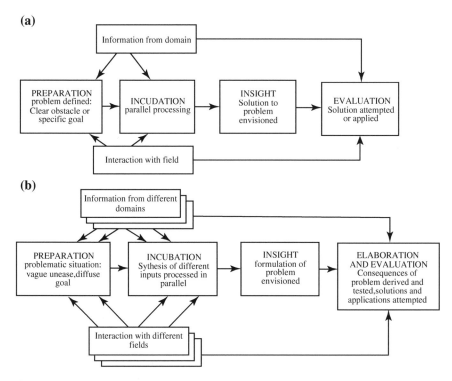

Fig. 7.1 The role of insight in the creative process. **a** Presented problem (normal, short-term).
b Discovered problem (revolutionary, long-term)

These two types of description of creative insight seem so different that they actually may represent two types of creative insight, resting at two extremes of a continuum. Although the creative process most likely involves a continuous range of time spans, in this chapter we will examine these extremes. To distinguish between these two ideal types, it might be useful to adopt the distinction developed by Getzels (1964) between presented problem solving and discovered problem finding. (See also Getzels and Csikszentmihalyi 1976. For a recent review of this literature, see Hoover 1990) The short time-frame process tends to occur when, a problem is known and preexisting in the domain and all that needs to be found is a solution to it. We will refer to this as a *presented problem-solving* process. The long time-frame process tends to occur when the nature of the problem to be solved is less clear; in fact, the problem itself may not be formulated until the moment of insight. Great creative breakthroughs, paradigmatic shifts, belong to this category. We will refer to this as a *discovered problem-finding process* (Fig. 7.1).

In both problem-solving and problem-finding narratives, the importance of social interaction is salient. Our interviews suggest that the four-stage perspective must be extended from the intrapsychic to the interpsychic level. If 99 % of the activity takes place in stages that are predominantly social—the preparation, evaluation, and elaboration stages—then the interpersonal aspect of the process must be seriously considered and, in fact, may be more significant than the intrapsychic aspects of creativity. The isolation that seems to accompany the incubation stage preceding the moment of insight may have obscured the observation that this part of the process serves to juxtapose and integrate information that derives from the domain and from the field and is hence interpsychic in origin.

To link the intrapsychic and interpsychic levels, we suggest postulating a conscious-subconscious interaction that parallels the interpsychic-intrapsychic dimension. Although conscious attention is limited in capacity and must be managed and directed constantly by the individual (James 1890; Broadbent 1958; Kahneman 1973; Hasher and Zacks 1979; Eysenck 1982; Csikszentmihalyi 1978, 1990b), several research traditions have suggested that subconscious mental processing may have a much greater capacity. Researchers from Freud to current cognitive scientists have argued that conscious awareness is the tip of the iceberg, with a significant amount of mental processing occurring beneath the surface. Recent society-of-mind theories have suggested that the subjective sense of a unified self is illusory and that the ego rests at the top of a complex network of progressively less complex, subconscious entities (Minsky 1985; Ornstein 1986). Such theories hypothesize that each of these subconscious entities acts as an independent mental processing unit, almost like a pseudoconsciousness, and these entities compete for a turn in consciousness. This competitive interaction results in the ego, or the experience of reflective self-awareness, as an emergent phenomenon (Dennett 1991).

If conscious attention is serial and limited, whereas the subconscious capacity of the mind is parallel and multiple, how can the individual coordinate them? If it is to result is a public product, everything that is in the subconscious must at some point pass through conscious awareness. All activities of daily life—not only creative insight—must involve a strategic balance of the strengths and weaknesses of the two: conscious awareness, which can be directed but is sequential (one at a time), and the subconscious, which cannot be directed but is parallel and has a much greater capacity. The paradox for the creative individual is somehow to direct this undirectable subconscious process so that useful insights result. In fact, many of our respondents claim that they have developed the ability to do just that: to control without controlling, indirectly to direct the subconscious mind.

Preparation

The preparation stage of the creative process involves many components. Essentially, it requires concentrating attention on a problematic issue—a need, a desire, a challenge, or a specific problem that requires solution—long enough to master and understand its parameters. Issues of motivation, cognition, and socialization all are involved. Hence, it can be said that Leonardo da Vinci prepared himself for his insights into the workings of nature—how the wind blows, how water flows, how birds fly—by an early interest in human anatomy, in mechanics, and in the structural composition of leaves and branches. Likewise, Darwin prepared himself for his insights into evolution through a childhood interest in collecting insects, the reading of geology, and the painstaking observations he made during the voyage of the *Beagle*. Curiosity, interest, access to information, and some impulse that sets questioning in motion are all part of the preparatory phase of the creative process.

The difference between presented problems and discovered problems at this stage of the process is that the former confront the person with a relatively clearly formulated problem within a normal scientific paradigmatic tradition (Kuhn 1962), whereas the latter confronts the person with a general sense of intellectual or existential unease outside a paradigmatic context. For instance, to increase the profitability of a firm by firing 20 % of the employees is a presented problem. The questions of who should be fired, when they should be fired, and how to fire them still need to be solved, but the problem itself is not in question. However, one can reject this perception of the problem and ask, "How can the profitability of the firm be increased?" This reformulation would lead to less of a presented problem-solving and more of a discovered problem-finding process. As this example suggests, a process of problem discovery usually yields a presented problem as an outcome. In other words, the problem-finding question, "How can profits be increased?" might yield the answer, "By firing 20 % of the employees," resulting in a presented problem to be solved.

Incubation

Given the importance of unconscious work in reaching creative insights, a key component of the process must be the filtering mechanism that determines which information will be passed from conscious awareness to the subconscious. The social influences of the domain and the field appear to act as the primary controlling mechanisms of the creative individual's subconscious. Through acculturation and apprenticeship in a given domain, the individual internalizes that domain's built-in assumptions and rules, much as Kuhn's paradigm constrains the thinking of individuals in a scientific field.

This internalized interpsychic, fundamentally social filtering mechanism may rest just beneath conscious awareness or perhaps on the boundary between conscious and subconscious processing.[1] Although the subconscious network cannot be manipulated directly by consciousness, the conscious creation and development of this filter (through education, mentoring or apprenticeship, or reading texts) can influence the subconscious network indirectly. This conscious manipulation takes

---

[1] Note the parallels with Mead's (1934) "generalized other" and with Vygotsky's (1978) descriptions of how social interactions are internalized to become cognitive processes. Our proposal is consistent with Vygotsky and Mead, particularly the latter's claim that each distinct social sphere of individual activity will result in a distinct "other".

place during the preparation stage and, in our interviews, the social dimension of this stage is crucial and includes apprenticeship, mentoring, solitary study, and interaction with fellow students.

One major difference between presented and discovered processes at the incubation stage appears to be the diversity of inputs that the latter includes. Revolutionary creative *insight*s seem to be based on the random convergence of ideas from different domains, usually facilitated by interaction with individuals from different fields. For example, Linus Pauling explains the origins of his insights into the mathematical representation of chemical bonds, which earned him a Nobel prize in chemistry, in terms of his original interest in the composition of matter inherited from his pharmacist father plus the chance exposure to the first wave of quantum mechanics at Cal Tech.[2]

In his case, incubation consisted in the combination of elements from the domains of quantum physics and chemistry, at the very least. Practically every respondent we interviewed seems to have combined information from more than one domain prior to the occurrence of a major insight.

The preceding discussion suggests a three-level mental model of the preparation and incubation stages of the creative process. This model is applicable to both presented problem-solving and discovered problem-finding creativity; however, because of the longer time frame, the model suggests that problem-finding creativity will make greater use of the subconscious and will combine information derived from more different sources.

Level 1: Conscious Attention (Serial Processing)

Certain stimuli or problematic issues are invested with attention. Choices are made in terms of the three components of the system model: the person, field, and domain, In other words, genetically programmed predilections, learned motives, socialized interests, and cultural values all enter into determining which stimuli or issues will be invested with attention. Only a few chunks of information can be attended to at any one time; thus, this level is characterized serial, directed-attention processing.

Level 2: Semiconscious Filters

A semiconscious filter determines what information is passed to the subconscious. This filter also is structured following the systems model: It is an internal mental image of the field-domain-person trichotomy, and it selects which information is

---

[2] This anecdote, and those that follow, are based on interviews collected for our ongoing project, Creativity in Later Life, sponsored by the Spencer Foundation.

viewed as relevant. Personality traits, such as curiosity, interest, intrinsic motivation, and flexibility, are also important at this level.

Level 3: Subconscious Processing Entities, or the Society of Mind

The distributed, parallel nature of this network of subconscious processing entities allows multiple chunks of information to be viewed simultaneously. Connections between ideas can be tested, perhaps in a subconscious generate-and-test fashion. Of the theorists discussed earlier, only Hadamard (1949) proposed a model in which this incubation stage is distinct from the preparation stage. We suggest that a Hadamard-like incubation takes place but in a parallel fashion: Rather than a Freudian unitary subconscious working on the problem, many smaller entities are interacting randomly and perhaps collectively working on many problems.

The Three Levels Functioning Synchronously

These three levels, in particular the semiconscious filters and the subconscious network, are developed and internalized through professional socialization. Once the individual is socialized into a field, the basic flow of information storage during the preparation stage is from conscious awareness, through the filter, into the subconscious network. This is, in effect, a mapping from diachrony to synchrony: Whereas ideas can be addressed only one at a time in consciousness, once they have passed to the subconscious, ideas that entered awareness In a serial fashion may be considered in parallel.

Insight

The two types of creative insight, presented and discovered, correspond to the well-known distinction first suggested by Thomas

Kuhn (1962) between normal science and revolutionary science (although we are, of course, speaking not only of scientific fields but of all fields of creative activity). So-called normal science consists of working within an accepted tradition, incrementally advancing the field with experiments and discoveries. In contrast, revolutionary science involves the creation of a completely new field, a new domain of activity. It is not simply an incremental advance but instead is a discontinuous leap to a new perspective, what Kuhn calls a new "paradigm." Our model suggests that creative revolutions involve the three-level subconscious process just described, resulting in a discovered problem-finding insight, whereas normal science can proceed as presented problem solving and may remain largely conscious. The small insights that seem to be a frequent part of everyday life are more like problem solving, whereas the revolutionary insights that change the course of history will he problem-finding insights.

Within our three-level model, insight is a type of information retrieval, the reverse of the information storage flow in the preparation stage. This reverse process begins in the subconscious: A particular combination or pattern that has emerged (randomly, undirected) from the subconscious network is strong enough to surface into consciousness. This is similar to Simonton's (1988a) description of how a stable chance configuration gets into conscious awareness. It is also reminiscent of Simon's (1977) suggestion that insight occurs through selective forgetting, a type of mental erosion during which good ideas remain whereas the bad ones simply erode away with time. Our theory suggests a more active subconscious process than Simon's. As similarities between ideas or configurations in different domains are recognized in the subconscious—such as that between geological and biological changes in the case of Darwin, or between subatomic quantum relationships and chemical bonds in Pauling's case—a new configuration combining the two emerges and filters into consciousness. Although in the popular conception, insight results from a specific stimulus (such as the apple that fell on Newton's head), we have not found descriptions of this sort in our interviews. The insights are always described as welling up from the subconscious, but there is never a mention of a specific external stimulus. Perhaps there is, nonetheless, a sort of internal stimulus, a subconscious event that causes a final, critical shift in the subconscious networks like the final shout that releases the avalanche.

Evaluation and Elaboration

In our four-stage model of creative insight, the evaluation and elaboration stage represents a reverse filtering of the insight, from the subconscious network into consciousness. Like the preparation stage, this process also is intricately bound up with the internalized social model of the field and domain. The ensuing elaboration of the insight is palpably social, as individuals develop their artistic or mechanical creation or communicate verbally with colleagues in an attempt to transfer their insight into an exogenous, interpsychic social object.

Figure 7.1 describes a simple linear process. In reality, most creative ideas, especially of a discovered land, are the result of multiple cycles of preparation, incubation, insight, and elaboration, with many feedback loops, the end result of which is a solution that may be either final or temporary, in which case the cycle may repeat itself again and again. A good example of the complexity of this process appears in Gruber's (1981) work on Darwin, which illustrates how the development of the evolutionary paradigm was the result of a lifetime spent elaborating the implications of an insight that was itself the result of a protracted series of partial understandings.

Narratives of Creative Insight

To illustrate concrete instances of creative insight, and especially the social contribution to their emergence, we will use data from our ongoing interview study. This study involves structured videotaped interviews of approximately 2 h duration with a sample of creative individuals. The respondents who are chosen meet the following criteria: (1) They are persons who have made a creative contribution to the natural sciences, the social sciences, the arts and humanities, or business or politics. (2) They are generally older than 60 years. (3) They are still involved actively either in the domain in which they had achieved fame or in a new domain. Currently, 60 interviews have been completed, and we anticipate a total sample of 100.

This chapter will draw on the content of nine interviews that have undergone preliminary analysis. The nine respondents will be identified as follows:

- Respondent A: environmental activist, organizer of special-interest groups, author of several books (female)
- Respondent B: physicist, holder of two Nobel prizes (male)
- Respondent C: banker, chief executive officer of one of the wealthiest and most influential financial conglomerates in the nation (male)
- Respondent D: mathematician and physicist (male)
- Respondent E: economist, poet, environmentalist (male)
- Respondent F: literary critic, author, rhetorician (male)
- Respondent G: ceramicist of international reputation (female)
- Respondent H: sculptor (female)
- Respondent I: physicist (male)

We will use representative quotations relevant to both presented and discovered processes and from each stage of these processes. The quotations were chosen to highlight the role of social factors at each stage.

Presented Problem Solving

As noted previously, respondents' narratives of moments of creative insight tended to fall into two types: those that seem more everyday and occur within four-stage cycles of short duration and those that are more exceptional, with a four-stage duration of up to several years. The former we have referred to as *presented problem-solving insights*. They involve relatively short incubation periods and a single domain and field, with a fourth stage of evaluation rather than elaboration. The problem-solving insights are more consistent with the popular uses of the term *insight*, which one finds in newspaper articles or in everyday conversation.

Several subjects described problem-solving insights. For example, the political activist, respondent A, described her daily routine as a period of work followed by "off time":

In the morning, that's when I really like intellectual activity, very finely focused intellectual activities. That's when I write, working at my desk, talking on the phone, and then after lunch is always a time where I like to slack off; maybe *snooze* for 15 min, maybe take a bike ride.... I mean, who knows? When you might suddenly have a terrific "Aha!" idea, I don't know! Mostly it happens to me when I'm gardening....or doing something steadying with my hands.... I develop a lot of my ideas in dialogue.

In the problem-solving narratives, the stages of preparation and evaluation occur within a day or two of the moment of creative insight. The incubation stage occurs over a period of a few hours, usually on a daily basis, and often in the morning. The evaluation stage occurs immediately after the insight enters consciousness: Because the individual is in a problem-solving mode, it is relatively easy to determine quickly whether the insight is appropriate to the given problem.

The following four sections address each of the four stages in turn, using quotations that are representative of the range of comments on that stage.

Preparation

In problem-solving narratives, some individuals focused on preparation as hard work on a problem which is more specific to that problem than to the domain at large. Others focused on hard work rather than domain influences.

Several of our interview subjects stated that to have creative ideas, you should attempt to have a large quantity of ideas and select from these the good ones. This is consistent with theories of ideational fluency (Milgram 1990) and Simonton's (1988a) argument that creativity is proportional to productivity. A businessman told us, "Quantity is very important...I only look for quantity of ideas, and finally the quality will come out." A chemist suggested that "you have a lot of ideas, and throw away the bad ones." Respondent C makes long lists of ideas and then is constantly reviewing the list to rank the ideas.

Respondent D described how collaboration is a key social aspect of the preparation stage, by using the metaphor of the open door.

> Science is a very gregarious business; it's essentially the difference between having this door open and having it shut. If I'm doing science, I have the door open. That's kind of symbolic, but it's true. You want to be all the time talking with people... it's only by interacting with other people in the building that you get anything interesting done; it's essentially a communal enterprise.

> Many of the nonscientists also spoke of the importance of collaboration, Respondent C's first impulse when a problem presents itself is to pick up the phone: "When I'm trying to get my mind around something new, I seek out people and talk to them." This is not restricted to a new problem: It is also part of respondent C's daily schedule; "I very much network the world; I travel; there [is]... probably a group of 40 people, maybe, that I stay in touch with;"

Incubation

As we hypothesized earlier, the incubation phase seems to be less of a factor in presented problem solving than it is in discovered problem finding. Nonetheless, many of the individuals we interviewed structured their day to include a period of solitary idle time that follows a period of hard work. The idle time may be in the afternoon, after a hard morning of preparation; or it may be in the morning, based on preparation from the night before. Respondent C schedules this time in the morning:

> [Starting at 5:30 AM] I typically try to work either at home or at the office, and that's when I do a good bit of my thinking, and priority setting... Typically get to the office about 6:30. I try to keep reasonably quiet time until 9:30 or 10. Then you get involved in lots of [interpersonal] transactions... I do my best work when I have some alone time.

A surprising number of the individuals we interviewed told us that they carefully structure their workday to include a similar period of idle time. Many of them told us that without this solitary, quiet time, they would never have their most important ideas. This daily idle time seems to be a period during which a problem-solving incubation stage may be at work. Several respondents keep their mind idle by engaging in repetitive physical activity on a daily basis. Respondent A compared the repetitive aspect of physical activities to a Zen practice:

> Generally, the really high ideas come to me when I'm gardening, or while I'm doing something steadying with my hands. You know, most people have chores, something quite repetitive.... The repetitive physical activities are really like a Zen practice, like the Zen monks sweeping the temple garden. And it's in that motion that you're in tune with the whole universe.

Insight

Almost without exception, our respondents told us that the daily problem-solving insights come to them during this idle time. This is consistent with the model we presented earlier, which suggests that insights will occur after a period of incubation. The banker, respondent C, carries a notepad with him everywhere he goes, and when he has an insight, he begins to write to himself: "It often happens when I'm sitting around a hotel room; I'm on a trip and nothing's going on. I sit and think. Or I'm sitting on a beach... and I find myself writing myself notes." Respondent D described his daily insights as coming while performing repetitive physical activity: "You don't know how it comes into your head. You're shaving, taking a walk." The economist, respondent E, has his insights during idle time either outdoors or in the bath:

> We have this little cabin...a beautiful little place...I do a lot of writing out there.... Ideas often, come to me in the bathtub. We have a little ritual in the morning; [my wife] takes a short bath, and then I have a 40- min bath and do some exercise.

Although most respondents described insights as occurring during a solitary idle time, several described how insights can be sparked by interaction. Respondent A emphasized the importance of dialogue in generating ideas:

> I develop lots of my ideas in dialogue. It's very exciting to have another mind that is considering the same set of phenomena with as much interest as one is. It's very exciting, the sparks, and dynamic interaction, and very much newer things, new ways of looking at things, that come out of those conversations.

However, respondent D warned us not to be misled by tins solitary moment: "That's something you do alone, but not for weeks alone, a few hours, and then you talk to somebody in the hall. So it's solitary but only in small chunks." Even in. the most solitary, private moment—the moment of insight itself—many creative individuals are aware of the deeply social nature of their creative process.

Evaluation

Many respondents discussed the act of rapidly evaluating an insight as it enters consciousness. They described the evaluation stage as the point at which the large number of ideas generated would be filtered and selected. This evaluation occurs spontaneously and is phrased in terms of whether the insight is both interesting and relevant. The literary critic, respondent F, described a recursive, social process of evaluation rather than an instant judgment:

> In all matters which entail evaluation, I think what we have to do is come to our own clear first impressions...yon enter into it as fully as you can, and you form a judgment, conscious or unconscious, expressed or not, and you talk to somebody, and they say you missed something, and you go back a second time, and sometimes you have a revelation the second time.

Respondent F had perhaps the most elaborate theory of how social interaction influences the evaluation stage of creativity, having coined his own term for collective creativity—*coduction*: In my last book I coined the term *coduction* for what we do when we evaluate literary works, and I think it might be extended to the kind of...recursive and...essentially sloppy, process. I wanted to have a term that had an air of respectability about it, with that *duction* part, and the *co* emphasized the fact that it has to be done communally, in the sense that you try out ideas, you listen to what other people have said, you then change your mind, come back, and do it again.

Respondent G, the ceramicist, described the stages of insight and evaluation in terms of playfulness and discipline:

> "I was playful in creating these things in my work—but I was completely disciplined in working in factories, working with my clients...It has to be produced, it has to be produced at a price, it has to be produced to the liking, of the foreman." Her concept of evaluation is fundamentally social.

Respondent C always involves people in the process of evaluation: "I'm a big talker. I will talk people through my ideas, bounce ideas off people."

Discovered Problem Finding

The second type of creative insight, *problem finding*, often is what researchers focus on when they study famous scientists or artists. These are the revolutionary insights that pave the way for pathbreaking new work or that integrate two fields which had never crossed paths. Because the psychological and social processes involved are much more elaborate than with problem-solving creativity, we will devote the bulk *of* our analysis to this type of insight.

In an extended narrative relating his groundbreaking work in quantum electrodynamics, the physicist, respondent D, described how he came to reconcile the approaches of two famous physicists, Feynman and Schwinger. Feynman had recently begun to use idiosyncratic diagrams to solve problems more quickly and as accurately as the complex equations of Schwinger. While Schwinger's equations had been rigorously proved and were accepted by physicists, Feynman's method was somewhat suspect, because no one had been able to integrate it with mainstream physics. Respondent D told us:

> The biggest event of my life, from a scientific point of view....this is what made me famous... I spent 6 months working very hard, to understand both of them [Feynman and Schwinger] clearly, that meant simply hard work of calculating. I would sit down for days and days with large stacks of paper...and at the end of 6 months, I went off on a vacation, took the Greyhound bus to California, spent a couple of weeks just bumming around in California....after 2 weeks in California, where I wasn't doing any work, just sightseeing, I got on the Greyhound bus to come back to Princeton and suddenly, in the middle of the night, when we were going through Kansas, the whole thing sort of suddenly became crystal clear, so that was sort of the big revelation for me, the eureka experience or whatever you like to call it, that suddenly the whole picture became clear...and the result was a theory that actually was useful. So that was the way it happened, sort of the big creative moment of my life. It wasn't, I don't think, particularly unusual; that's the way it happens. You have to do 6 months of very hard work first and get all the components bumping around in your head, and then you have to be idle for a couple of weeks, and them—ping—it suddenly falls into place.... Then I had to spend another 6 months afterward working out the details and writing it up and so forth That was my passport into the world of science.

The moment of creative insight occurs during an idle period just after a long period of hard work and must be followed by another long period of hard work. The following four sections address each of the stages in turn, using quotations that are representative of the range of comments on that stage.

Preparation

Almost all respondents emphasized the importance of the preparation stage to the subsequent creative insight. In narratives about problem-finding on a long time scale, preparation was discussed in terms of apprenticeship to a field, learning the basic rules and principles of the domain. Many respondents described this type of preparation, particularly the social and collaborative aspects. Of those who discussed this, all but one were physical or social scientists. The single nonscientist was the sculptor, respondent H, who described the importance of keeping current with other artists' work: "There is no one who goes to museums and looks at objects and looks at artworks and looks at sculpture and looks at paintings more *than* do artists." A chemist summarized the approach of the scientists: "Study the more fundamental sciences...learn in the university the more fundamental subjects that are harder to study by oneself."

In addition to the preparation involved in learning a domain, preparation can also take the form of constant daily work in a domain, over a long period of time. Respondent H described the work preceding creative inspiration: "Before you can do such a spontaneous thing, you must have done hundreds of them...that doesn't come without work." Respondent D described this work as a struggle: "You have to describe it as a sort of struggle....I have always to force myself to write...it's awfully hard to get started...you may work very hard for a week producing the first page.... Without that preliminary forcing and pushing probably nothing would ever happen." On several occasions, respondent C described the importance of preparation as a sort of "domain awareness": "I happen to read broadly, and I very consciously build a very broad spectrum of activities, because I enjoy it. I'm innately curious, but I also think that the real key, at the most senior levels of companies, is to have a perspective." Respondent G described the primary importance of social factors in her life. She began to make pottery through a series of historical accidents; she had been pursuing a career as a painter. She says, "There was always something happening at the time of my life that influenced where I was going or where I lived—so you can't take my life as a life that was based on my decision alone. It had also to do with the fact that I was curious to see the world." She says you must "first decide what life you want and then fit in your profession." Despite a career distinguished by constant innovation, she continually emphasizes the importance of cultural tradition: "Tradition is your home in designing... you can' only work in your own tradition. Everything I did in my whole life, no matter how different it was, was always based on traditional expectations." She also talked about the culturally constructed notion of aesthetic value: "*In* pottery, anything that is attractive... has to have an aspect of obviousness This aspect of obviousness has something to do with a common culture... everybody wants, to be different...this doesn't work." Although the artist's daily work schedule involves more isolation than the scientist's, it is still guided by internalized social norms.

Incubation

Most of the narratives related to problem-finding insight described it as occurring during an extended period of idle time, such as a vacation or sabbatical, in contrast to the daily idle time scheduled in by many respondents who described problem-solving insights. Once again, we see the problem-solving process expanded in time in the problem-finding process. Most respondents had rich, well-developed metacognitive theories of the importance of "off time." Respondent D began his interview by emphasizing the importance of being idle: "I'm fooling around not doing anything, which probably means this is a creative period.... I think that people who keep themselves busy all the time are generally not creative, so I'm not ashamed of being idle."

Respondent E described three sabbaticals, each 1 year long, which he views as the three most creative periods of his life: "These 3 years away were very creative, getting away from the humdrum, getting into a new environment; Stanford, Jamaica, Japan."

Respondents D, H, and I all made interesting observations about their own internal processes of incubation. They believe that the creative process requires an incubation period during which a subconscious idea is continually developed:

> The creative process is very largely unconscious.... Somewhere in your mind, there is a great variety of things, disconnected fragments of ideas and thoughts and symbols and so forth. The creative process is somehow just shaking and sorting these until somehow a combination fits together and makes sense, (respondent D)

> You have these ideas, and then you work on them. As you work on them, you get new ideas.... One makes the other one come out, it's as though creatures come out. If you don't work on it, they hide in there.... Something has begun to work, and you continue it, you feel the singing inside you. (respondent H).

> I would say that scientific intuition is more sort of half-conscious knowledge, where you can see connections between things where a connection is not obvious, almost unconsciously, almost like a dream, (respondent I).

In discussions of the incubation phase, we have found that artists feel the need for solitude more strongly than scientists. The sculptor, respondent H, referred to Thomas Mann in describing the necessity of a period of solitary, hard work:

> There are many times when you go down to your studio and nothing comes... it might be weeks... and suddenly, you don't know how...but you've been, working on things, and you suddenly say, "Oh, hey, I want to do one thing." So what that means to me is you don't leave that studio...and suddenly you say, "Oh, I have *this* idea."

However, even this respondent emphasized the importance of visiting museums and feedback from other artists while creating, and she stressed the importance of daily discussion with her husband, an active collaborator.

Insight

Almost every respondent described moments of discovered problem-finding insight. The descriptions of the moment of creative insight were the richest, most elaborate portions of the narrative. Based on the narratives, these insights always occur during a period of incubation, such as a vacation, a sabbatical, or a long trip. Respondent C remarked that the major creative insights of his career always come while he is on vacation, often while on the beach. An example was his well-known "memo from the beach," which outlined the structure of the first consumer *banking* enterprise, in 1974:

> I was on a vacation, and I started out saying, "I'm sitting on a beach thinking about the business," and it went on for 30 pages. And it turned out to be the blueprint. I didn't sit down and say, "I'm gonna write a blue-print;" I said, "I'm sitting on the beach thinking" and I sort of thought through the business in a systematic way... and I shared it with my colleagues.

A more recent insight, leading to a corporate reorganization in the 1980s, occurred while he sat on a bench in Florence: "In September I had been kind of tired... and I had gone to Italy for a week, just gotten away.... I'd get up early in the morning, and I'd wander around, and I sat on a park bench, between 7 in the morning and noon.... I had a notebook, and I wrote myself long essays on what was going on and what I was worried about." These essays turned out to contain more than 80 % of the content of a 2-year reorganization plan.

Respondent F described the creative insight as almost peripheral to the social importance of the endeavor: "The feeling is an epiphenomenon of the importance of the experience itself—I guess a sense of trying to save the world, working with people. Everything I've mentioned has been communal, except reading." As noted earlier, even reading, although solitary, involves an interaction with the domain of activity, a form of communication with other individuals in the field. Respondent F described his first important insight as a confluence of personal and social factors: "If I were coming up through the department now, I probably wouldn't have thought of that.... It was a combination of the way of analysis then and the way I was then.... When you look back 25 years later, [your insight] is much less original than you thought, and more a product of the time."

Several creativity researchers have described a polarity between two types or styles of creativity, which we can refer to as *analytical creativity* and intuitive *creativity* (following Simonton 1988a).[3] Martindale (1990) refers to the two poles respectively as *conceptual* and *primordial* creativity. Perhaps the most appropriate dimension to characterize the narratives just cited would be Freud's distinction between *primary-process* cognition and *secondary-process cognition.* Many of the insights we have described represent periods in which primary-process cognition is

---

[3] See Martindale (1990, pp. 56–57) for a quick review of theories that include such a dichotomy, starting with Nietzsche's well-known distinction between Apollonian and Dionysian creativity.

dominant. In contrast, descriptions of the preparation stage (and of the entire presented problem-solving process) tend to indicate that secondary-process cognition is dominant.

Elaboration

The problem-finding narratives of insight included a fourth stage of elaboration, in contrast to the evaluation that follows a problem-solving insight. Elaboration of the problem-finding insight includes developing it into a complete solution and communicating it to other individuals in the field. Respondent D emphasized the importance of the subsequent elaboration to the insight itself: "For this shaking and sorting process (of creative insight) to work, there has to be an outlet. Something to write or compose... and I write for a particular person, audience, and not just for myself." Respondent H repeatedly emphasized the hard work that follows an insight, which she calls a *germ*:

> You have a few good ideas, your head begins to swim for a few minutes, you get excited, you have a "moment," and you nuke your model, and then for weeks and months afterwards, you just work on it....

It's like being a mason, or being a carpenter half the time. That germ of an idea doesn't make a sculpture that stands up So the next stage is the hard work.

This respondent proceeded to describe the period of communication with the field that follows this hard work: "To show, you must know galleries...you must get it out in the open; you can't keep it in the studio."

Respondent A emphasized the importance of implementing and communicating insights; she conceives of her role in life as "altering the cultural DNA" by introducing her ideas into the larger culture:

> What I am very interested in and very concerned with is to get my ideas out there, so I get very excited when my ideas are understood and published.... (After *you* have the idea for a new organization), how do you compress the idea into logic, and into a program of behaviors, which will allow that organization to act powerfully as a new piece of DNA that you're splicing into the dominant culture, that will replicate?

As noted previously, it is respondent D's contention that "it's only by interacting with other people in the building that you get anything interesting done; it's essentially a communal enterprise." In developing the first application of quantum mechanics to chemistry, respondent B described a period of elaboration following his insight; this resulted in a series of papers that, by communicating the insight to chemists, advanced the field of chemistry and resulted in his receipt of the Nobel prize. The banker, respondent C, also emphasized the importance of elaboration by characterizing his work as involving two types of activities: making decisions and getting things done. This pair corresponds to the balance between the solitude of insight and the need for social interaction to elaborate the insight, to make it useful.

Of all subjects, only respondent E claimed to have insights that did not need further elaboration. His writing habits involve speaking in written prose style into a Dictaphone for later transcription, which allows him to generate complete books in a matter of days. He rarely edits the material afterward, describing the process thus: "The last 9 days I was there [in California], I dictated the book a chapter a day and revised it very little actually. I'd been thinking about it for over a year, and it just came through. It was like having this intellectual orgasm, it just comes [laughs]."

Discussion

The narratives of creative insight summarized in the preceding sections are not inconsistent with current psychological theories of the creative process. However, there are several ways in which these narratives diverge from the standard models. First, we have identified two variants of the four stages: (1) discovered problem finding, characterized by a narrative structure of long preparation, long incubation, insight, and elaboration, and (2) presented problem solving, characterized by a narrative structure of hard work, short incubation, insight, and evaluation. Contemporary stage theories of creativity have not explored this distinction.

Second, previous models tend to focus on psychological processes, neglecting the influence of the domain, the paradigm containing prior research results and defining what types of work are appropriate, and the field, the group of researchers and administrators who make up the discipline. In both problem-solving and problem-finding narratives, interactions with members of the field are described at the stages of both preparation and evaluation or elaboration, and involvement with the culturally constituted domain is discussed with reference to preparation, incubation, and evaluation or elaboration. These interviews provide support for our proposed psychological model, in which internalized representations of the concerns of the field and the problems of the domain are involved in the moment of insight itself.

Third, several of the subjects described a creative process in which hard work and insight were coincident processes; rather than one big insight, many smaller ones continuously occurred during the stage of hard work. Respondent F described a creative process that is spread out:

> [My creative periods] tend to be sort of spread out rather than moments of actually clear illumination. I've had a few, where at a specific moment in time, I said, "Now that's what I'm looking for," and "Now I know," but generally speaking, it's a matter of hard work and steady progress rather than moments of total transformation and clarity.

Processes of creativity such as these are difficult to accommodate within the four-stage model. Perhaps for these individuals, the stages occur on such a short time scale that they are practically simultaneous.

In a fourth variant of the model, several respondents describe a dialectic process alternating between work and idle time, in which the elaboration following one insight or period of idling also functions as the preparation for the next. The sculptor, respondent H, described the process as a dialectic, continually switching between hard work and insight: "You have these ideas, and then you work on them. And as you work on them you get new ideas. Because one complements the other, one makes the other one come out."

Evaluating the psychological models against the narrative material from these interviews results in an expanded, richer perspective on the stages of the creative process. These models are helpful in understanding the narratives, but they need to be expanded to account for the influence of social factors noted in the interviews. Our interviews also suggest that theoretical issues surrounding the distinction between problem solving and problem finding need to be addressed. Finally, variants of the four-stage model in which the stages seem to blend together, or in which work and idle time alternate in a dialectic pattern, need to be more fully elaborated.

Conclusion

What do these results suggest about understanding the process of insight, at least as it takes place in the context of creative processes? We believe the following conclusions can be drawn:

- Insight is part of an extended mental process. It is based on a previous period of conscious preparation, requires a period of incubation during which information is processed in parallel at a subconscious level, and is followed by a period of conscious evaluation and elaboration.
- The length of this process depends on whether the insight is embedded in a presented problem-solving process or in a discovered problem-finding process. Problem solving may cycle in a period as short as a few hours, whereas problem finding may take a year or more.
- At every stage, the process that comes before and after the insight is heavily dependent on social interaction. This takes the form, of face-to-face encounters and of immersion in the symbolic system of one or more domains.
- Problem-finding insights are characterized by the synthesis of information derived from more than one symbolic domain. These domains may be as far apart as DNA chemistry is from social norms or as close as two neighboring branches of mathematics.
- To achieve such a problem-finding synthesis, the following prerequisites must be met: (1) thorough knowledge of one or more symbolic domains; (2) thorough immersion in a field that practices the domain; (3) focus of attention on *a* problematic area of the domain; (4) ability to internalize information relevant to the problematic area; (5) ability to let the relevant information interact with

information from other domains at a subconscious level where parallel processing takes place; (6) ability to recognize a new configuration emerging from this interaction that helps resolve the problematic situation; and (7) evaluation and elaboration of the insight in ways that arc understandable and valuable to the field.

From these considerations, it follows that problem finding insights are unlikely to occur under the following conditions:

- The absence of a strong interest, curiosity, or intrinsic motivation that drives the person to commit attention to a problematic area in a domain. *A person who is not intrinsically motivated has no incentive to push* beyond *generally accepted boundaries of knowledge.*
- The absence of a thorough grounding in at least one symbolic domain, presumably as apprentice to an expert, and not having experienced the colleagueship of other expert apprentices. *Creative insights* typically *involve the integration of perspectives from more than one domain.*
- The absence of interaction with other individuals who are experts in the domain or in potentially relevant other domains. *At every stage of the process, the stimulation and feedback of peers is necessary* to *select and evaluate potential insights.*
- A schedule in which a person is always busy, goal-directed, involved in conscious, rational problem-solving. *Incubation is facilitated by* periods *of idling, leisure, and involvement in activities such as* walking, *gardening, driving* (i.e., activities that require some attention but are automated enough to permit subconscious processes to work just below the threshold of awareness).
- A person's lack of the opportunity or inclination to test the insight and to develop its implications. *A person must be particularly in touch with the field at the stage of evaluation and elaboration; otherwise, the insight is likely to have no effect beyond the individual.*

The narrative data analyzed in this chapter also have many implications for current creativity theory. The influence of social factors at each stage of the creative process needs further attention. Individual differences in the experience of the creative process—such as the dialectic process between hard work and insight, or continuous periods that combine work, insight, and elaboration—could result in a fuller, more accurate theory of creative insight.

If the creative process occurs in both long and short time frames, as both a social and a psychological process, then the relationship between the two should be explored. The pragmatists, including James (1890), Dewey (1938), and Mead (1934), suggested that mental processes were a reflection of social processes. The psychological model we have presented is an elaboration of this position, with the creative individual having internalized the domain of activity. If it is not simply a coincidence that creative processes on these time scales display a similar staged processual pattern, then it would be interesting to explore why and how these parallels exist. Perhaps the psychology of creativity is, in fact, the social process of creativity, absorbed and internalized by those individuals whom we call *creative*.

Although we have chosen to focus on a subset of our respondents in this chapter, the entire sample of creative individuals spoke at length on the subject of creativity. Their descriptions of their own careers and working styles were articulate and complete and are consistent with the accounts reported here. The material in these interviews is interesting as narrative data and as autobiographical descriptions that the respondents use to help structure their experience. For these individuals, interactive social factors are perceived as fundamental to their creativity, and these factors are salient in our interviews. The narratives are examples of how individuals can develop rich, elaborate stories about the events that bring them fame, success and, most important, satisfaction in life.

Acknowledgment This research was supported by a grant from the Spencer Foundation.

References

Barron, F. (1988). Putting creativity to work. In R. J. Sternberg (Ed.), *The nature of creativity* (pp. 76–98). Cambridge: Cambridge University Press.

Broadbent, D. E. (1958). *Perception and communication*. New York: Pergamon Press.

Campbell, D. T. (1960). Blind variation and selective retention in scientific discovery. *Psychological Review, 67,* 380–400.

Csikszentmihalyi, M. (1978). Attention and the holistic approach to behavior. In K. S. Pope & J. S. Singer (Eds.), *The stream of consciousness* (pp. 335–358). New York: Plenum.

Csikszentmihalyi, M. (1988). Society, culture, and person: A systems view of creativity. In: R.J. Sternberg (ed.) *The nature of creativity* (pp. 325–339). Cambridge: Cambridge University Press.

Csikszentmihalyi, M. (1990a). The domain of creativity. In: M.A. Runco, R.S. Albert (eds.) *Theories of creativity* (pp. 190–212). Newbury Park: Sage Publications.

Csikszentmihalyi, M. (1990b). *Flow: the psychology of optimal experience*. New York: HarperCollins.

Csikszentmihalyi, M., & Rathunde, K. (1990). Wisdom: an evolutionary interpretation. In: R.J. Sternberg (ed) *The nature of wisdom*. New York: Cambridge University Press.

Dennett, D.C. (1991). Consciousness explained. Boston: Little Brown.

Dewey, J. (1938). Experience and education. New York: Macmillan.

Epstein, R. (1990). Generativity theory and creativity. In: M.A. Runco, R.S. Albert (eds.) *Theories of creativity* (pp. 116–140). Newbury Park, CA: Sage Publications.

Eysenck, M.W. (1982). *Attention and arousal*. Berlin: Springer.

Feldman, D.H. (1988). Creativity: dreams, insights, and transformations. In: R.J. Sternberg (ed.) *The nature of creativity* (pp. 271–297). Cambridge: Cambridge University Press.

Getzels, J.W. (1964). Creative thinking, problem-solving, and instruction. In: E.R. Hilgard (ed.) *Theories of learning and instruction (sixty-third yearbook of the National Society for the Study of Education)* (pp. 240–267). Chicago: University of Chicago Press.

Getzels, J. W., & Csikszentmihalyi, M. (1976). *The creative vision*. New York: Wiley.

Ghiselin, B. (1952). *The creative process*. New York: Mentor.

Gruber, H.E. (1981). Darwin on man: a study of scientific creativity. Chicago: University of Chicago Press. (Original work published 1974).

Gruber, H.E., & Davis, S.N. (1988). Inching our way up Mount Olympus: the evolving-system approach to creative thinking. In: R.J. Sternberg (ed.) *The nature of creativity* (pp. 243–270). Cambridge: Cambridge University Press.

Hadarnard, J. (1949). *The psychology of invention in the mathematical field*. Princeton: Princeton University Press.

Harrington, D.M. (1990) The ecology of human creativity. A psychological perspective. In: M.A. Runco & R.S. Albert (eds.) *Theories of creativity* (pp. 143–169). Newbury Park: Sage Publications.

Hasher, L., & Zacks, R. T. (1979). Automatic and effortful processes in memory. *Journal of Experimental Psychology, 108*, 356–388.

Hoover, S. M. (1990). Problem finding/solving in science: Moving toward theory. *Creativity Res J, 3*(4), 330–332.

James, W. (1890). *Principles of psychology* (Vol. 1). New York: Henry Holt.

John-Steiner, V. (1992). Creative lives, creative tensions. *Creativity Res J, 5*(1), 99–108.

Kahneman, D. (1973). *Attention and effort*. Englewood Cliffs: Prentice Hall.

Kuhn, T. (1962). *The structure of scientific revolutions*. Chicago: University of Chicago Press.

Langley, P., & Jones, R. (1988). A computational model of scientific insight. In: R.J. Sternberg (ed.) *The nature of creativity* (pp. 177–201). Cambridge: Cambridge University Press.

Martindale, C. (1990). *The clockwork muse: the predictability of artistic change*. New York: Basic Books.

Mead, G. H. (1934). *Mind, self, and society*. Chicago: University of Chicago Press.

Milgram, R.M. (1990). Creativity. An idea whose time has come and gone? In: M.A. Runco, & R.S. Albert (eds.) *Theories of creativity* (pp. 215–233). Newbury Park: Sage Publications.

Minsky, M. (1985). *The society of mind*. New York: Simon and Schuster.

Ohlsson, S. (1984). Restructuring revisited: an information processing theory of restructuring and insight. *Scandinavian Journal of Psychology, 25*, 117–129.

Omstein, R. (1986). *Multimind*. Boston: Houghton Mifflin.

Perkins, D.N. (1988). The possibility of invention. In: R.J. Sternberg (ed.) *The nature of creativity* (pp. 362–385). Cambridge: Cambridge University Press.

Poincaré, H. (1913). *The foundations of science*. New York: The Science Press.

Runco, R. A. (1990). Implicit theories and ideational creativity. In M. A. Runco & R. S. Albert (Eds.), *Theories of creativity* (pp. 234–252). Newbury Park: Sage Publications.

Shrady, M. (1972). *Moments of insight*. New York: Harper & Row.

Simon, H.A. (1977). Boston studies in the philosophy of science: Vol. 54. Models of discovery. Boston: Reidel.

Simonton, D. K. (1988a). *Scientific genius: a psychology of science*. Cambridge: Cambridge University Press.

Simonton, D. K. (1988b). Creativity, leadership, and chance. In R. J. Sternberg (Ed.), *The nature of creativity* (pp. 386–426). Cambridge: Cambridge University Press.

Sternberg, R. J. (1988). A three-facet model of creativity. In R. J. Sternberg (Ed.), *The nature of creativity* (pp. 125–147). Cambridge: Cambridge University Press.

Torrance, E.P. (1988). The nature of creativity as manifest in its testing, In R.J. Steinberg (Ed.), *The nature of creativity* (pp. 43–75). Cambridge, England: Cambridge University Press.

Vygotsky, L. S. (1978). *Mind in society: the development of higher psychological processes*. Cambridge: Harvard University Press.

Woodman RW, Schoenfeldt LF (1989) Individual differences in creativity: an interactionist perspective. In: Glover JA, Ronning RR, Reynolds CR (eds) Handbook of creativity. New York: Plenum.

Chapter 8
Creativity and Genius: A Systems Perspective

Mihaly Csikszentmihalyi

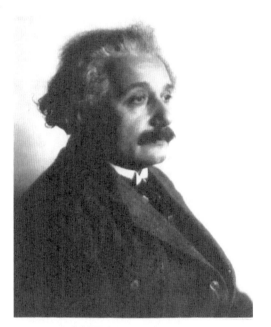

ALBERT EINSTEIN

M. Csikszentmihalyi, *The Systems Model of Creativity*,
DOI: 10.1007/978-94-017-9085-7_8,
© Springer Science+Business Media Dordrecht 2014

Introduction

The title of this volume, *Genius and the mind*, suggests that one should look for the explanation to the mysteries of genius inside the human cranium. My goal in this chapter will be to argue that while the mind has quite a lot to do with genius and creativity, it is not the place where these phenomena can be found. The location of genius is not in any particular individual's mind, but in a virtual space, or system, where an individual interacts with a cultural domain and with a social field. It is only in the relation of these three separate entities that creativity, or the work of genius, manifests itself. In popular usage, 'genius' is sometimes used as a noun that stands by itself, yet in reality it appears always with a modifier: musical genius, mathematical genius, scientific genius, and so forth. Genius cannot show itself except when garbed in a concrete symbolic form.

The attribution of genius is not based on any precise criterion; it depends on a consensus of peers. Generally genius is attributed to a person who can perform with ease feats that even the experts in a given field can achieve only with great difficulty. In science, some of the central criteria for which genius is attributed include exceptional memory, fast calculation, original insights, and perhaps more than anything else, the ability to see problems from unusual perspectives. A leading astronomer gives a good summary of the traits that lead to the attribution of genius in describing her teacher, George Gamow:

> Gamow was a fascinating person to work with...not just because he was so brilliant...he truly belongs in the genius class... No amount of my attempting to follow him would have made it possible for me to think the way he thought. He just could raise questions that had not been raised before... Some people have some kind of intuition about how the universe works... Maybe that is what you mean when you say 'genius'. People that take these enormous leaps, (see end note 1).

This ability to 'take enormous leaps' is probably grounded in some peculiarity of the nervous system. Perhaps it is a function of that superabundance of glial cells in the left inferior parietal lobe found in the autopsy of Einstein's brain (Gardner et al. 1996, p. 135). But to tell the truth, at present there is no firm evidence on which to base a structural, or even a functional explanation of genius. In other words, there is no anatomical evidence about differences in brain structure, and there are no measures of thought processes that differentiate geniuses from ordinary mortals, except anecdotal accounts and the direct evidence of superior accomplishments.

At this point in the state of knowledge, it seems more useful to examine genius not as an intra-psychic phenomenon, but as a historical process which takes place in a social and cultural context. And instead of genius, I shall focus on the creative process, which is a much more broadly researched area. Although not all geniuses produce creative works, and not all creative achievements involve genius, the overlap between these two concepts is large enough to treat them as closely related.

Creativity research in recent years has been increasingly informed by a systems perspective. Starting with the observations of Stein (1953, 1963), and the extensive data presented by Dean Simonton showing the influence of economic, political, and social events on the rates of creative production (Simonton 1988, 1990), it has become more and more clear that variables external to the individual must be taken into account if one wishes to explain why, when, and where new ideas or products arise and become established in a culture (Gruber 1988; Harrington 1990). A good example of this trend can be seen in the recent special issue of the *Creativity Research Journal* and the debate surrounding its lead article (Kasof 1995), which claims that 'creativity' and 'genius' are purely social attributions without any objective basis. We need to believe in the existence of special gifts, of exceptionally gifted individuals, and so we select successful individuals who possess certain likely characteristics (such as good luck, or the ability to overcome obstacles), and attribute to them the disposition of 'genius'.

The particular systems approach developed here is not that extreme. It has been described before and applied to historical and anecdotal examples, as well as to data collected to answer a variety of different questions (Csikszentmihalyi 1988b, 1990; Csikszentmihalyi et al. 1993; Csikszentmihalyi and Sawyer 1995; Feldman et al. 1994). In the present context, I will expand the model more rigorously, and develop its implication for a better understanding of how the work of genius can be studied.

Why Do We Need a Systems Approach?

Like most psychologists, when I started studying creativity over 30 years ago, I was convinced that it was a purely intra-psychic process. I simply assumed that one could understand creativity with reference to the thought processes, emotions, and motivations of individuals who produced novelty. But each year the task became more frustrating. In our longitudinal study of artists, for instance, it became increasingly clear that some of the potentially most creative persons stopped doing art and pursued ordinary occupations, while others who seemed to lack creative personal attributes persevered and eventually produced works of art that were hailed as important creative achievements (Csikszentmihalyi 1990; Csikszentmihalyi and Getzels 1988; Getzels and Csikszentmihalyi 1976). To use just a single example, young women in art school showed as much, or more creative potential than their male colleagues. Yet twenty years later, not one of the cohort of women had achieved recognition, whereas several in the cohort of men were successful.

The same situation holds in science. As Sir Francis Darwin said long ago, '...in science the credit goes to the man who convinces the world, not to the man to whom the idea first occurs' (Darwin 1914). New ideas in any discipline—from technology to religion—are very common; the question is, will they make a difference? And to make a difference, one must be able to 'convince the world', and have the idea become part of the cultural heritage of humankind.

Confronted with this situation, one can adopt one of two strategies. The first one was articulated by Abraham Maslow and involves denying the importance of public recognition (Maslow 1963). It is not the outcome of the process that counts in his opinion, but the process itself. According to this perspective a person who re-invents Einstein's formula is as creative as Einstein was. A child who sees the world with fresh eyes is creative; it is the quality of the subjective experience that determines whether a person is creative, not the judgment of the world. Although I believe that the quality of subjective experience is the most important dimension of personal life, I do not believe that creativity can be assessed with reference to it. It is a question, in the words of the Bible, 'to render unto Caesar the things which are Caesar's (Matthew 22:21). If creativity is to retain a useful meaning, it must refer to a process that results in an idea or product that is recognized and adopted by others. Originality, freshness of perceptions, divergent thinking ability are all well and good in their own right, as desirable personal traits. But without some form of public recognition they do not constitute creativity, and certainly! not genius. In fact, one might argue that such traits are not even necessary for a creative accomplishment.

In practice, creativity research has always recognized this fact. Every creativity test, whether it involves responding to divergent thinking tasks or whether it asks children to produce designs with coloured tiles, is assessed by judges or raters who weigh the originality of the responses. The tacit assumption is that an objective quality called 'creativity' is revealed in the products, and that judges and raters can recognize it. But we know that expert judges do not possess an external, objective standard by which to evaluate 'creative' responses. Their judgments rely on past experience, training, cultural biases, personal values, idiosyncratic preferences. Thus whether an idea or product is creative or not does not depend on its own qualities, but on the effect it is able to produce in others who are exposed to it. Therefore it follows that what we call creativity is a phenomenon that is constructed through an interaction between producer and audience. Creativity is not the product of single individuals, but of social systems making judgments about individuals' products.

A second strategy that has been used to accommodate the fact that social judgments are so central to creativity is not to deny their importance, but to separate the process of creativity from that of persuasion, and then claim that both are necessary for a creative idea or product to be accepted (Simonton 1988, 1991, 1994). However, this stratagem does not resolve the epistemological problem. For if you cannot persuade the world that you had a creative idea, how do we know that you actually had it? And if you do persuade others, then of course you will be recognized as creative. Therefore it is impossible to separate creativity from persuasion; the two stand or fall together. The impossibility is not only methodological, but epistemological as well, and probably ontological. In other words, if by creativity we mean the ability to add something new to the culture, then it is impossible to even think of it as separate from persuasion.

Of course, one might disagree with this definition of creativity. Some will prefer to define it as an intra-psychic process, as an ineffable experience, as a subjective event that need not leave any objective trace. This is especially so in our days, when creativity is seen by many as the last admirable quality for which human beings can legitimately take credit and therefore something that must be preserved at all costs in its own aura of mystification. But any definition of creativity that aspires to objectivity will have to recognize the fact that the audience is as important to its constitution as the individual to whom it is credited.

An Outline of the Systems Approach

Thus, starting from a strictly individual perspective on creativity, I was forced by facts to adopt a view that encompasses the environment in which the individual operates. This environment has two salient aspects: A cultural, or symbolic aspect which here is called the domain; and a social aspect called the field. Creativity is a process that can be observed only at the intersection where individuals, domains, and field's interact.

The domain is a necessary component of creativity because it is impossible to be a genius, at least by the definition used here, in the absence of a symbolic system. Original thought does not exist in a vacuum. It must operate on a set of rules, of representations, of notations. One can be a creative carpenter, cook, composer, chemist, or clergyman because the domains of woodworking, gastronomy, music, chemistry, and religion exist and one can evaluate performance by reference to their traditions. Without rules there cannot be exceptions, and without tradition there cannot be novelty.

Creativity occurs when a person makes a change in a domain, a change that will be transmitted through time. Some individuals are more likely to make such changes, either because of personal qualities, or because they have the good fortune to be well-positioned with respect to the domain—they have better access to it, or because of social conditions that allow them free time to experiment. For example, until quite recently the majority of scientific advances were made by men who had the means and the leisure—clergymen like Copernicus, tax collectors like Lavoisier, or physicians like Galvani—men who could afford to build their own laboratories and concentrate on their thoughts. All of these individuals lived in cultures with a tradition of systematic observation of nature, and a tradition of record-keeping and of mathematical symbolization which made it possible for their insights to be shared and evaluated by others who had equivalent training.

But most novel ideas will be quickly forgotten. Changes are not adopted unless they are sanctioned by some group entitled to make decisions as to what should or should not be included in the domain. These gatekeepers are what we call here the field. The term 'field' is often used to designate an entire discipline or kind of endeavour. In the present context, however, I want to define the term in a more narrow sense, and use it to refer only to the social organization of the domain—to the teachers, critics, journal editors, museum curators, agency directors, and foundation officers who decide what belongs to a domain and what does not. In physics, the opinion of a very small number of leading university professors was enough to certify that Einstein's ideas were creative. Hundreds of millions of people accepted the judgment of this tiny field, and marvelled at Einstein's creativity, without understanding what it was all about. It has been said that in the United States ten thousand people in Manhattan constitute the field in modern art. They decide which new paintings or sculptures deserve to be seen, bought, included in collections and therefore added to the domain.

In creativity research the field usually consists of teachers or graduate students who judge the products of children or other students. It is they who decide which test responses, mosaics, or portfolios, are to be considered creative. In this sense it is true that creativity tests can measure creativity—as long as it is recognized that what is meant by 'creativity' here is acceptance by the field of judges. Such creativity, while part of the domain of creativity research, may have nothing to do with creativity in any other domain. At every level, from Nobel Prize nominations to the scribbles of 4-year olds, judges are busy assessing new products and deciding whether or not they are creative—in other words, whether they are enough of an improvement to be included in a domain.

The systems model is analogous to the model that scholars have used to describe the process of evolution. Evolution occurs when an individual organism produces a variation which is selected by the environment and transmitted to the next generation (see for example Campbell 1976; Csikszentmihalyi 1993; Mayr 1982). The variation which occurs at the individual level corresponds to the contribution that a person makes to creativity; the selection is the contribution of the field, and the transmission is the contribution of the domain to the creative process. Thus creativity can be seen as a special case of evolution; it is to cultural evolution as mutation, selection, and transmission of genetic variation are to biological evolution.

In biological evolution it makes no sense to say that a beneficial step was the result of a particular genetic mutation alone, without taking into account environmental conditions. For instance, a genetic change that improved vision may contribute little to the evolution of a nocturnal species, whereas a change that enhanced hearing would be beneficial to it. Moreover a genetic mutation that cannot be transmitted to the next generation is also useless from the point of view of evolution. The same considerations apply to creativity when the latter is seen as the form evolution takes at the cultural level.

The Cultural Context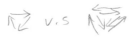

What we call creativity always involves a change in a symbolic system that has a counterpart in a mental structure. A change that does not affect the way we think, feel, or act will not be creative. Thus genius presupposes a community of people

According to this definition, creativity of student might not be valued. Yet students' work actually also challenge the gatekeeps, changing their perception.

who share ways of thinking and acting, who learn from each other and imitate each other's actions. It helps to think about creativity as involving a change in memes, or the units of imitation that Dawkins (1976) suggested were the building-blocks of culture. Memes are similar to genes in that they carry instructions for action. The notes of a song tell us what to sing; the recipes for a cake tells us what ingredients to mix and how long to bake. But whereas genetic instructions are transmitted in the chemical codes we inherit on our chromosomes, the instructions contained in memes are transmitted through learning. By and large we learn memes and reproduce them without change; when a new song or a new recipe is invented, then we have creativity.

Memes seems to have changed very slowly in human history for a very long time. One of the earliest memes was the shape that our ancestors gave to the stone tools they used for chopping, carving, scraping, and pounding. The shape of these flint blades remained almost unchanged during the Palaeolithic, or Old Stone Age, for close to a million years—99.5 % of human history. It is not until about 50000 years ago, in the Upper Palaeolithic, that humans began to use new tools: blades specialized for performing specific functions, and even tools for making other tools. The first change in the meme of the tool took almost a million years; once this first step was taken, however, new shapes followed each other in increasingly rapid succession. For thousands of generations, men looked at the stone blades they held in their hands, and then reproduced one exactly alike, which they passed on to their children. The meme of the tool contained the instructions for its own replication. But then someone discovered a more efficient way of chipping stone blades, and a new meme appeared, which started reproducing itself in the minds of men, and generating offspring, that is new tools that had not existed before, which were increasingly different from their parent.

The meme of a flint scraper or a flint axe is part of the domain of technology, which includes all the artifacts humans use to achieve control over their material environment. Other early domains were those of language, art, music, religion, each including a set of memes related to each other by rules. Since the recession of the last Ice Age about 15000 years ago, memes and corresponding domains have of course proliferated to an extent that would have been impossible to foresee only a few seconds earlier in evolutionary time. Nowadays the single domain of technology is subdivided into so many subdomains that no single individual can master even a minute fraction of it.

Cultures as Symbolic Domains

It is useful in this context to think about cultures as systems of interrelated domains. This is not to claim that culture is nothing but a system of interrelated domains; after all, there are over a hundred different definitions of culture being used by anthropologists, and no single definition can be exhaustive. The claim is simply that in order to understand creativity, it is useful to think of culture in this way.

It then follows that cultures differ in the number of domains they recognize, and in the hierarchical relationship among domains. For example in Western cultures, philosophy tended to develop out of religion, and then the other scholarly disciplines separated out of philosophy. For a long time religion was the queen of disciplines, and it dictated what memes could be included in different domains. Now scholarly domains are much more autonomous, although it could be claimed that mathematics has become the benchmark by which other domains are judged.

The multiplication and gradual emancipation of domains has been one of the features of human history across the planet. For a long time almost every aspect of cultural thought and expression was unified in what we would call a religious domain. Art, music, dance, narrative, proto-philosophy, and proto-science were part of an amalgam of supernatural beliefs and rituals. Now every domain strives to achieve independence from the rest, and to establish its own rules and legitimate sphere of authority.

It is usually the case that a domain with time develops its own memes and system of notation. Natural languages and mathematics underlie most domains. In addition there are formal notation systems for music, dance, logic; and other less formal ones for instructing and assessing performance in a great variety of different domains. For instance Piaget (1965) gave a very detailed description of how rules are transmitted in a very informal domain: that of the game of marbles played by Swiss children. This domain is relatively enduring over several generations of children, and it consists in specific names for marbles of different sizes, colour, and composition. Furthermore, it consists in a variety of arcane rules that children learn from each other in the course of play. So even without a notation system, domains can be transmitted from one generation to the next through imitation and instruction.

Creativity as Change in Domains

Typically, the memes and rules that define a domain tend to remain stable over time. It takes psychic energy to learn new terms and new concepts, and in so far as psychic energy is a very scarce and necessary resource (Csikszentmihalyi 1988b), and provided that the old terms and rules are adequate to the task, it makes sense for domains to remain stable. Thus the Egyptian civilization, for example, seems to have suffered no ill effects for intentionally keeping its religion, art, technology, and political system unchanged for several thousands of years.

The common belief is that if creativity is rare, it is because of supply-side limitations; in other words, because there are few geniuses. The truth seems to be that the limits to creativity lie on the demand-side. If there is too little creativity, it is because both individually and collectively we cannot change our cognitive structures rapidly enough to recognize and adopt new ideas. For example, each year about 100,000 new books are published in the United States alone. Assuming they all contain new ideas, how many of them will be read by enough people to change the culture? At the last census, about 500,000 individuals claimed to be artists. Even if they all produced exceptionally creative works, how many of them could we pay attention to, and remember? Surveys suggest that the average American can name fewer than two living artists.

A good example of how difficult it is to overcome the inertia that protects traditional memes is the history of the metric system. Before the metric system was adopted, weights and measures were not translatable into one another, and differed from culture to culture. The metric system was a perfect expression of rationalism, and it was introduced in France in the late eighteenth century as a way to make measurement simpler and more comparable. In this sense, the 'metre' was a very creative new meme that saved much time and needless mental effort. By 1875 this new system had been adopted by almost every European nation, and then by the rest of the world. Even Great Britain capitulated in the second half of the twentieth century. But in the United States the system is still resisted, partly because there is too much money invested in the older, more awkward system, and partly because it would take too much mental effort to learn the new system.

Domains tend to change when one culture is exposed to the memes of another, usually equally advanced but different culture. Thus ancient Greece, being at the cross-roads of trade between the North and the South, and between the East and the West, was influenced by ideas and practices converging from the Asiatic steppes and from Egypt, and from Europe as well as Persia and the Middle East. In Europe, similar melting pots for ideas arose later in Venice, Florence, Burgundy, the Hanseatic ports and the great sea-faring nations such as Portugal, Spain, England, and the Netherlands. Another source of change comes from conflicts between or within cultures; as Simonton has documented, social unrest is typically linked with the adoption of new memes (Simonton 1990).

Creativity is the engine that drives cultural evolution. The notion of 'evolution' does not imply that cultural changes necessarily follow some single direction, or that cultures are getting any better as a result of the changes brought about by creativity. Following its use in biology, evolution in this context means increasing complexity over time. In turn complexity is defined in terms of two complementary processes (Csikszentmihalyi 1993, 1996). First, complexity means that cultures tend to become differentiated over time—they develop increasingly independent and autonomous domains. Second, the domains within a culture become increasingly integrated; that is, related to each other and mutually supportive of each other's goals by analogy to the differentiated organs of the physical body that help each others' functioning.

In this sense, creativity does not always support cultural evolution. It generally contributes to differentiation, but it can easily work against integration. New ideas, technologies, or forms of expression often break down the existing harmony between different domains, and thus might, at least temporarily, jeopardize the complexity of a culture. The separation of physics from the tutelage of religion accomplished by Galileo's discoveries ushered in an era of tremendous differentiation in science, but at the expense of a corresponding loss of integration in Western culture. Presumably, if the evolution of culture is to continue, creative insights will in the future restore the interrelation between the currently divergent domains, thus temporarily restoring the complexity of the culture, at least until new steps in differentiation again sunder it apart.

What Characteristics of Domains Enhance Creativity?

According to this perspective, at any given point in time domains differ from one another (or from the same domain at earlier and later times) in terms of how easy it is to make a creative contribution to them. We shall review some of these characteristics below.

One obvious factor is the stage of development that the domain has attained. There are times when the symbolic system of a domain is so diffuse and loosely integrated that it is almost impossible to determine whether a novelty is or is not an improvement on the *status quo*. Chemistry was in such a state before the adoption of the periodic table, which integrated and rationalized knowledge about the elements. Earlier centuries may have had many potentially creative chemical scientists, but their work was too idiosyncratic to be evaluated against a common standard. Or conversely the symbolic system may be so tightly organized that no new development seems possible; this resembles the situation in physics at the end of the last century, before the revolution in thinking brought about by quantum theory. Both of these examples suggest that before a paradigmatic revolution, creativity is likely to be more difficult. On the other hand, the need for a new paradigm makes it more likely that if a new viable contribution does occur despite the difficulty, it will be hailed as a major creative accomplishment.

At a given historical period, certain domains will attract more gifted young people than at other times, thus increasing the likelihood of creativity. The attraction of a domain depends on several variables: its centrality in the culture, the promise of new discoveries and opportunities they present, and the intrinsic rewards that working in the domain gives. For instance, the Renaissance in early fifteenth century Florence would have not happened without the discovery of Roman ruins which yielded a great amount of new knowledge about construction techniques and sculptural models, and motivated many young people who otherwise would have gone into the professions, to become architects and artists. The quantum revolution in physics at the beginning of this century was so intellectually exciting that some of the best minds for several generations flocked to physics, or applied its principles to neighbouring disciplines such as chemistry, biology, medicine, and astronomy. Nowadays similar excitement surrounds the domains of molecular biology and computer sciences. As Kuhn (1962) remarked, potentially creative young people will not be drawn to domains where all the basic questions have been solved and therefore appear to be boring, offering few opportunities to experience the intrinsic and extrinsic rewards of solving important problems.

A domain with clear rules, where novelty can be evaluated objectively, with a rich and complex symbolic system, and a central position in the culture, will be more attractive than one lacking such characteristics.

Domains also vary in terms of their accessibility Sometimes rules and knowledge become the monopoly of a protective class or caste, and no-one else is admitted to it. Creative thought in Christianity was renewed by the Reformation, which placed the Bible and its commentaries in reach of a much larger population that had previously been excluded by an entrenched priestly caste. The enormously increased accessibility of information available on the Internet might also bring about a new peak in creativity across many different domains, just as the printing press did over four centuries ago.

Finally some domains are easier to change than others. This depends in part on how autonomous the domain is from the rest of the culture, or from the social system that supports it. Until the seventeenth century, it was difficult to be creative in Europe in many branches of science, since the Church had a vested interest in preserving the *status quo*. In Soviet Russia, the Marxist-Leninist dogma took precedence over scientific domains, and many new ideas that conflicted with it were not accepted. The most notorious case, of course, was Lysenko's application of the Lamarkian theory of evolution to the development of new strains of grain. This theory was considered to be more 'Marxist' than the Darwinian-Mendelian paradigm. Even in our time, some topics in the social (and even in the physical and biological) sciences are considered less politically correct than others, and are given scant research support as a consequence.

The Social Context

Even the most individually-oriented psychologists agree that in order to be called creative, a new meme must be socially valued. Without some form of social valuation it would be impossible to distinguish ideas that are simply bizarre from those that are genuinely creative. But this social validation is usually seen as something that follows the individual's creative act, and can be, at least conceptually, separated from it. The stronger claim made here is that there is no way, even in principle, to separate the reaction of society from the person's contribution; the two are inseparable. As long as the idea or product has not been validated we might have originality, but not creativity.

Nowadays everyone agrees that van Gogh's paintings show that he was a very creative artist. It is also fashionable to sneer at the ignorant bourgeoisie of his period, for failing to recognize van Gogh's genius and letting him die alone and penniless. The implication, of course, is that we are much smarter, and if we had been in their place we would have loved van Gogh's paintings. But we should remember that a 100 years ago those canvases were just the hallucinatingly original works of a sociopathic recluse. They became creative only after a number of other artists, critics, and collectors interpreted them in terms of new aesthetic criteria, and transformed them from substandard efforts into masterpieces.

Without this change in the climate of evaluation, van Gogh would not be considered creative even now. But would he have been creative anyway, even if we didn't know it? In my opinion, such a question is too metaphysical to be considered part of a scientific theory. If the question is unanswerable in principle, why ask it? The better strategy is to recognize that in the sciences as well as in the arts, creativity is as much the result of changing standards and new criteria of assessment, as it is of novel individual achievements. Having adopted such a convention, it becomes easier to understand how new memes are accepted in the domain, and in the culture (see note 2).

Who Decides What Is Creative?

The recognition that culture and society are as involved in the constitution of creativity as the individual may set the course of investigation on the right footing, but it certainly does not answer all the questions. In fact, it brings a host of new questions to light. The major new question this perspective reveals is; 'Who is entitled to decide what is creative?' According to the individual-centred approach, this issue is not problematic. Since it is assumed that creativity is located in the person and expressed in his or her works, all it takes is for some 'expert' to recognize its existence. So if some kindergarten teachers agree that a child's drawing is creative, or a group of Nobel Prize physicists judge a young scientist's theory creative, then the issue is closed, and all we need to find out is how the individual was able to produce the drawing or the theory.

But if it is true, as the systems model holds, that attribution is an integral part of the creative process, then we must ask', 'What does it take for a new meme to be accepted into the domain? Who has the right to decide whether a new meme is actually an improvement, or simply a mistake to be discarded? How can creativity be influenced through the attributional process?'

In the systems model, the gatekeepers who have the right to add memes to a domain are collectively designed as the field. Some domains, such as Assyrian languages and literature, may have a very small field consisting of a dozen or so scholars across the world. Others, such as electronic engineering, may include many thousands of specialists whose opinion would count in recognizing a viable novelty. For mass market products such as soft drinks or motion pictures, the field might include not only the small coterie of product developers and critics, but the public at large.

In some domains it is almost impossible to do novel work without access to capital. To build a cathedral or to make a movie requires the collaboration of people and materials, and these must be made available to the would-be creative artist. Not surprisingly, creativity in the arts and sciences has flourished histori-cally in societies that had enough surplus capital to finance experimental work. For

example, the masterpieces of Florence were built with the interest that accumulated on the ledgers of the city's bankers throughout Europe; the masterpieces of
Venice were the fruit of that city's seagoing trade. The Dutch painters and scientists took off after Dutch merchants began to dominate the sea lanes. As
resources accumulate in one place, they lay down the conditions for innovation.

Occasionally fields become extensions of political power, responsible to society
at large. For instance, the works of Renaissance artists were not evaluated by a
separate aesthetic field, but had to pass muster from ecclesiastical authorities.
When Caravaggio painted his vigorously original portrait of St Matthew in a
relaxed pose, it was not accepted by the Prior of the church that had commissioned
it because it looked too un-saintly. In the Soviet Union, specially trained party
officials had the responsibility of deciding which new paintings, books, music,
movies, and even scientific theories were acceptable, according to how well they
supported political ideology.

Some of the most influential new ideas or processes seem to occur even though
there is no existing domain or field to receive them. For instance, Freud's ideas had
a tremendous diffusion even before there was a domain of psychoanalysis, or a
field of analysts to evaluate them. Personal computers were widely adopted before
there was a tradition and a group of experts to judge which were good, which were
not. But the lack of a social context in such cases is more apparent than real. Freud
was immersed in the domain of psychiatry, and simply expanded its limits until his
conceptual contributions could stand on their own as a separate domain. The first
field of psychoanalysis was composed of medical men who met with Freud to
discuss his ideas, and were convinced by them to the point of identifying themselves as practitioners of the new domain. Without peers and without disciples,
Freud's ideas might have been original, but they would not have had an impact on
the culture, and thus would have failed to be creative. Similarly, personal computers would not have been accepted had there not been a domain, in this case
computer languages, that allowed the writing of software and therefore various
applications; and an embryonic field, that is people who had experience with
mainframe computers, with video games, and so on, who could constitute themselves as a field of 'experts' in this emerging technology.

In any case, the point is that how much creativity there is at any given time is
not determined just by how many original individuals are trying to change
domains, but also by how receptive the fields are to innovation. It follows that if
one wishes to increase the frequency of creativity, it may be more advantageous to
work at the level of fields than at the level of individuals. For example, some large
organizations such as Motorola, where new technological inventions are essential,
spend a large quantity of resources in trying to make engineers think more creatively. This could be a good strategy, but it will not result in any increase in
creativity unless the field, in this case management, is able to recognize which of
the new ideas are good, and has ways for implementing them, that is including
them in the domain. Whereas engineers and managers are the field who judge the
creativity of new ideas within an organization such as Motorola, the entire market
for electronics becomes the field that ultimately evaluates the organization's

products. Thus at one level of analysis the organization is the entire system, with innovators, managers, and production engineers as its parts; whereas at a higher level of analysis the organization becomes just one element of a broader system including the entire industry.

Characteristics of Fields that Enhance Creativity

Fields vary on a variety of dimensions, such as the extent to which they are autonomous. Some fields can make judgements about creativity irrespective of the society in which they are embedded, whereas others do little more than mediate public opinion. The autonomy of a field is to a certain extent a function of the codification of the domain it serves. When the domain is arcane and highly codified, like Assiriology or molecular biology, then the decision as to which new meme is worth accepting will be made by a relatively small field. On the other hand in the domains of movies or popular music, which are much more accessible to the general public, the specialized field is notoriously unable to decide which works will be creative. For the same reasons, creativity is much more ephemeral in the arts compared to the sciences. Works of art that seemed to shine with originality to audiences at the beginning of this century may seem trite and pointless to us. It is instructive to compare the list of Nobel Prize winners in literature against that of the winners of the science prizes; fewer of the writers from years past are now recognized as creative compared with the scientists.

Another important dimension along which fields vary is the extent to which they are open or closed to new memes. The openness of a field depends in part on its internal organization, in part on its relation to the wider society. Highly hierarchical institutions, where knowledge of the past is greatly valued, generally see novelty as a threat. For this reason churches, academies, and certain businesses based on tradition seek to promote older individuals to leadership positions, as a way of warding off excessive change. Creativity is not welcome in fields whose self-interest depends on keeping a small cadre of initiates performing the same routines, regardless of efficiency; some of the trades unions come to mind in this context.

In addition to autonomy and openness, there are many other features of a field that will make it either more or less likely to stimulate the acceptance of new memes. One of the most important ones is access to resources. A field is likely to attract original minds to the extent that it can offer scope for experimentation, and promises rewards in case of success. Even though, as we shall see, individuals who try to develop domains are in general intrinsically motivated—that is, they enjoy working in the domain for its own sake—the attraction of extrinsic rewards such as money and fame are not to be discounted.

Leonardo da Vinci was one of the most creative people on record in terms of his contributions to the arts and the sciences, and constantly moved during his lifetime from one city to another, in response to changing market conditions. The leaders of

Florence, the Dukes of Milan, the Popes in Rome, and the King of France waxed and waned in terms of how much money they had to devote to new paintings, sculptures, or cutting-edge scholarship. As their fortunes changed, Leonardo moved to wherever he could pursue his work with the least hindrance.

The great flowering of impressionism in Paris was in part due to the willingness of the new middle classes to decorate their homes with canvasses. This in turn attracted ambitious young painters from every corner of the world to the banks of the Seine. The first beneficiaries of the new affluence were academic painters, but as their craft became so perfect it became boring. Subsequently, new photographic techniques made life-like pictures no longer unique, benefiting those painters who broke with tradition and introduced new memes.

How central a field is in terms of societal values will also determine how likely it is to attract new persons with an innovative bent. In the present historical period, bright young men and women are attracted to a range of often contrasting domains, all of which, however, have widespread ideological and/or material support. Some might be attracted to computer sciences because they provide the most exciting new intellectual challenges; some to oceanography because it might help to save the planetary ecosystem; some to currency trading, because it provides access to financial power, and some to family medicine, because it is the new medical speciality in demand. Any field that is able to attract a disproportionate number of bright young persons is more likely to witness creative breakthroughs.

Societal Conditions Relevant to Creativity

We have already considered some of the societal conditions that make a field more responsive to novel ideas. It is useful, however, to focus more explicitly on the traits of societies that facilitate the entire creative process, including all three elements: the domain, the field, and the person.

As mentioned earlier, other things being equal a society that enjoys a material surplus is in a better position to help the creative process for several reasons. It makes information more readily available, it allows for a greater rate of societal differentiation and experimentation, and it is better equipped to reward and implement new ideas. A subsistence society has fewer opportunities to encourage and reward novelty, especially if it is expensive to produce. Only societies with ample material reserves can afford to build great cathedrals, great universities, great scientific laboratories. Even the composition of music, the writing of poetry, or the painting of pictures seems to require a market where subsistence needs are not primary. But it seems that there is often a lag between social affluence and creativity, and the impact of wealth may take several generations to manifest itself. So the material surplus of nineteenth century America was first absorbed by the need to build a material infrastructure for society (canals, railways, factories), before it was invested in supporting novel ideas, such as the telephone or the mass production of cars and planes.

A further and more controversial requirement might be that an egalitarian society is less likely to support the creative process than one where relatively few people control a disproportionate amount of the resources, especially in relation to the arts. Aristocracies or oligarchies may be better able to support creativity than democracies or socialist regimes, simply because when wealth and power are concentrated in a few hands, it is easier to use part of it for risky and 'unnecessary' experiments. The development of a leisure class often results in a refinement of connoisseurship that in turn provides more demanding criteria by which a field evaluates new contributions.

Societies located at the confluence of diverse cultural streams can benefit more easily from that synergy of different ideas which is so important for the creative process. It is for this reason that some of the greatest art, and the earliest science, developed in cities that were centres of trade. The Italian Renaissance was in part stimulated by the Arab and Middle Eastern influences that businessmen and their retinues brought into Florence and the seaports of Venice, Genoa, and Naples. The fact that periods of social unrest often coincide with creativity is probably due to the synergy that results when the interests and perspectives of usually segregated classes are brought to bear on each other. The Tuscan cities supported creativity best during the fourteenth and fifteenth centuries, a period in which noblemen, merchants, and craftsmen fought each other bitterly, and when every few years a good portion of the citizenry was banished.

But it is not enough to be exposed to new ideas, it is also important to be interested in them. There have been societies with great resources at the confluence of trade routes where new ideas have been shunned. In Egypt, for example, a unique burst of creativity resulted in astonishing accomplishments in architecture, engineering, art, technology, religion, and civic administration. Following this, the leaders of society apparently agreed that the best policy was to leave well enough alone. Thus most of Egyptian art for several thousand years was produced in a few central workshops supervised by priests or bureaucrats, relying on universally binding rules, common models, and uniform methods. '...originality of subject-matter,' writes the sociologist of art Arnold Hauser 'was never very much appreciated in Egypt, in fact was generally tabooed, the whole ambition of the artist was concentrated on thoroughness and precision of execution...' (Hauser 1951, p. 36).

Whether a society is open to novelty or not depends in part also on its social organization. For instance, a farming society with a stable feudal structure would be one where tradition counts more than novelty, whereas societies based on commerce, with a strong bourgeois class trying to be accepted by the aristocracy, have usually favoured novelty. Whenever the central authority tends towards absolutism, it is less likely that experimentation will be encouraged. Chinese society is another good example of a central authority supported by a powerful bureaucracy that resisted the spread of new ideas for centuries. Despite enormous early cultural advances, and a great frequency of creative individuals, Chinese authorities believed that the uses of gunpowder for weapons, or of movable type for the printing of books, were bad ideas. Of course, they might have been right. Nevertheless, currently China is trying to catch up as fast as possible with the new ideas that in the past they had elected politely to ignore.

The Creative Person

When we get to the level of the person in creativity research, we are immediately on more familiar ground. After all, the great majority of psychological research assumes that creativity is an individual trait, to be understood by studying individuals. A recent analysis of doctoral dissertations on the topic found that six out of ten theses written by psychology Ph.Ds in 1986 were focused on individual traits (Wehner et al. 1991) and none dealt with the effects of culture and social groups. Cognitive processes, temperament, early experiences, and personality were the most frequently studied topics.

The systems model makes it possible to see the contributions of the person to the creative process in a theoretically coherent way. In the first place, it brings to attention the fact that before a person can introduce a creative variation, he or she must have access to a domain, and must want to learn to perform according to its rules. This implies that motivation is important—a topic already well understood by scholars in the field of creativity. But it also suggests a number of additional factors that are usually ignored; for instance that cognitive and motivational factors interact with the state of the domain and the field.

Second, the system model reaffirms the importance of individual factors that contribute to the creative process. People who are likely to innovate tend to have personality traits that favour breaking rules, and early experiences that make them want to do so. Divergent thinking, problem finding and all the other factors that psychologists have studied are relevant in this context.

Finally, the ability to convince the field about the virtue of the novelty one has produced is an important aspect of personal creativity. The opportunities one has to get access to the field, the network of contacts, the personality traits that make it possible for one to be taken seriously, the ability to express oneself in such a way as to be understood, are all part of the individual traits that make it easier for someone to make a creative contribution.

But none of these personal characteristics is sufficient, and probably they are not even necessary; conservative and unimaginative scientists have made important creative contributions to science by stumbling on important new phenomena. Primitive painters like le Douanier Rousseau or Grandma Moses, who were trying to be traditional but could not quite paint realistically enough, have been seen as having contributed creatively to the history of art. At the same time, it is probably true that those who can master a domain, and then want to change it, will have a higher proportion of their efforts recognized as creative. So we now review briefly the characteristics of such persons.

Accessing the Domain

In order to bring about a novel change, a person has to have access to the information contained in a given domain. How much access a person has depends on two sets of factors: one external and structural, the other subjective and internal. The external factors include the amount of cultural capital a person can dispose of, and the domain-related roles available in the social environment. Cultural capital consists of the educational aspirations of one's parents, the non-academic knowledge one absorbs in the home, and the informal learning that one picks up from home and community. Moreover, it involves learning opportunities which include schooling, mentoring, exposure to books, computers, museums, musical instruments, and so forth. Domain- related roles are those opportunities for expressing one's creative potential that vary from culture to culture, from social class to social class, and from historical epoch to epoch. For example, whether a person will be able to study physics or music long enough to be able to innovate in it depends in part on whether there are laboratories or conservatories in which one can practice and learn state-of-the-art knowledge in the particular domain.

Whether people will avail themselves of existing knowledge does not depend only on these external, structural factors. It depends also, perhaps more, on subjective traits such as curiosity, interest, and intrinsic motivation. At this point we do not know to what extent such dispositions are inherited and form part of a person's temperament, and to what extent they are learned and cultivated in the early family environment. In either case, the fact is that traits such as curiosity and motivation vary considerably between people. For instance one of the subjects of our study, Manfred Eigen, was drafted into the German air defence out of high school, at age 15. He was taken to Russia to man an anti-aircraft battery on the Eastern front, and at the end of World War II he was taken prisoner by the Soviet troops. He escaped from the prisoner of war camp and walked for over 500 miles without money or food, evading Russian soldiers, until he reached the doors of the University of Gottingen. Here he was resolved to study science, having heard that Gottingen had the highest reputation in the field. The University had not reopened yet after the war, but when it did the young Eigen was admitted even without his High School diploma. He went to work with a vengeance, received his doctorate at age 23, and by 1967—at age 40—his discoveries in chemistry had earned him a Nobel prize.

This example shows the extent to which internal factors like curiosity and determination can compensate for the lack of structural opportunities. There are similarities to the ways in which Michael Faraday (described in Chap. 5 by Michael Howe) overcame obstacles in his determination to become a scientist. It would have been easy for Eigen to resign himself to the lack of educational opportunities in the prison camp, or in post-war Germany—in which case it would have been impossible for him to contribute creatively to science. However, it should be added that his curiosity and determination seem, at least in part, to be the result of the cultural capital he had accumulated in his early years. Eigen's father was a musician, and he grew up in a family where culture was held in high esteem, where children were expected to be proficient in a variety of subjects, and where training in music and science was provided as a matter of course. By the age of 15, when he was drafted into the Army, Eigen's desire to access the domain of science was so firmly established that the enormous obstacles in his way scarcely slowed down his progress. Nevertheless, if for example he had been taken to a Siberian gulag, or if Germany had been prevented from rebuilding its scientific infrastructure, it is probable that Eigen would not have been able to overcome this lack of opportunity.

Producing Novelty

Being able to access a domain is indispensable but certainly not sufficient, for a person to make a creative contribution. He or she must also have the ability and inclination to introduce novelty in the domain. It is convenient to divide the personal qualities that help the production of novelty into four kinds: innate ability, cognitive style, personality, and motivation.

Innate ability refers to the fact that it is easier to be creative if one is born with a physical endowment that helps to master the skills required by the domain. Great musicians like Mozart seem to be unusually sensitive to sounds from the earliest years, and artists seem to be sensitive to colour, light, and visual shapes even before they start practising their craft. If we extend the definition of creativity to domains such as basketball—and in principle there is no reason for not doing so— then it is clear that a creative player like Michael Jordan benefits from unusual physical co-ordination. At this point, we know very little about the relationship between brain organization and the ability to perform in specific domains. It would not be surprising, however, to discover that interest or skill in certain domains can be inherited, as suggested by David Lykken in Chap. 2. Howard Gardner's postulate of seven or more separate forms of intelligence (Gardner 1983, 1993) also seems to support the notion that each of us might be born with a propensity to respond to a different slice of reality, and hence to operate more effectively in one domain rather than another. Many of the subjects in our study displayed unusual early abilities that were almost at the level of the child prodigies described by Feldman (1986). On the other hand, a roughly equal number of individuals who achieved comparable creative contributions appeared to have rather undistinguished childhoods, and were not recognized as exceptional until early adulthood.

Clearly very little is known as yet about the relationship of central nervous system structures and creativity, although many claims are being made these days with limited support. For instance, cerebral lateralization research has led many people to claim that left-handers or ambidextrous individuals, who are presumed to be using the right side of their brains more, are more likely to be creative. Left-handers are apparently over-represented in such fields as art, architecture, and music. Many exceptional individuals from Alexander the Great to Leonardo da

Vinci, Michelangelo, Raphael, Picasso, Einstein were all left-handers (Coren 1992; Paul 1993). Suggestive as such trends might be, there is also evidence that left-handers are much more likely to be prone to a variety of unusual pathologies (Coren 1992, pp. 197–220). Thus whatever neurological difference handedness makes might not be directly linked to creativity, but rather to deviancy from the norm that can take either a positive or a negative value.

The most salient attributes of the cognitive style of potentially creative individuals appear to be divergent thinking (Guilford 1967) and discovery orientation (Getzels and Csikszentmihalyi 1976). These are, of course, some of the most thoroughly researched dimensions of creativity to be found in the psychological literature. Divergent thinking, usually indexed by fluency, flexibility, and originality of mental operations, is routinely measured by psychological tests given to children, and shows modest correlations with childish measures of creativity, such as the originality of stories told or pictures drawn (Runco 1991). Whether these tests also relate to creativity in 'real' adult settings is not clear, although some claims to that effect have been made (Milgram 1990; Torrance 1988). Discovery orientation, or the tendency to find and formulate problems where others have not seen them, has also been measured in selected situations, with some encouraging results (Baer 1993; Runco 1995). As Einstein and many others have observed, the solution of problems is a much simpler affair than their formulation. Anyone who is technically proficient can solve a problem that is already formulated, but it takes true originality to formulate a problem in the first place (Einstein and Infeld 1938).

Some scholars dispute the notion that problem finding and problem solving involve different thought processes. For example, the Nobel-prize winning economist and psychologist Herbert Simon has claimed that all creative achievements are the result of normal problem-solving (Simon 1985, 1988). However, the evidence he presents is based on computer simulation of scientific breakthroughs. This is not relevant to the claim, since the computers are fed pre-selected data, logical algorithms, and a routine for recognizing the correct solution—all of which are absent in real historical discoveries (Csikszentmihalyi 1988a, c).

The personality of creative persons has also been exhaustively investigated (Barron 1969, 1988). Psychoanalytic theory has stressed the ability to regress into the unconscious while still maintaining conscious ego controls as one of the hallmarks of creativity (Kris 1952). The widespread use of multi-factor personality inventories suggest that creative individuals tend to be strong on certain traits such as introversion and self-reliance, and low on others such as conformity and moral certainty (Csikszentmihalyi and Getzels 1973; Getzels and Csikszentmihalyi 1976; Russ 1993). Some examples of this approach are provided by Robert Albert in his evaluation of the mathematicians Srinivasa Ramanujan and G. H. Hardy (Chap. 6).

There is a long tradition of associating creativity with mental illness, or genius with insanity (Jacobson 1912; Lombroso 1891). Recent surveys have added new credence to this tradition by demonstrating rather convincingly that the rate of various pathologies such as suicide, alcoholism, drug addiction, and institutionalization for nervous diseases is much higher than expected in certain 'creative' professions, such as drama, poetry, music, and so forth (Jablow and Lieb 1988;

Jamison 1989; Martindale 1989; Richards 1990). These results, however, only demonstrate that some fields, which in our culture get little support, are associated with pathology either because they attract persons who are exceptionally sensitive (Mitchell 1972; Piechowski 1991), or because they can offer only depressing careers. They may have little or nothing to say about genius itself. Another perspective on these issues is provided by Gordon Claridge in Chap. 10.

One view this author has developed on the basis of his studies is that creative persons are characterized not so much by single traits, but rather by their ability to operate through the entire spectrum of personality dimensions. So they are not just introverted, but can be both extroverted and introverted depending on the phase of the process. When gathering ideas a creative scientist is gregarious and sociable; when he starts working, he might become a secluded hermit for weeks on end. Creative individuals are sensitive and aloof, dominant and humble, masculine and feminine, as the occasion demands (Csikszentmihalyi 1996). What dictates their behaviour is not a rigid inner structure, but the demands of the interaction between them and the domain in which they are working.

The importance of motivation for creativity has long been recognized. If one had to bet on who is more likely to achieve a creative breakthrough—a highly intelligent but not very motivated person, or one less intelligent but more motivated—one should always bet on the second (Cox 1926). Because introducing novelty in a system is always a risky and usually unrewarded affair, it takes a great deal of motivation to persevere. One recent formulation of the creative person's willingness to take risks is the 'economic' model of Sternberg and Lubart (1995).

In order to want to introduce novelty into a domain, a person should first of all be dissatisfied with the *status quo*. It has been said that Einstein explained why he spent so much time on developing a new physics by saying that he could not understand the old physics. Greater sensitivity, naiveté, arrogance, impatience, and higher intellectual standards have all been adduced as reasons why some people are unable to accept the conventional wisdom in a domain, and feel the need to break out of it.

Values also play a role in developing a creative career. There are indications that if a person holds financial and social goals in high esteem, it is less likely that he or she will continue long enough braving the insecurities involved in the production of novelty, and will tend to settle for a more conventional career (Csikszentmihalyi et al. 1984; Getzels and Csikszentmihalyi 1976). A person who is attracted to the solution of abstract problems (theoretical value) and to order and beauty (aesthetic value) is more likely to persevere.

Perhaps the most salient characteristic of creative individuals is a constant curiosity, an ever renewed interest in whatever happens around them. This enthusiasm for experience is often seen as part of the 'childishness' attributed to creative individuals (Csikszentmihalyi 1996; Gardner 1993). Another way of describing this trait is that creative people are intrinsically motivated. A recurrent refrain among them goes something like this, 'You could say that I worked every day of my life, or with equal justice you could say that I never did a lick of work in my life.' In other words, work and enjoyment are so deeply intertwined that they cannot be disentangled.

How these patterns of cognition, personality, and motivation develop is still not clear. Some may be under heavy genetic control, while others develop under the conscious direction of the self-organizing person. In any case, the presence of these traits is likely to make a person more creative if the conjunction with the other elements of the system—the field and the domain—happen to be propitious.

Convincing the Field

To make a creative contribution, a person must not only be able to produce a novelty in the domain, but must also be able to present the novelty in such a way that the field will accept it as an improvement over the *status quo*, and thus worth including in the canon of the domain. If this does not happen, the novelty is likely to disappear from the record without affecting human consciousness any further. There are exceptions, as when a painting or a theory that had been ignored in the author's lifetime is rediscovered posthumously. In such cases what changes is not the creative contribution, but the field or the domain that receives it. As the totality of the system changes with time, a painting or theory that was simply different may become 'creative', or vice versa. In most cases, however, the author's own actions will help determine whether the novelty is accepted or not.

Every model of the creative process recognizes that after the phases of preparation, incubation, and insight there must follow a phase of elaboration during which the novel idea or product is polished and prepared for public scrutiny. For a scholar this might involve many months of hard work readying an article for publication; for an inventor it involves building a prototype that will pass the scrutiny of the patent office; for an artist it might involve convincing a gallery or a collector that a canvas is worth exhibiting. This phase of the creative process is often the least appealing, and it involves skills and behaviours that are often at variance with the preceding phases. For instance if the beginning of the creative process involves a great deal of flexibility, idiosyncrasy, and divergent thinking, its end requires convergent thinking, social skills, and sheer endurance. It is partly for this reason that the creative personality includes opposite dimensions; the creative process requires opposite personality traits.

In our longitudinal study of artists, it became apparent that the kind of young people who in art school were considered to be the most promising embodiments of the 'artist', had a great deal of trouble once they left college. Art teachers rewarded students who were highly original, reclusive, abrasive, unconcerned about material rewards and success. But after graduation, such students had a very hard time getting public support for their work. They antagonized the 'field' of critics, gallery owners, and collectors, and pretty soon found themselves without contacts or commissions. At that point most of them lost heart and took up some other occupation, refurbishing old houses, customizing cars, starting a plumbing company, thereby forfeiting any claims to changing the domain. The young artists who left their mark on the world of art tended to be those who in addition to originality also had the ability to communicate their vision to the public, often resorting to public relations tactics that would have been abhorrent in the pure atmosphere of the art school. It is interesting that in the analysis presented by Andrew Steptoe in Chap. 11, the more successful artists of the Italian Renaissance also appear to have coupled creativity with social and diplomatic skills.

This is how George Stigler, a winner of the Nobel prize in economics, expressed this requirement in his interview for our study:

> I've always looked upon the task of a scientist as bearing the responsibility for persuading his contemporaries of the cogency and validity of his thinking. He isn't entitled to a warm reception. He has to earn it, whether by the skill of his exposition, the novelty of his views …Everybody has to sooner or later say, unless he's insane, 'I have to accept the judgement of the people around me. I can't say I'm great if everybody else says I'm not.' Or if I do say it and don't bring it to fruition, I am clearly a romancer or a utopian, not an active participant in my society.

In order to persuade one's contemporaries, it is important for a person to be able to internalize the rules of the domain and the opinions of the field, so that one can anticipate its judgements and avoid having to beat one's head against a wall. Practically all creative individuals say that one advantage they have over their peers is that they can tell when their own ideas are bad, and that they can immediately forget the bad ideas without investing too much energy in them. Linus Pauling, the winner of two Nobel prizes, was asked at his sixtieth birthday party how he had been able to come up with so many epochal discoveries. 'It's easy', he is said to have answered, 'You think of a lot of ideas, and throw away the bad ones'. To be able to do so, however, implies that one has a very strong internal representation of which ideas are 'good' and which are 'bad', a representation that matches closely the one accepted by the field.

An extremely lucid example of how a person internalizes the system is given by the inventor Jacob Rabinow, who has 250 patents on a variety of very different inventions. In addition to being a prolific inventor himself, he is also prominent in the field, because he works for the patent office, and hence decides which inventions by other individuals deserve recognition. In describing what it takes to be an original thinker, Rabinow mentions first the importance of what I have called the *domain*:

> So you need three things to be an original thinker. First, you have to have a tremendous amount of information—a big database if you like to be fancy. If you're a musician, you should know a lot about music, that is, you've heard music, you remember music, you could repeat a song if you have to. In other words, if you were born on a desert island and never heard music, you're not likely to be a Beethoven. You might, but it's not likely. You may imitate birds but you're not going to write the Fifth Symphony. So you're brought up in an atmosphere where you store a lot of information.

So you have to have the kind of memory that you need for the kind of things you want to do. And you do those things which are easy and you don't do those things which are hard, so you get better and better by doing the things you do well, and eventually you become either a great tennis player or a good inventor or whatever, because you tend to do those things which you do well and the more you do, the easier it gets, and the easier it gets, the better you do it, and eventually you become very one-sided but you're very good at it and you're lousy at everything else because you don't do it well. This is what engineers call positive feedback. The small differences at the beginning of life become enormous differences by the time you've done it for 40, 50, 80 years as I've done it. So anyway, first you have to have the big database.

Next, Rabinow brings up what the person must contribute, which is mainly a question of motivation, or the enjoyment one feels when playing (or working?) with the contents of the domain:

> Then you have to be willing to pull the ideas, because you're interested. Now, some people could do it, but they don't bother. They're interested in doing something else. So if you ask them, they'll, as a favor to you, say: 'Yeah, I can think of something.' But there are people like myself who *like* to do it. It's fun to come up with an idea, and if nobody wants it, I don't give a damn, it's just fun to come up with something strange and different.

Finally he focuses on how important it is to reproduce in one's mind the criteria of judgement that the field uses:

> And then you must have the ability to get rid of the trash which you think of. You cannot think only of good ideas, or write only beautiful music. You must think of a lot of music, a lot of ideas, a lot of poetry, a lot of whatever. And if you're good, you must be able to throw out the junk immediately without even saying it. In other words, you get many ideas appearing and you discard them because you're well trained and you say, 'that's junk.' And then you see the good one, you say, 'Oops, this sounds interesting. Let me pursue that a little further.' And you start developing it.... And by the way, if you're not well trained, but you've got ideas, and you don't know if they're good or bad, then you send them to the Bureau of Standards, National Institute of Standards, where I work, and we evaluate them. And *we* throw them out.

Conclusion

It is certain that those who are interested in the phenomenon of genius will continue to focus on the. individual and his or her thought processes. After all, the unique qualities of those whose mind takes 'enormous leaps' are so attractive that we can't curb our curiosity about them. What the present chapter seeks to accomplish, however, is to point out that genius cannot be recognized except as it operates within a system of cultural rules and it cannot bring forth anything new unless it can enlist the support of peers. If these conclusions are accepted, then it follows that the occurrence of genius is not simply a function of how many gifted individuals there are, but also of how accessible the various symbolic systems are, and how responsive the social system is to novel ideas. Instead of focusing exclusively on individual geniuses, it will make more sense to focus on communities that may or may not nurture genius. In the last analysis, it is the community and not the individual who makes genius manifest.

Notes

1. This quote and the subsequent ones are taken from interviews conducted by the author with 100 creative individuals in the context of a study supported by the Spencer Foundation.
2. The parameters of the systems model are very simple, but difficult to understand. Its implications are so counter-intuitive that most people exposed to the model dismiss it out of hand, even before they have a chance to reflect on it. A typical objection is the following caveat from one of the reviewers of this volume: 'My only criticism concerns the author's consistent confusion of creativity with the recognition and acceptance of creativity. Is the universe still there if no humans are around to recognize its existence? ...Was Herman Melville not a genius until a critical mass of individuals began to really like *Moby Dick?* If so, how many people did it take to recognize him as a genius before he became one...' I would love to be able not to confuse creativity with its recognition and its acceptance. But how would I go about it? Unfortunately, as a scientist, I must resign myself to observe creativity only after it has been recognized. There is no other way to do it. For creativity, unlike the universe, is not a physical entity that would exist even if humans were not around to recognize its existence. The first obstacle in the way of understanding the systems model is to think that creativity is a 'natural kind'—something on the order of atoms or molecules. My contention is that if no humans had ever existed, and all of Shakespeare's works were to miraculously materialize on a distant planet, no entity in the universe would know whether they were 'creative'—for they would lack the essential element of human response. This argument is not the same conundrum that George Berkeley proposed almost three centuries ago, when he asked whether there would be a sound in the forest if a tree fell, and no one was there to hear it. If by 'sound' we mean the vibrations of molecules in the air, then certainly there is sound regardless of human presence. But the same argument does not hold for creativity, which is a judgement people make of certain ideas or products, and which therefore cannot exist without people.

   The reviewer proceeds with the rhetorical question: 'Was Melville not a genius ...?' The answer is 'No'. If a critical mass of individuals had not begun 'to really like *Moby Dick*' then the reviewer would not have used Melville as an example, and the readers could not have understood the reviewer's reference. In other words, whether Melville is or is not a genius as long as he is unrecognized is a metaphysical question which cannot be answered in empirical terms. The reason the question can be asked in the first place is that a critical mass has already identified Melville as a genius. 'How many people does it take ...to recognize him as a genius' is an empirical question, and one of the purposes of the systems model is to begin answering it.

Acknowledgement The research reported herein was supported by a grant from the Spencer Foundation.

References

Baer, J. (1993). *Creativity and divergent thinking*. Hillsdale: Lawrence Erlbaum.

Barron, F. (1969). *Creative person and creative process*. New York: Holt Rinehart and Winston.

Barron, F. (1988). Putting creativity to work. In R. J. Sternberg (Ed.), *The nature of creativity* (pp. 76–98). Cambridge: Cambridge University Press.

Campbell, D. T. (1976). Evolutionary epistemology. In D. A. Schlipp (Ed.), *The library of living philosophers: Karl Popper* (pp. 413–463). La Salle: Open Court.

Coren, S. (1992). *The left-handed syndrome: the causes and consequences of left-handedness*. New York: The Free Press.

Cox, C. (1926). *The early mental traits' of three hundred geniuses*. Stanford: Stanford University Press.

Csikszentmihalyi, M. (1988a). Motivation and creativity: toward a synthesis of structural and energistic approaches to cognition. *New Ideas Psychology, 6*, 159–176.

Csikszentmihalyi, M. (1988b). Society, culture, person: a systems view of creativity. In: R.J. Sternberg *The nature of creativity*, pp. 325–39. Cambridge: Cambridge University Press.

Csikszentmihalyi, M. (1988c). Solving a problem is not finding a new one: a reply to Simon. *New Ideas Psychology, 6*, 183–186.

Csikszentmihalyi, M. (1990). The domain of creativity. In M. A. Runco & R. S. Albert (Eds.), *Theories of creativity* (pp. 190–212). Newbury Park: Sage Publications.

Csikszentmihalyi, M. (1993). *The evolving self: a psychology for the third millennium*. New York: HarperCollins.

Csikszentmihalyi, M. (1996). *Creativity: flow and the psychology of discovery and invention*. New York: HarperCollins.

Csikszentmihalyi, M., & Getzels, J. W. (1973). The personality of young artists: an empirical and theoretical exploration. *British Journal of Psychology, 64*, 91–104.

Csikszentmihalyi, M., & Getzels, J. W. (1988). Creativity and problem finding. In F. G. Farley & R. W. Neperole (Eds.), *The foundations of aesthetics, art, and art education* (pp. 91–106). New York: Praeger.

Csikszentmihalyi, M., & Sawyer, K. (1995). Shifting the focus from individual to organizational creativity. In C. M. Ford & D. A. Gioia (Eds.), *Creative action in organizations* (pp. 167–172). Thousand Oaks: Sage Publications.

Csikszentmihalyi, M., Getzels, J.W., & Kahn, S.P. (1984). Talent and achievement: a longitudinal study of artists. A report to the Spencer Foundation. Chicago: The University of Chicago.

Csikszentmihalyi, M., Rathunde, K., & Whalen, S. (1993). *Talented teenagers: the roots of success and failure*. New York: Cambridge University Press.

Darwin, F. (1914). *The Galton lecture*. London: The Eugenic Society.

Dawkins, R. (1976). *The selfish gene*. Oxford: Oxford University Press.

Einstein, A., & Infeld, L. (1938). *The evolution of physics*. New York: Simon and Schuster.

Feldman, D. (1986). *Nature's gambit: child prodigies and the development of human potential*. New York: Basic Books.

Feldman, D., Csikszentmihalyi, M., & Gardner, H. (1994). *Changing the world: a framework for the study of creativity*. Westport: Praeger.

Gardner, H. (1983). *Frames of mind: the theory of multiple intelligences*. New York: Basic Books.

Gardner, H. (1993). *Creating minds*. New York: Basic Books.

Gardner, H., Komhaber, M. L., & Wake, W. K. (1996). *Intelligence: multiple perspectives*. Fort Worth: Harcourt Brace.

Getzels, J. W., & Csikszentmihalyi, M. (1976). *The creative vision: a longitudinal study of problem finding in art*. New York: Wiley.

Gruber, H. (1988). The evolving systems approach to creative work. *Creativity Research Journal, 1*, 27–51.

Guilford, J. P. (1967). *The nature of human intelligence*. NewYork: McGraw-Hill.

Harrington, D. M. (1990). The ecology of human creativity: a psychological perspective. In M. A. Runco & R. S. Albert (Eds.), *Theories of creativity* (pp. 143–169). Newbury Park: Sage Publications.

Hauser, A. (1951). *The social history of art.* New York: Vintage Books.

Jablow, H. D., & Lieb, J. (1988). *The key to genius: manic-depression and the creative life.* Buffalo: Prometheus Books.

Jacobson, A. C. (1912). Literary genius and manic depressive insanity. *Medical Record, 82,* 937–939.

Jamison, K. R. (1989). Mood disorders and patterns of creativity in British writers and artists. *Psychiatry, 52,* 125–134.

Kasof, J. (1995). Explaining creativity: the attributional perspective. *Creativity Research Journal, 8,* 311–366.

Kris, E. (1952). *Psychoanalytic explorations in art.* New York: International Universities Press.

Kuhn, T. S. (1962). *The structure of scientific revolutions.* Chicago: The University of Chicago Press.

Lombroso, C. (1891). *The man of genius.* London: Walter Scott.

Martindale, C. (1989). Personality, situation, and creativity. In R. R. J. Glover & C. R. Reynolds (Eds.), *Handbook of creativity* (pp. 211–232). NewYork: Plenum.

Maslow, A. H. (1963). The creative attitude. *The Structuralist, 3,* 4–10.

Mayr, E. (1982). *The growth of biological thought.* Cambridge: Belknap Press.

Milgram, R. M. (1990). Creativity: an idea whose time has come and gone? In M. A. Runco & R. S. Albert (Eds.), *Theories of creativity* (pp. 215–233). Newbury Park: Sage Publications.

Mitchell, A. R. (1972). *Schizophrenia: the meaning of madness.* New York: Taplinger.

Paul, D. (1993). *Left-handed helpline.* Manchester: Dextral Books.

Piaget, J. (1965). *The moral judgment of the child.* New York: The Free Press.

Piechowski, M. J. (1991). Emotional development and emotional giftedness. In N. Colangelo & G. A. Davis (Eds.), *Handbook of gifted education* (pp. 285–306). Boston: Allyn and Bacon.

Richards, R. (1990). Everyday creativity, eminent creativity, and health. *Creativity Research Journal, 3,* 300–326.

Runco, M. A. (1991). *Divergent thinking.* Norwood: Ablex.

Runco, M. A. (Ed.). (1995). *Problem finding.* Norwood: Ablex.

Russ, S. W. (1993). *Affect and creativity.* Hillsdale: Lawrence Erlbaum.

Simon, H.A. (1985). Psychology of scientific discovery. Keynote presentation at the 93rd annual meeting of the American Psychological Association, Los Angeles, CA.

Simon, H. A. (1988). Creativity and motivation: a response to Csikszentmihalyi. *New Ideas Psychology, 6,* 177–181.

Simonton, D. K. (1988). *Scientific genius.* Cambridge: Cambridge University Press.

Simonton, D. K. (1990). Political pathology and societal creativity. *Creativity Research Journal, 3,* 85–99.

Simonton, D. K. (1991). Personality correlates of exceptional personal influence. *Creativity Research Journal, 4,* 67–68.

Simonton, D. K. (1994). *Greatness: who makes history and why.* New York: Guilford.

Stein, M. I. (1953). Creativity and culture. *Journal of Psychology, 36,* 311–322.

Stein, M. I. (1963). A transactional approach to creativity. In C. W. Taylor & F. Barron (Eds.), *Scientific creativity* (pp. 217–227). New York: Wiley.

Sternberg, R. J., & Lubart, T. I. (1995). *Defying the crowd: cultivating creativity in a culture of conformity.* New York: The Free Press.

Torrance, E. P. (1988). The nature of creativity as manifest in its testing. In R. J. Sternberg (Ed.), *The nature of creativity* (pp. 43–75). Cambridge: Cambridge University Press.

Wehner, L., Csikszentmihalyi, M., & Magyari-Beck, I. (1991). Current approaches used in studying creativity: an exploratory investigation. *Creativity Research Journal, 4,* 261–271.

Chapter 9
The Social Construction of Creative Lives

Carol A. Mockros and Mihaly Csikszentmihalyi

Introduction

Researchers who study creativity often concede that cultural norms and practices influence the development and expression of creativity. Nevertheless, the degree to which such forces influence expressions of ability and creativity is generally underestimated. For the most part, attention is focused on how cognitive factors or other individual characteristics such as personality, values, problem-finding orientation, and motivation contribute to the appearance of creativity and eminence. Such an orientation only peripherally addresses how historical, social, and cultural environments impact various life experiences and expressions of creativity.

Recently theorists have begun to recognize the importance of looking at creativity in terms of interacting multiple systems (e.g., Albert 1990; Csikszentmihályi 1988, 1990; Feldman and Goldsmith 1986; Gruber 1980, 1981, 1982; Gruber and Davis 1988; Simonton 1988; Tannenbaum 1987; Walters and Gardner 1986). The systems in question are comprised of individuals, fields, and domains, as well as the social and cultural forces that impact these subsystems. Systems theory offers a framework by which multiple forces and complex processes involved in attaining high levels of creativity and eminence may be analyzed. According to systems theory, discussed in greater detail elsewhere (e.g., Csikszentmihályi 1988, 1990) creativity should be viewed as a part of a complex dynamic system of feedback in which novel ideas and acts may result in creativity only in the context of an interaction with a symbolic system inherited from previous generations, and with a social system qualified to evaluate and accept the novelty. In this model, creativity is not an attribute of individuals, but of social systems making judgments about individuals.

Reproduced with permission from C. Mokros and M. Csikszentmihalyi, in A. Montouri & R. Purser (Eds.) Social Creativity, Vol. 1. Creskill, NJ, © 2000, Hampton Press.

Most theorists agree that people are considered creative if they have been recognized by experts as having contributed something of original value to the culture. Over a century ago Galton (1869) suggested that eminence is partially determined by others who are expert and experienced enough to appreciate and judge the performances or results. Hence, before any novelty can be considered creative, appropriately qualified judges must assess the ideas and products as likely to produce a lasting impact on the domain. In this way, accomplishments become recognized as valuable and innovative after they have received social recognition either from the larger society, or from a specialized field. The field is responsible for acknowledging and legitimizing the efforts of *potentially* creative individuals as well as deciding what ideas *get* incorporated into the domain. Although the field provides the context for activity in the domain, the domain itself, comprised of the structured or organized body of knowledge, exists independently of people and serves to transmit information to individuals. For instance, the domain of music contains the various notations systems, styles of compositions, and past musical masterpieces. A creative musician is one who, working within the symbolic system of music, produces a new composition that the field (other musicians, conductors, critics, recording executives, etc.) deems worthy of adding to the domain. The more a person's work changes the existing domain, the more that person will be considered creative.

Although fields are necessary to insure that poor ideas and products are not too easily assimilated into domains, they may also constrain growth and development by being too conservative. In any case, the complexity and diversity of eminent and creative adult lives suggests the need for a more thorough understanding of how social relationships, institutions, and cultures provide a context for stimulating and judging creative efforts.

This chapter examines how individuals develop through an interaction with social institutions, norms, and rules. In addition, it considers some of the ways fields and domains determine progress via historical, educational, professional, and cultural systems and practices that impact which ideas and knowledge are deemed relevant and valued. We intend to present several basic theoretical assumptions that influence the expression of creativity. In particular, we focus on how social and cultural norms and practices contribute to the apparent absence of eminent and creative women in virtually every field. Examples and documentation based on narrative data gathered from a study of creativity in later life are used to illustrate how socializing mechanisms and personal priorities and values contribute to expectations, choices, decisions, personal perceptions, and attitudes regarding career related abilities, goals and aspirations. These, in turn, ultimately determine how far and how high a potentially eminent life will go. The ideas that follow have implications for theories of creativity by indicating how social and cultural norms and practices influence the expression of creativity for both men and women.

Creativity in Later Life Project

The strength and full impact of a creative piece of work is often not recognized by the field until after the creator is dead; as a result, samples of living geniuses are hard to come by. On the other hand, studying contemporary geniuses allows us to gain relatively equivalent information on all individuals that would not be possible using exclusively biographic information of historical figures. As a result, 6 years ago, with the assistance of the Spencer Foundation, we began a research study to learn more about creative lives, and about the current attitudes and work habits of individuals who, at a stage of life when most people are preparing for retirement, are vigorously involved in important new activities. The project called "Creativity in Later Life", involved interviewing persons over 60 years of age who have made significant contributions to a domain.

Sample

The selection of individuals to interview was based on three general criteria: (a) Subjects are at least 60 years old: (b) there is consensus among experts in the field who recognize the subjects work as original and having significantly impacted the domain: (c) the population of subjects is distributed across gender, general area of expertise, and geographical/cultural background. The four main areas of expertise are Natural Science, Social Science. Arts and Humanities, and Business, Media, and Politics. These domain categories are not mutually exclusive, as some individuals will have worked within several disciplines. The goal of the original study was to interview 100 individuals. Thus far, 91 interviews have been completed.

The process of selecting our interviewees involved several stages. Names were acquired through (a) published records of prestigious awards such as Nobel Laureates and Pulitzer prize winners, (b) recommendations of other experts in the field, and (c) sources such as books and articles that recognize the significant work of various individuals. Following the acquisition of a group of 10–20 names, short biographies were gathered and read by the research team to determine the relative eminence of individuals. Based on this information, the research team made judgments about which subjects to pursue. At this stage potential subjects received a brief letter and consent form explaining the nature of the project and requesting their participation in the study. If subjects responded affirmatively, subjects were contacted and an interview date was arranged. If subjects did not respond to the initial request, a follow-up letter was sent. When possible, subjects who had not responded to the follow up letter were contacted by phone. At this point, if we were unsuccessful at making contact, no further attempts were made to acquire their participation.

Among those who were kind enough to participate in our interviews were several Nobel-Prize-winning scientists such as Linus Pauling, Rosylyn Yallow, John Bardeen, Hans Bethe, Jerome Karle and Manfred Eigen; Pulitzer Prize winners such as C. V. Woodward; the eminent German poetess Hilde Domin and the Italian writer Grazia Livi: and the innovative CEOs of Motorola (Robert Galvin) and Citibank (John Reed).

The sample on which we are drawing for this chapter consists of 12 women and 17 men. For purposes of identification, the sample has the following characteristics:

Women (12)

F1   Psychologist, author. Created an influential theory of personality development

F2   Social scientist. Pioneered the study of aging. Past president, Gerontological Society; recipient Kleemeier Award, Brookdale Award

F3   Sociologist, educator, author. Recipient Lentz peace prize, National Woman of Conscience Award

F4   Mathematician, computer expert, politician. Executive Board, Association of Women in Science. First woman elected a fellow of the American Nuclear Society

F5   Astronomer. Past director Association University Research in Astronomy; past president Committee on Galaxies, International Astronomical Union

F6   Chemist. Recipient Lifetime Achievement Award Women in Science and Engineering; past president, American Crystallographic Association

F7   Historian. Writer of screenplays. Past president, American Historical Association

F8   Visual artist. Winner of many prizes, works in the permanent collections of the Library of Congress, Denver Art Museum, Museum of Contemporary Art

F9   Sculptor. Widely exhibited sculptor, facilitator of intellectual and cultural exchanges

F10   Editor of one of the most distinguished European newspapers

F11   Ceramicist. Work exhibited in the New York Museum of Modem Art and elsewhere. Owner-manager of mass-produced quality ceramic factory

F12   Physicist, Medical researcher. Winner of Nobel Prize

Males (17)

M1   Physicist. Winner of two Nobel Prizes

M2   Historian. Winner of Pulitzer Prize

M3   Physicist. Winner of Nobel Prize

M4   Physicist, author. Winner Einstein and Niels Bohr Prizes

M5   Physicist, author. Recipient Max Planck Medal and National Medal of Science

M6   Lawyer, author, sociologist

M7   Historian, author Winner National Book Award

M8   Psychologist. Former Cabinet member

M9   Physicist, historian of science, author. Recipient R. A. Millikan medal

M10   Physicist, literary author. Fellow of the Royal Society and the National Academy of Sciences

M11   Historian, educator, author. Past president American Historical Association
       and American Philosophical Society
M12   Pediatrician, activist, author, U.S. Presidential candidate
M13   Biologist, educator, ecological activist, politician. Recipient Newcomb
       Cleveland prize. First Humanist International Prize
M14   Medical researcher, author, philanthropist. Decorated Legion of Honor,
       Robert Koch medal, Presidential medal of Freedom
M15   Chemist, activist. Winner of two Nobel Prizes
M16   Economist, educator. Recipient of Distinguished scholarship in Human-
       ities; Corecipient of International Peace Research Award
MI7   Chemist. Winner of Nobel Prize

Interviews

The primary method of data collection was a semistructured interview. The
semistructured interview format allowed for some flexibility and variability with
regard to responses. The interviews were videotaped and lasted approximately 2 h.
The interview protocol was designed to address several broad issues concerning the
creativity of eminent older adults. It consisted of four primary groups of questions.
These included *Career and life priorities,* related to interests, obstacles, and goals;
relationships with other people, which inquired about the nature of various social
interactions with mentors, colleagues, and family; *working habits and insights,*
which attempted to elicit information about how individuals come up with and
solve problems; and *attentional structures and dynamics,* which involved how and
on what individuals spend time. A sample of the specific questions in each of the
four categories include: Of the things you have done in your life, of what are you
most proud? Has there been a specific person or persons in your life who have
influenced or stimulated your thinking and attitudes about your work? Can you
describe your working methods? If we would have spoken to you 30 years ago,
what different views of the world and yourself would you have had? Supplementary
sources of information on the eminent adults included published books and articles
containing autobiographical and biographical information on the subjects.

Creative Women

Some important differences concerning how social and cultural influences impact
creativity emerged as soon as we began to compose lists of potential interviewees.
When the study was initially proposed, we intended to interview equal numbers of
eminent men and women. In soliciting names for participants we perused anthologies
of people who have made major accomplishments, and won distinguished prizes

(e.g., Nobel Laureates, Pulitzer Prizes) as well as inquired with experts within each field. It quickly became clear, however, that we were going to have great difficulty locating eminent and creative women. Moreover, the women who consented to be interviewed were not comparable to many of the men in terms of their renown or apparent creativity. Indeed, a brief glance at history, science, or literature texts reveals that few eminent women are listed as having made major contributions to a domain. Even in disciplines that are traditionally associated with women such as teaching and cooking it is unusual to find female principals, superintendents, or head chefs. Although all sorts of reasons have been offered to explain why this should be so, little attention has been paid to understanding the effects of this state of affairs an the development of future cohorts of creative men and women.

A combination of explanations may explain why it is difficult to locate highly creative older women. The lack of eminent women may be due to the fact that their abilities haven't been appropriately recognized by educational and professional institutions, or that they haven't had adequate opportunities to develop their ability, or that they are not encouraged to develop the skills and abilities necessary to achieve eminence in a domain, or that they have different definitions and expectations of success, or perhaps their mental orientation differs from that of the people who are in charge of dispensing recognition? Each of these reasons may be rooted in sociocultural limitations inherent in the ways we socialize young children into the world and young adults into a field, as well as how we promote adult achievement in later life.

Social norms and values determine whether a person will become eminent. Expectations influence whether talent is noticed, appreciated, and nurtured. The remainder of the chapter illustrates how cultural expectations influence the development of creative identities, and account for the differential between the number of eminent men and women represented in various fields.

The Interaction Between Self-Constructions and Social Systems

High levels of self-confidence have been found to help eminent individuals to seek out opportunities for continuing advancement in a field. Creative achievement depends on a combination of important personal qualities including skills, ego strength, a sense of purpose, and the ability to mobilize and productively orchestrate aspects of one's life. These skills are necessary to sustain a committed, enduring career. In addition, a strong willingness to take risks coupled with high degrees of self-motivation and discipline are also characteristic of highly eminent and creative individuals (Albert 1990; DeGroot 1965; Getzels and Csikszentmihályi 1976; Gruber 1986). Cox (1926) found that intelligence in the standard "IQ" sense did not appear to be the hallmark of future achievement as much as perseverance in work and confidence in one's abilities. In any case, self-motivation and confidence are considered essential to the development of creativity and eminence.

But where do motivation and confidence come from? And how are they are developed within an individual? It appears that there is a dialectical relationship between the development of the creative person and the social influences that determine which abilities are valued and reinforced. Through direct and indirect feedback from parents, teachers, peers, colleagues, authority figures, and media sources, some people are encouraged and validated for their ability. These fortunate individuals often notice their own abilities because they have been noticed, labeled, or validated by others. Future demonstrations of ability become subsequently affected by increasing the availability of opportunities and networks of relevant people. Conversely, obstacles, impediments, restrictions, or the lack of opportunities and positive external affirmation for one's interests and abilities will generally produce negative attitudes about one's self-concept and competence. In light of this, it follows that the development of self and ability are fundamentally social processes determined by cultural norms, values, and expectations. Hence, attempts to understand the development of confidence and eminence in adulthood requires a deeper understanding of the ways competent behavior, definitions of success, and pedagogical strategies are influenced by other people throughout the life span.

The Early Socialization of Creative and Eminent Individuals

The systems model suggests that the key issues that will determine whether a young person will have a chance to develop in a creative direction—in addition to innate ability. Exceptional development rests on whether: (a) there is a domain appropriate to a child's talent available in the culture (i.e., if the culture is ignorant of mathematics, a math-talented child cannot become a creative mathematician); (b) the domain is accessible (caste, gender, social class, or ethnic origin may prevent some children from being exposed to a given domain); (c) the society supports involvement in the particular domain; and (d) the child is perceived by the representatives of the field as suitable for training in the domain.

The field operates through processes of social selection and social interaction. Selection mechanisms determine the values and abilities people are allowed and expected to cultivate, as well as the opportunities available for developing these abilities. Social interactions involve the communication of expectations, attitudes, strategies, and direction as well as the provision of guidance and support, to develop. It is through both social selection and social interactions that young children receive the opportunities and the affirmation that contributes to the development of early ability and talent. Numerous biographical studies have revealed that individuals who have made great accomplishments received critical supports as key stages in their early development (Albeit and Runco 1987; Bloom 1985; Cox 1926; Feldman and Goldsmith 1986; Goertzel and Goertzel 1962; Gruber 1986; Holloway 1986; Kanigel 1986; Ochse 1990; Roe 1953; Simonton 1983, 1986, 1988; Zuckerman 1977).

For young talented children, the commitment of parents, teachers and other adults is crucial to the development of self-concept and confidence. In particular, talent in the child may be of less importance than parental encouragement. Adults responsible for the early development of creative individuals devote a great deal of time and energy to their children's development (Bloom 1985; Cox 1926; Csikszentmihályi et al. 1993; Goertzel and Goertzel 1962; MacKinnon 1978; Ochse 1990; Pariser 1991; Roe 1953; Simonton 1988; Zuckerman 1977). They often help children develop habits of practice, discipline, and attention to detail and both implicitly and explicitly transmit values such as commitment, critical thinking, learning, and achievement. In addition, adults organize, stimulate, and facilitate the learning process via the provision of academic opportunities to work with appropriate teachers and mentors during early childhood. Parents themselves often have personal interests and drive toward intellectual and creative achievement. In this way they serve as models of the work ethic and are likely to emphasize the importance of doing one's best.

Although parents are generally thought to be the primary influences on children's development, other relatives and teachers contribute to developing abilities and aspirations by encouraging and supporting talent. Teachers often identify and recognize the ability and interests of talented young people and may subsequently nurture or encourage the development of these abilities by talking to the child and his or her parents, about it. They also provide the child with materials, exercises, or experiences that facilitate the development of talent. In any case, families and early teachers are instrumental for providing opportunities and experiences that introduce talented youth to the field. Likewise, they support and encourage talent development by affirming ability and interests during early childhood. This early social support and encouragement contributes to the development of self-confidence and subsequent independence.

The Differential Socialization of Boys and Girls

The literature on the social influences leading to gender differences with respect to aspirations and achievements among the gifted and talented is extensive. Only a cursory discussion of these differences will be given here. Research has looked at factors that influence academic success and productivity as well as career decisions among gifted and talented youth (Astin 1974; Bloom 1985; Fox 1977; Hollinger 1985, 1986; Holloway 1986; Kerr 1985; Solano 1983; Tomlinson-Keasey and Burton 1992). Most of this research focuses on the attitudes, aspirations, and achievements of young boys and girls in mathematics and science. The findings show that during elementary school by most measures girls tend to be intellectually equal or superior to boys. Over time, however, girls' achievements progressively fall off as compared to boys. As girls mature, their talent and giftedness become sources of conflict, whereas for young boys the cultivation and expression of ability is a source of pride and generally enhances their overall image of themselves. This may be due to the fact that girls are not encouraged to develop their interests, talent, and abilities. A critical component of attaining eminence in this culture involves the development of a specified identity that allows a person to differentiate oneself from others, and develop independence and autonomy in one's field of endeavor.

Research has found that boys generally evaluate themselves more positively when they identify themselves as being more competitive, autonomous, and independent. Girls, on the other hand, root self-concepts more in dependency, and relational competencies and values. As a result, competition and independence may have more favorable effect on men's identity development than women's. Our culture partly defines creativity and eminence with characteristics and qualities that are appropriate for males and somewhat inappropriate for females. Cultivating and expressing independence and competitiveness may be difficult for women because it interferes with priorities and attitudes toward work.

Studies have found that parents and teachers respond differently to achievement and intellectual competence in boys and girls (Helson 1990; Hollinger 1985, 1986; Holloway 1986; Solano 1983). In general, given similar external accomplishments or scholastic achievements, the ability of boys is recognized as superior to that of girls. In addition, young boys are affirmed for their progress and ability, whereas the accomplishments of girls are either ignored or discouraged by significant adults. Likewise, boys' early academic and artistic choices tend to be more readily supported by parents and teachers. In addition, parents and teachers generally select a particular child in which they invest their time and energy. They locate educational opportunities that will serve the child identified as best suited to take advantage of the opportunities. The chosen child receives intense socialization in the field. In general, girls are less likely to be the chosen child by parents or teachers. In this way, the processes of socializing girls involves an increasing negation of intellectual and creative goals that may interfere with the development of their identities. Although this assumption has not been adequately studied, much of the literature suggests that young girls actively choose to forgo academic success and intellectual achievements when social and personal values and expectations of behavior conflict with the development of a positive (feminine) sense of self.

As young children, both the men and women in our sample of eminent individuals received recognition and encouragement from adults. Virtually all eminent people discuss the importance of someone else who believed in what they were doing and encouraged them at some time in their lives. In this way, young people invariably benefit from the encouragement of an adult. Nonetheless, as young boys, the men were more often the chosen child in the families:

> I was not considered very bright. My brother was older than I and I never felt I was treated quite as well. I was a girl, and I think this had a profound impact on the way we were treated. I came from this very intellectual family and everybody was supposed to be at least a university professor if not a medical doctor. I was not considered the gifted child in the family. So maybe being a second class citizen took the seriousness out of my ambitions [F11].

> I had a sister who was smarter than I in school. She was younger and she pushed me. The relationship between my sister and I was not totally smooth because I did better than she in

academic life and her subsequent career has not been as happy as mine. She said she was
not pleased with the fact that I left her behind [M7].

The majority of the men received support and encouragement as children from
a parent or family member:

Both my parents were valedictorians of their classes. So, I had very strong parental model
and example of accomplishment and ambition which pervaded my childhood. My parents
never put overt pressure on me to do anything I did not want to do, but I think it's also true
that they expected superior performance from me and they got it, I think breaking the
parental bond for me was very difficult because they were very kind to me and certainly
did all that they could to facilitate my life [M7].

My father was the dean of the medical school and very busy. Still, he encouraged me by
frequently giving me extra math problems to do [M1].

They left me complete freedom to do my stuff which was science. And neither of them
was a scientist but they understood what it was about [M10].

My mother was very strong and had a lot of courage. She would always tell me,
"understand this, even the angels cannot do any better than their best" [M11].

My parents always supported me, although sometimes they were not in agreement. They
thought it was important I get in touch with what I wanted to do. They supported my
scientific interests by buying books or giving me money for instruments even though they
themselves were not very interested in science. My mother had a strong influence on me,
not in science, she didn't understand much about science, but in art and music. She loved
me very much. I didn't have a lot of worries as a child [M5].

Typically in the evening the family would be sitting around the living room, everybody
with his book or homework … my father was very interested in science … but he was
limited in how he could get around because he had a family to support… One of his
motto's was that "there is nothing that cannot be done better" … (they gave) encouragement of being behind me… "… That a boy! Go after it" [M4].

I had an aunt and uncle who were intellectuals. My uncle kept an eye on me and
encouraged me to move in intellectual directions. So I was lucky that way. My father
wanted me to become a radio repairman. But, my uncle made it clear that I should go to
college [M13].

Many people, including various neighbors encouraged me and helped me accomplish what
I wanted accomplish, which was to learn more about chemistry [M15].

Although most of the women were not overtly discouraged, they rarely received the
affirmation or encouragement for their early interests, performance, and achievements comparable to that received by the men. Here are some typical accounts:

I joined the *Amateur Astronomers,* which was an adult organization in Washington and
(father) would come to meetings with me. I think he thought it was improper for a young
girl to go off…. My father thought I should become a mathematician—do something more
practical—he was afraid I would never be able to make a living as an astronomer….
Maybe my mother would have liked me to have been more social. I really preferred to read
and to study and was not really interested in an active social life [F5].

My father was a lawyer and then a judge…. I don't think my mother had a particular
direction she wanted me to go. I think my father wanted me to be a probation officer or

something like that, to be helpful to a judge.... He liked me, but he had very sexist ideas about the professions, and he didn't quite approve of my being a psychologist [F1].

My parents wanted me to be a school teacher [F12].

I wanted to be a chemist and that threw my parents. My mother thought I would be a teacher and my father thought I would be a lawyer. They didn't really know what my interest in chemistry would lead to [F6].

My father was a mechanical engineer. I remember when I was interested in going into mechanical engineering and he told me—and that was the only time he ever said anything to me one way or another about what to do—and he said, "Well, if you are a women going into mechanical engineering you will end up filing blue prints. Don't do that." [F4]

My family was very middle class and bourgeois and always doing the right things. No one in my family considered for one second that I would be anything except a wild girl. Everybody always thought I was imaginative and wild, but they did not encourage it They were absolutely upset, terrified and horrified that I wanted to study theater. It was like being a street walker to them. I think they wanted me to be quietly married off somewhere [F9].

Adults outside the family often perpetrated the same differential treatment of boys and girls. Young girls received considerably less encouragement and affirmation from teachers than the men did as boys.

I skipped from grade 3 to 7 and took High School algebra at age 10. In seventh grade I worked closely with a mathematics teacher at the University High School. My early intellectual interests in math and later academic success are due to this teacher's interest and encouragement [M1].

I always scored well on exams in school. I got a scholarship to high school, and had excellent teachers who helped me get a scholarship to Oxford [M16].

I was told right from the beginning that I would have to work harder, twice as hard as anybody else (due to antisemitism). But my teachers thought I was bright enough and it would be worthwhile [M13].

When I came upon obstacles I don't think I took them very seriously, I just felt that the people who presented obstacles did not understand that I really wanted to be an astronomer. And, I tended to ignore them or dismiss them.... In general I think there was just a lack of support. I always met teachers who told me—in college, in graduate school—to... go and find something else to study... they didn't need astronomers... I wouldn't get a job... I shouldn't be doing this, and I really just dismissed all that I just never took it seriously. I just thought they didn't understand [F5].

I went to the counseling center and a counselor told me that psychology was too mathematical for me.... He based that on my college aptitude test.... Still, apparently I knew enough to get good grades, but he decided on the basis of my exam that math was too hard for me [F1].

Many women find out that they haven't got the background for math or science because they copped out early on. Also, I think when children get into high school and there are lots of social activities, and women seem to spend their time watching men do sports. Like cheerleaders. They themselves don't participate in the competitions as much [F4].

I have not had a formal education. I went to school, but I never attended university. I went to university, but only to occasional lectures [F10].

I knew my parents were sacrificing to send me to college. So, I thought I'd better get something out of it. In fact, that is the reason I went into math. I felt it was something for which my parents were getting their money's worth. It was hard and I felt I was learning a lot [F4].

Not surprisingly, such differential reinforcement leads to particular attitudes about one's potential, and often negative consequences for the subsequent professional goals of girls. Again, however, it should be pointed out that despite differential treatment, gifted girls were more like gifted boys than they were like average girls in their interests, abilities, and aspirations. Moreover, eminent women frequently demonstrate a great deal of self-confidence, autonomy, and independence in pursuing their goals. Many describe social influences that helped them develop self-confidence and counteract standard messages and expectations of female achievement and performance. In particular, as is discussed later, women often received considerable support from their husbands. In addition, eminent women mathematicians and scientists talk about having performed well and received attention, encouragement, and affirmation from parents and early teachers:

I was in high school by the time I was 11. That was because we lived in a small town and nobody knew what to do with a bright child so they just kept on pushing me up a grade [F2].

After I graduated from high school I went on to a university in Detroit and by some quirk in scheduling my chemistry course was with the chemical engineers and I was the only girl. I was good at it, and the teacher soon singled me out as the one who got 100s on the tests. I graduated from college when I was 19. I got my PhD a month after my 22 birthday [F6].

I was 15 when entering college [F1].

What distinguishes eminent women from their peers may lie in the fact that they *did* receive encouragement and recognition for their early abilities. The fact remains, however, that the social environment does not consistently reward and encourage intellectual rigor and curiosity in young girls. Cultural norms are generally less antagonistic to developing profitable characteristics for men's success and achievement. As a result, men more frequently encounter relationships that support their intellectual and creative efforts, These social mechanisms not only lead to girls' decreased interest and motivation, but also to a decrease in the opportunities that are available to them during the early stages of their careers. Moreover, unless young girls are exposed to someone who encourages and supports their interests it is unlikely they will persevere given the opposing messages on identity development as well as impending constraints on educational opportunities.

Adulthood and Professional Socialization

The construction of a creative life is a complex developmental process that occurs over the life span (Albert 1983, 1990; Bloom 1985; Csikszentmihályi 1988; Feldman and Goldsmith 1986; Gruber 1980, 1981, 1986; Tannenbaum 1987). Young adulthood is often the time during which one's "purpose" begins to form. At this time, people formulate a personal vision or dream for their life (Erikson

1950; Gergen 1990; James 1990; Levinson et al. 1978; Roberts and Newton 1987; Stewart 1977; Terman and Oden 1959). For both men and women, career choices are often defined by interpersonal needs. The dominant issues surrounding identity formation for young men generally center around professional goals, aspirations, and achievements (Levinson et al. 1978; Valliant 1977). As a result, it is important to understand how people make personal and professional choices when examining this portion of the life span.

Socializing experiences during adulthood also have a profound impact on people by validating or invalidating competencies. For this reason, the mobilization of critical segments of the field is important as young people continue to develop their personal and professional aspirations. For young adults, professional institutions, mentors, and spouses are the chief socializing agents. Just as teachers and parents provide instrumental support, encouragement, and opportunities for talented children, during young adulthood, mentors and spouses function similarly. We turn now to a discussion of the ways young adults are reinforced and socialized into professional communities; in particular, the way the field defines and develops the attitudes, abilities, and people it perceives to be beneficial to the domain.

Mentors

During young adulthood, people generally benefit from relationships that endorse a more highly developed, domain-specific self-concept. At this time, identity development occurs in the context of identifying with role models within the career and work context. At the same time, hierarchical training systems indoctrinate young people into a field. The mentor-apprentice relationship transmits information, knowledge, and skills from one generation to the next. Professional communities have long recognized the value of mentor-apprentice relationships in cultivating ability (Kanigel 1986; Kram 1985; Simonton 1978, 1984; Zey 1984, Zuckerman 1977). People who do well in senior positions have often been guided and taught by a mentor.

Not surprisingly, mentor relationships are often one of the most important relationships during young adulthood. A mentor can be a teacher, supporter, guide, protector, and counselor for a young adult as he or she enters the adult world of work. Mentors play a critical role in helping negotiate both personal and professional issues. They contribute to the development of young people by building self-confidence, affirming and encouraging their abilities, and helping them develop a stronger and clearer professional identity. For some, mentors help increase self-confidence by expressing or demonstrating faith in the apprentice, whereas for others mentors specifically and directly communicate positive feedback regarding performance or life circumstances. In this way, mentors effect a fundamental transformation in the way young people perceive themselves, their value, their potential, their careers, and their relationship to the field and domain.

Generally, a less important aspect of the apprenticeship revolves around teaching specific substantive knowledge; rather, the value of the relationship stems from seeing how mentors operate, think, find, and solve problems. In this way, the principal benefits of apprenticeships include exposure to procedures and standards of work as well as inner processes of thought. Thus, although apprenticeships provide the beginner with access to the overt aspects of developing skills through close collaborations with mentors, novices learn dimensions of knowledge that are not formally articulated.

Good mentors offer young students the freedom and expertise needed to cultivate problem-finding abilities. Likewise, they help recognize innovative ideas that may be tested and pursued. In this way they serve as gatekeepers in deciding what ideas and projects are worthy of being pursued as well as those that are inappropriate or not likely to come to fruition. Mentors often provide a safe, secure environment in which novel ideas can be developed, nurtured, and experimented with. In addition, they advance young people in an organization by teaching specific skills or strategies of work and problem solving, providing them with opportunities, sponsoring them, challenging them, and protecting them from negative gossip and feedback. At the same time, mentors use their position and influence to raise the visibility and credibility of the young person while providing insight into effective ways to function within an organization or system. Hence, mentor-apprentice relationships contribute to the development of ability, self-confidence, as well as positions and credibility within the Geld.

Zuckerman (1977) demonstrated that both apprentices and masters are engaged in a motivated search to find and work with scientists of talent. For the Nobel Laureates, both self-selection and social selection enlarge opportunities for further work that, in turn, opens up additional opportunities. In choosing an apprentice, the mentor makes judgments and assessments about his or her perceived skills in the field. In this way, the promotion of young people is not based on current performance but on perceived potential, which is highly subjective. At the same time, those perceived to be lacking the skills necessary to succeed will be overlooked as useful and valued apprentices.

In selecting apprentices, many senior people look not so much for a good worker as for a replica of themselves. In this way, the selection processes are biased toward people who display characteristics or attitudes similar to those the mentors possessed as young people. Women and minorities in business, for example, are automatically perceived to be less competent in managerial, leadership, and technical skills. As a result, opportunities to be apprenticed to top executives often do not exist.

Among our eminent adults the value and importance of having mentors were often discussed:

> Young people should try to get personal contact with scientists at the university. Talk to them and work with them. Thai's the way to learn. Not by just taking courses. The apprenticeship is very important in science [M5].

When you are young I think personal encounters with others are especially important [M7].

People can grow beyond their fears or early low self-estimates of their worth during midlife if they get the affirmation. They may get the affirmation on their own *or* with the help of a mentor who brings out what is in them [M8].

What you need in teachers is to have people you can go to, like friends when you have a problem. Graduate school is tough, people need support; moral support and encouragement from teachers [F5].

I think having a sponsor helps. Somebody who recognizes your work and pushes you forward. I think the kind of recognition you get with, for example the National Academy depends on having somebody there to push you. It's such a Byzantine system. You have to have somebody who will push for you [F1].

I think women need to have women who are role models and people who are doing things, not just looking on from the audience, bat participating [F4].

By all means it is important to try to be an apprentice to an artist. Being an apprentice is a very very very, basic and important element of education. It is important because it is not learning the facts of making art. Working with a person who is creative and you become part of their body. You begin to learn that way. You learn what it is about studio discipline and also being an artist is not just making art. It is keeping books and being a business person. You learn about that. You learn how tough it is to work with dealers and what it means to have shows [F8].

Men and Women in Mentor Relationships

Although mentors play a significant role in the development of creative individuals during the formative years of their careers, men and women do not have similar experiences with teachers and mentors. In the past, research has suggested that women and men have different needs with respect to mentors (Jeruchim and Shapiro 1992). Whereas men seek mentors who are useful to their career advancement, women seek mentors who teach them how to live their lives. At the same time, both young men and women establish mentor relationships for different reasons, at different times, and with different expectations. It appears, for example, that women who have received support and basic affirmation for their abilities and competence as children, may have fewer personal, emotional needs as young adults. At the same time, if a young man has not had sufficient early affirmation and has not developed an inner sense of direction and purpose, he may need a mentor who can offer these things rather than (or in addition to) career and professional guidance.

For the most part, however, men and women have different experiences with mentors. Most of our women cannot point to a particular person in the field who influenced them during the early stages of their careers; rather, they indicate that many people influenced their development For example, in one woman's case numerous undergraduate teachers encouraged her ability and interests and thereby contributed to her self-confidence in the field:

Almost all of the teachers I had at Vassar were female... and they were very good... and maybe from them I acquired some of this self-confidence [F5].

Women also discuss not having been significantly influenced by anyone during the early years of their careers:

> I don't remember modeling myself after anyone, even as a child. I have been asked this often and I have thought about it so it must be true. I can never come up with anybody who influenced me in an overt sense [F2].

> Well, I didn't really have (an advisor), I mean it was during the war years and it would have been... although our ideas were antithetical. So I think technically it was... but he wasn't too much interested in the kind of thing I was interested in... so I just did my own thing [F1].

> He (graduate advisor) was a fascinating person to work with but my relationship to him as a graduate student was really not very close.... I don't think he had an enormous influence on me professionally [F5].

> I don't know if I had a role model or not, I don't remember one [F4].

> I don't think I can find a single person who particularly influenced my style, I can't think of anybody [F11].

> At the University of Michigan I enjoyed most of the professors but they were a little distant. I don't think that I had any bad experiences. I had indifferent experiences, so (to them) if I survived that was fine. No obstacles were put in my way. I didn't have bad personal relations with others. They were nonexistent in some ways, but if I did my work, it was OK. Most of what kept me going were my own personal interests [F6].

> I was put into my place by my master. I had to wear waterproof pants and a red kerchief. He took me to nice houses to set ovens to show that my job as an apprentice was not an elegant one.... I did not identify with him. I played out my role [F11].

Many of male respondents, on the other hand, had significant influential teachers and mentors during the early years of their careers. In addition, their mentors were often highly eminent figures in the field such as Niels Bohr, G. H. Hardy, and Richard Feynman.

> He was a critical role model who introduced me to the history of science and technology in China. My relationship with him led to my initial interest and entry into the field [M16].

> My relationship with him (Bohr) was absolutely wonderful. He was somebody who kept his eye on the ball and depended so much on talking with others to clarify issues. If he couldn't talk he was lost...and he had a great sense of proportion [M4].

> I had essentially undivided attention from a great mathematician... we would go for long walks around the country side in Cambridge and talk about all kinds of things... and his style in mathematics was quite influential.... I mean that is the way I think and do mathematics. He had what was a kind of meat-grinding approach to mathematics. He would get a hold of a problem and put it through the grinder and just grind it very, very small. Out of it would come a theorem or whatever it was that he was trying to prove.... From time to time I would write things to him which led to my first published work, so I have felt very much indebted to him [M10].

> When I went to Columbia, I wasn't admitted.... But one of my relatives got me in.... I was going to stay at Columbia as a graduate student, a professor of mine called me in one day when I was about to start graduate work. He said, "You're going to Harvard.... I've arranged for you to become a graduate student...." I hadn't applied... that's how I got to Harvard. He was a very bright man, who was enormously devoted to his work. But on top

of that, he was somebody who labored very hard to explain why he was so interested in the work. And you knew damn well that he was somebody who felt that what he was doing was important. It was important for me to understand why he thought it was important. Also, this was a guy with a keen interest in social and political problems. I was a student in his course. What I learned was the importance of data, intellectual discipline, and rigorously dealing with information, but on top of that, being interested in it. That is, having an emotional link to the process [M13].

When I was young there were several important individuals.... They taught me a great deal. In part my views about teaching come from the man I did my dissertation with. He wanted me to be myself, and I suppose I modeled myself partly after him.... He himself was a very famous historian and had some very good ideas. He continued to have new notions and ideas as long as he was alive. The place that he kept his ideas alive was in his writing. He was a man who was trying to think things through [M7].

I had one (mentor) when I was a graduate student. He did me an invaluable service by reading my book manuscript, taking it seriously and helping me improve it. He also influenced me in many ways by his vigor and his example [M2].

I don't think my curiosity was developed or encouraged until I met him my senior year in college. He was 10 years older in age but he was really light years older than I. He saw more in me than I saw in myself. He gave me a sense of the wider range of possibilities. I felt very marginal and unconnected although visible and active. He gave me a sense of possibility and I feel very fortunate for that. Also the combination of challenging me and respecting me was just extraordinary. I think it was be who helped me also appreciate a broader way of thinking [M6].

My PhD supervisor in experimental physics was P. W. Bridgman, who is very well-known and really the father of operationalism. One of my very dear professors, for whom I was a teaching fellow, and later became a colleague was Philipp Frank. I was lucky that as a graduate student 1 was allowed to sit in on a shop club of people like Norbett Weiner, Giorgio de Santillana, Bridgman and Frank, and others. They would have discussions and internal fights. I was allowed to help out with the group. And although I was the secretary, I was almost treated as an equal [M9].

In 1933 I heard the Institute for Advanced Study was opening at Princeton with Einstein and other notables. I had a couple of years of graduate work but I didn't have a PhD, so I decided to go to graduate school at Princeton. I was at Princeton for two years. At Princeton I worked under Eugene Wigner. He was one of the pioneers in the field who taught the first generation. He had much broader interests. I was Wigner's second student [M1].

In any case, mentor relationships not only cultivate self-confidence and ability, but also influence choices, opportunities, and experiences relevant for career advancement. It may be that a lack of eminent women in different fields is a result of social selection mechanisms that reduce women's access to professional mentors early in their career. This point is illustrated well by two women:

At some level 1 think the system is kind of a self-fulfilling prophecy. The people that you give the opportunities tend to develop [F5].

The management is still almost all male and they talk to each other. A lot of the news about what opportunities are available at the laboratory does not even filter down. I think all of the people making the decisions and policies and doing the hiring are men. Their friends are men and they talk to men [F4].

Among the eminent adults, several individuals articulate how the field tends to discriminate against women during the early stages of their career:

Yes, I'm sure for a long time I was not taken seriously because I was a woman, but I was really so naive that I didn't know or didn't even know enough to think about it [F5].

Professionally people who have succeeded see themselves as the model for how to succeed. That is, if you are the chairman of the department and male and attended a particular type of college and post doc, you see this as a program for success. Consciously or unconsciously you think this is the recipe for success. If someone comes in with a different kind of background, it is hard to believe he or she will be as successful.... Being female is a slight disadvantage because women look different, and talk in a softer voice.... I think people look upon people who are most similar to them as potentially most successful. If you are a minority or foreign, I think you are perceived as having less potential to be successful [F5].

Differences between men and women are built in from the biology and all of the socialization. It takes a special kind of support and fortitude for women to deal with that. And there are an awful lot of casualties. There is a lot of wasted talent, and probably more often with women because you have to have very subtle and longstanding encouragements to rise in a field [F2].

Women's letters of recommendation often talk about whether they're attractive or not attractive, or whether they get along with people, while men's discuss their ability and achievements [F5].

The little children used to say, "Auntie... are you an uncle or an auntie?" because I had those pants on and they had never seen a women in pants. I had to carry the pots on a big plank to the other side of the road. The little children used to throw things at me [F11].

It was completely out of the ordinary for a young lady from a good family to go there. This was a slimy sort of place. It was not where young ladies made pottery [F11].

In another instance, when asked about female students one eminent male physicist talked about how his professional association with a female graduate student was limited because fellow colleagues and students often gossiped about their relationship when they saw them together:

I can recall, to my shame, that I had to look... and here I was on the Princeton campus, as if I were not always going around in her company because there were colleagues there that were rather old-fashioned [M4].

Although men in positions of authority are often reluctant to work with young women, some women are able to work well with male mentors. Nevertheless, these relationships may lack the emotional and social support for issues that are salient and significant to women's identity development and needs:

It might be possible that a supportive male could fill that role, but I am not sure he would want to. Also, I don't know many women or young girls who would feel comfortable with that. What young people need is to have people like friends they can go to when they have a problem [F5].

At the same time, young women rarely have the opportunity to work with eminent women because very few women are in senior positions. In addition, if a woman is able to find a female mentor, she is likely to have less power than a male mentor. Women also tend to be overextended as they struggle to balance family and career commitments. Because of this, eminent women may simply not have the time or energy to invest in the careers of young people. Not only are distinguished women scarce, they may often find themselves overwhelmed by young people who need support and counsel:

> I am often the first women in the department and I make it my business to get to know all of the young women. There have been episodes where after a few months I really felt that the emotional drain was almost more than I could bear. These women really had no one else to calk to *so they told me* all their troubles.... At this particular place women just came out of the woodwork, from all departments, because there were just so few women around. Yet here were a group of brilliant men, and every time they hired a faculty member they did not see the need for hiring a women. Had they seen the need, given approximately equal professional scientific qualifications and the fact that you had to support your women students, being female would have been an important requirement. But having men making the decisions and doing the hiring meant that having someone support women graduate students never became an important part of the job description [F5].

> There are still very few women here. There are some divisions that do not have any women. We would have women come in as post docs and they would be there a very short time. While they were there they would often be the only woman in their department and they would not see other women during the day [F4].

In any case, whether a result of different expectations or ideas of men and women's competence or the result of social biases and constraints on the development of ability, by and large, women have less access to mentors than do men.

Spouses as Social Influences

In addition to mentors, spouses play a significant role in helping creative achievement during adulthood. Unfortunately, until now little research has explored how spouses influence the professional lives of eminent individuals. Research has generally focused on the social support provided by parents and teachers. Spouses, however, can be very helpful both at early and later, more prominent, stages of one's career. They can provide encouragement, emotional and financial support, and a peaceful home environment conducive to full concentration on professional goals. The literature also shows that spouses function differently for men and women with regard to the developing aspirations, goals, and achievements.

Wives, for example, play a supportive role more consistently for the husbands' goals and aspirations (Droege 1982; Furst 1983; Mockros 1993; Roberts and Newton 1987; Terman and Oden 1959). When there is a conflict between husbands' and wives' goals, it is almost always the wife who makes the sacrifice (Droege 1982; Furst 1983). According to Levinson et al. (1978) the "special woman" in a man's life is the one connected to his "dream." Her significance lies in part in her ability to help facilitate the achievement of his dream. Our interviews corroborate previous research regarding gender differences between husbands and wives of eminent individuals. As is the case with mentors, men and women do not receive the same type of support from a spouse. Men rarely talk about having made a decision to move or not move because of family obligations; they make decisions that are best for their own career. Moreover, their families subsequently support these decisions. For the men wives generally provide emotional support and encouragement:

I am married to a college classmate of mine. We have been married 50 years. I couldn't have done what I have done if she hadn't been the type of person that she is. She is understanding, cooperative, long suffering, loyal and terribly terribly good. I remember several of my colleagues at various institutions have said, "John you can do what you do because you have the kind of wife that you have." She never said "Well I want more of your time, or I want... or we should do this... we should do this we should... don't bother with that... why do you have to write that?' That is what some fellows are faced with. I never faced that. She never raised a question about anything like that. She was a librarian at the law school here and would send me my expenses as I needed them. I stayed and I broke the back of that book up there. In *my* view she had as much to do with making me as I did. And therefore there is nothing too good for her. And whatever benefits we have derived from what I have done, she shares in them equally. I could not possibly have done what I have done, as large or as small, without her and the kind of sensitivity, and understanding, cooperation and loyalty that she has provided. I don't mind talking about it to all of the world [M11].

My wife was very helpful. She was interested in what I was doing. She was not a scholar herself but she was sympathetic and supportive. She gave me emotional support. She was somebody to rely on. And she would often go on these trips with me and take notes. I enjoyed having her along [M2].

My wife has very much influenced my life and made me happy. Before I was married, I never was very happy. I had happy times, moments, weeks, but since I got married I am more or less continually happy. It is just her being there. We talk a lot over meals and we take long walks together. She has made my life settled, happy, and easy [M3].

Oh, she's terrific. She has good sense, good judgment. She has often been left with the problem of looking after things. That has been a lot of responsibility. She has also backed me up and tried to get me to steer in a good direction. She generally has good judgment about people and who I should devote time to and who I shouldn't.... She supports me. Right now, for example, I don't have a grant from the National Science Foundation, but I still have a secretary and I can't let her work for nothing so I pay her, expecting that someday I may get some money back. My wife goes along with that [M4].

I found a wonderful wife. We had a wonderful, harmonic marriage, and raised a family, with great children. There was rarely any conflict. That's very important because conflicts really take away from your work because you worry about them. Your mind wanders and you can't think about your scientific problem if you are worrying about your personal problems and whether your wife will run away with somebody else. In a good marriage both sides know what the other is interested in. and they know it is important to leave time for it. I guess I was very lucky in this regard [M5].

I've been privileged to have a wife who has not had a job. That's meant that part of her life has been involved with mine. She has enjoyed academic ethnography and when we visited colleges she has gone to classes, and enjoyed meeting people and making reports. We have enjoyed being a team, in fact one of the books that gives me pleasure is the diaries we kept when we were in Japan [M6].

I had very great luck in my family. My wife always agreed that it was worthwhile having me do what I wanted to do when it came to writing books and she went to great lengths to allow me to do so. Having a good wife is important. A wife who is supportive in the immediate family setting. I am sure that is absolutely important. It is like having bad health, it can disrupt you terribly [M7].

I've been married 57 years. I have a very strong family orientation. I have two daughters, who are now in mid-life, and their children four grandchildren. We're a very close unit and that is important to me. I think it's an important counterbalance, particularly to an active professional life or bang successful [M8].

As a hobby I was editing a journal I founded. In fact my wife figures in this because she was an editor then and knew about editing. The two of us adopted this journal as a family hobby…. I stopped by and the woman in charge of this group was very interested, not so in much in me as in my wife. I think she had a lot in common with my wife, so she invited me to come the following year [M9].

When my wife and I came here we decided we would try to implement it…. The major method developed for the work (for which he won the Nobel Prize) came from my wife. I had a lot of input from her. It was the practical aspect she offered. She was very helpful in something called *bridging*. On the one hand you have ideal theoretical mathematics and on the other hand you have the real world of finite and approximate data that you get. The particular scheme we were working with was very complex. She had a real talent for finding criteria that would enable us to find a pathway to the solution. She has a marvelous talent for solving complex structures. Through the 60s, for all intents and purposes she did practically all of the major structures [M17].

By contrast, the literature suggests that husbands are more of an obstacle to the fulfillment of an achievement-oriented career woman's dream (Roberts and Newton 1987). Although our eminent women were not thwarted by their husbands, the majority still built their careers around their husbands' plans. They describe how they went to (or stayed at) a particular university or geographical location in order not to interfere with their husband's career:

This wasn't a very congenial place for me…. I mean I would have been happy at the University of California, but then I got married and so… [F1].

Of course I stayed because my husband was fixed. He was in the world of business…. For example, I never took a year off and went to the think tank although I was invited. He couldn't leave his business career… and in that sense we were stabilized with his career…. I didn't go on the job market or respond to job change because I was not geographically mobile [F2].

I'll tell you another obstacle and though it did not remain an obstacle, it was during the early years of our marriage. My husband was already very famous when we met. I was 10 years younger. I got tired of going to conferences with him because he was surrounded by people and I would be standing there in limbo without anything to do. The way I dealt with that was simply to create other spaces, and choose activities so that I wasn't left standing on the periphery of his circle [F3].

I met my future husband and we decided to get married. That's why I came back to the lab. I really came back because of that. I didn't think commuting would make a very stable marriage [F4].

Well, the first obstacle would have been to find a professional position after getting the PhD. As we already mentioned during lunch, it was difficult for both a husband and wife to get a good position in the same city [F6].

Given the time in history, it is not surprising that the husband's career tended to take precedence over the wife's. Most women did not express bitterness about these decisions, rather they felt fortunate to have had a successful career and a husband who supported their career interests. As we probed to find out how women's husbands were supportive, it quickly became clear that "support" is defined relative to one's own cohort rather than current social norms and expectations of a "supportive" husband. People's identities are tied to their assessment and comparison of themselves in relation to their peers. At this time in history, the husbands' attitudes and behavior toward their wives' careers was indeed very unusual. The women often describe how their husband "allowed" them to work after they had made adequate arrangements for the care of the children and the household. In addition, they often supported their efforts to balance family and career responsibilities;

> My husband said, "I want you to be content and I want the kids to be properly cared for and I know you share that, and so I don't have to worry about that. After that do as you like. I mean if you want to be away half of a day from the house, or all day, fix it up" [F2].

> He was very supportive when we had children. Still, although in some sense he helped enormously much of the burden fell on me. I still was the person who had to shop and cook and get the kids to school. He still took my career very seriously. He took care of the kids when I went off observing. He encouraged me to go to meetings when I was invited and it just seemed impossible to leave [F5].

> I had awful good backing in my husband. He has always been supportive. It was very difficult in the beginning. Mostly, there were just so many things pushing against me and if he hadn't kept telling me to keep working, I probably would have given up. When my son was born they wanted me to quit because they had no policy for when you have children. At that time all of the women's magazines were talking about latch-key children and that you should stay home with your children.... I just couldn't take all of that. My husband was the one who really encouraged me. He said, "you let house go... you wouldn't be happy", so he went out and hired someone. Even my sister was saying she would take my son if I didn't want him. My husband was very very supportive all of the time [F4].

Indeed, most women had the primary responsibility for the children and running of the home. No husband made a radical personal career sacrifice or attended to the child care and household responsibilities.

Compared to their female peers, however, the women in our sample regarded themselves as extremely fortunate to have had a husband who not only allowed them to work, but also conveyed interest and encouragement to them regarding their career. The biographies of eminent women such as Marie Curie, Margaret Mead, and Georgia O'Keefe confirm the narratives of our women regarding their husband's provision of psychological support as well as professional encouragement, inspiration, and help for his talented and ambitious wife. These data suggest that eminent women often receive the affirmation and assistance from a husband that many men receive from a professional mentor (Kerr 1985; Mockros 1993; Roberts and Newton 1987). Husbands frequently encourage their wives careers help them make valuable connections to other professionals in the field, as well as in some cases collaborate with them:

He encouraged me all along. He bad a PhD a few years before I did and he just knew my work was very important to me. He encouraged me all along the way. He was very supportive of my work. For a number of years I really did not know another astronomer. It was he that I talked to every night. He never annoyed me with his work but I must have annoyed him nightly with my work.... Probably the greatest role he played was in encouraging and listening in a professional sense. Also, I really knew no astronomers and scientists so the physicists that I got connected with were those I knew through ray husband. So, very early in my career a lot of the connections came from him [F5].

I think my husband is the brightest man who ever lived, as far as mathematics go. He and I worked together a lot. He did the mathematical analyses and I did the programming. We worked together. We complement one another. I am someone who could check his ideas and see what was not quite right. He is someone who is probably not quite as detailed as I was. I check things many times. He is more likely to think of things out in left field and I am more of the detail person [F4].

Of course, my husband was my teacher. I learned a lot from him regarding the whole field and how to go into it as a professional. That is partly because he was one of the founders of the field. Although we didn't collaborate I learned a lot from our conversations. Since we are in the same field there has been a very rich interaction between us [F3].

Although for the most part husbands rarely made radical career sacrifices for their wives, a few women talked about how their husbands made some provisions for their careers. These included either taking a position at a place that would also be beneficial for the wife's career or having a marital relationship in which the husband and wife each had personal and professional freedom and ted a relatively independent life.

Several women were separated from their husband for months at a time while they each pursued career opportunities and interests. Some also thought that marrying relatively late in life was significant in determining the course of their career and subsequent success. In any case, even though many creative women did prioritize their children and family above career advancement, few had marital relationships that would be considered conventional for the time. Even by today's standards, the attitudes and support of their husband was considered beneficial for a woman's careen.

My husband and I and the kids spent a year at the University of California—San Diego, where the Burbidges were a very important influence. It was 16 years after my PhD. I had four children and I was really ready to get back into astronomy. My husband had received a National Science Foundation Senior Post-Doctoral fellowship and decided to go to La Jolla because he knew I could do astronomy there [F5].

My husband was most anxious I carry on my career and realized there were only so many hours in the day [F6].

My husband is not here. He teaches at Toronto. We often talk on the phone in the morning before work. Then, on the weekends we are always together [F7].

We are both artists. We went to graduate school together. He has been extremely sup-portive. For the last 15 or 20 years now we spend a great deal of time separated. We have a place in Massachusetts, and I have a loft in New York. We decided a long time ago that the best way to maintain our relationship, both personal and professional, was to have separate lives and interconnect when we felt like it. So sometimes I go up for a weekend.

He lives in Massachusetts and I live in New York. I have a free life which is supported by his. He also has a free life. We just feel we have been able to maintain that and get along. We have what I would call a perfect marriage. I spend summers up there because I love the garden. When I am there he goes out West to go fishing. So, we have never been with each other all that much. It works out because I don't really think that at a certain stage, at least for a woman, it would have been possible for me to do what I have done without living by myself and pursuing my work by working every day and following *my* own schedule. I spent years as a mother and a wife and those years were very formative and important. When my daughter went to college, though, I began to really live as an individual. It is not something everybody can do. Most men would not have put up with me for a minute [F8].

I think my husband and I give each other a lot of space. In the winter time he is at Harvard and I am here. Originally when we built the addition onto the house including his study and my studio, my husband wanted to make them connecting so we could talk to each other during the day. I didn't think I wanted do that because although I loved seeing him, I didn't when I was working. We will see each other in the evening. I am quite sure he likes to see me, but he wants to be left alone when he works. So we have separate buildings and we go to our separate places. I think it is important to be left alone. In the summertime when our lives are much closer together, we have separate cabins. In one cabin my husband does his writing and in one cabin I do my work. So we see each other in the morning and sometimes in the late afternoon we meet for a sandwich. It works perfectly well. But I am fortunate. I guess we are both a little fortunate since we both understand the need to be left alone when one is thinking through things and really enveloped by the work [F9].

I wasn't married and I did not have children for many years. I can't imagine being able to have a career like this with a family. I know today my younger female colleagues are very tired. It is very hard. I married very late. Looking back, when I started it was my ambition to be very good. But. I realize today I lived like a nun for the first 10 years of my career. In privacy and seclusion [F10].

It should also be pointed out that for some women husbands provide the financial support that allows them to pursue their creative interests without the pressure of having to support the family. This allows them relatively more flexibility and freedom to take risks in their professional endeavors because the family does not depend on their salaries:

I had a situation in which I didn't have to be accountable for an idea, or something rested on it. I did not have a big investment in becoming successful or having to make money and I think I was reflecting my husband's attitudes. He would say, "Do what you want to do", and nothing hung on it [F2].

It is interesting that in advising young people about their futures and careers, no men specifically refer to the importance of their wives, but as one woman pointed out:

The advice… to a young woman, and probably a young man as well, is to marry the right person, because if you don't marry the right person it will not work, and that's a shame, that's a tragedy. You have to make decisions really early in life if you get married very early and the decision you make about who you will marry is going to influence an enormous amount of your later life [F5].

Hence, although both men and women's careers benefit from the encouragement of a spouse, given the overt and covert educational and social barriers women face regarding academic and professional success, establishing eminence for a woman may be more contingent on whether she has a supportive spouse.

Colleague Interaction and Collaboration

Professional socialization does not end with entry into the field. For many adults, the field continues to be significant to the development of eminence. The importance of interacting with colleagues has often been overlooked in the literature. Nonetheless, colleague interaction and collaboration undoubtedly influences productivity and eminence by facilitating both problem finding and problem solving. Given that no one is an expert in all aspects of a domain, it is important to read about and discuss the ways one's own work may be informed by others in the field. Numerous eminent individuals stress the importance of actively maintaining professional networks and relationships with colleagues. Interestingly, many creative individuals discuss the necessity of being intellectually autonomous and independent, yet most are also eloquent about the professional environments facilitating the expression of their creativity:

> It is only by interacting with other people that you get anything interesting done.... I was in an advantageous position of being familiar with both of them (two eminent colleagues) and I got to know and work with each of them [M10].

> Usually ideas grow slowly, they're like flowers that have to be tended by reading, and talking with people... if you don't kick things around with people you are out of it. Nobody, I always say, can be anybody without others around [M4].

> I was able to do creative work collaborating with other people. Most of my work is collaborative. That's how you find out how to do something which hasn't been done before. Collaboration is extremely important. First of all, it prevents you from making mistakes because another guy can correct you. In addition, there is a division of labor. One person may be better in mathematics, while the other may be better in other things. In this way we complement each other.... I myself, have collaborated on several important papers. My collaborator was certainly a better mathematician than I, but I think I had a better overview of the problem. And this is how we can help each other [M5].

> A colleague of mine and I were working very closely together and the arguments went back and forth.... This is an instance in which he had a very different expertise than I and I have a certain background that he does not have. This is a case in which two quite different fields of research are brought together, not to be compared but so that parts of one can be integrated with parts of the other [M17].

> Traveling, lecturing, and consulting does take me away from my work but it also keeps me in touch with the professional community. I get a certain stimulus from listening to other people and thinking about what they say [M7].

> By that time my colleague... had joined us and was working on something.... I phoned him and told him that it looks like the problem is solvable. He agreed and then the deck was clear. You see, there was so much in the literature that said this was not solvable. I ran it off to him to see if he could see something that I couldn't. He said no. Now that was encouragement [M18].

> As you interact with the scientific community you get ideas that are very interesting. You can have them in your head for years until you get the opportunity to do it [M18].

> I often learned from contemporary historians with whom I work and lived. Colleagueship is important because of the values derived from them.... I have numerous colleagues I talk to

and I show my work to. I ask for criticism and receive good suggestions. The recent changes and conclusions for the different editions of my book come largely from criticisms. I think that the worst mistake a historian can make is to be indifferent to or contemptuous of what is new. There is nothing permanent in history, it is always changing [M2].

I think one needs colleagues. But they can be invisible colleagues, they don't have to be here. They can be the books one reads. They can be people that one knows about but doesn't necessarily know, face-to-face. I've always looked for colleagues and I found them in different ages, and fields. They thought they depended on me but I also depended on them. One docs need a network of people to be connected with, and it's better if they're living, and if you have commensal times together, but it's not essential [M6].

Out of it came this contact with Campbell and after a long conference we hit it off very well. He introduced me to some people in Switzerland that might want to hear about my work in science. The amazing thing was that you could really try out your ideas with this very rich and wonderful group of people. I used this group to formulate my ideas and to set them forth, There was no audience anywhere else at that time [M9].

I knew one very fine executive. He was the head of a great corporation. He told me he was an inventor and was very interested in new technology. He said he wanted to work for NASA. At the time I was On pretty good terms with the President. I called him and before you knew it he was in charge of what was then the beginning of the space shuttle [M8].

Bell Labs has a pretty outstanding group. The theorists talked among themselves and it was a very exciting time to be there. There was great enthusiasm for quantum theory [M1].

Again, women do not report similar experiences with regard to collaboration and the influence of colleagues. By and large, they discuss having been relatively more isolated than the men:

I didn't have a job in the department until I was 55 years old. We came here in 45, so I have been on the outside all those years. I was never really part of anything. I just did my own thing. I taught courses, but I didn't have tenure. I didn't have a position in the university. I wasn't integrated into the department.... I didn't have a lot of colleagues. I haven't had a lot of students and the closest I ever came to the mainstream was serving on a committee. I've just hung on by my fingernails [F1].

There are still very few women here. There are some divisions that still do not have any women. I don't know why the number of women participating in the group has dropped. I don't know if it is because women are so busy with their careers and homes and they don't have time. We had women come in as post docs who would only be there a very short time. While they were there they would often be the only woman in their department and they would not see any other women during the day [F4].

For a number of years I did not know another astronomer or scientist.... I still work in a very personal way and I make all of the decisions myself. I do all of the observing myself. It takes me a long time and I think it is because I don't have graduate students and colleagues working with me... so it is hard [F5].

There are a lot of connections, career-type connections I didn't have when the children were little because I had two main things, the children and my writing.... I wasn't much part of the university community at that point. So, granted, in terms of career context, the children may have been a drawback [F7].

I can't say that I belonged to a group of artists or anything [F11].

After I got involved in the structure field I was a bit apprehensive since I was outside of the biochemical community. I had nobody to talk to. I mean, the National Institute of Health is 35 miles away.... It has worked out OK, but... [F6].

Regarding early career development and mentors, some women discuss overt discrimination in connection with colleagues and rules within professional institutions. Needless to say, peers and colleagues are central to professional development throughout adulthood. As a result, women's relative lack of peer interaction inhibits productivity and the development of their careers.

Colleague Affirmation and Approval

Aside from professional collaboration with others, people are also frequently influenced by unsolicited feedback, including affirmation and criticism from either the field or the larger society. Aging and intellectual functioning are related to the social interaction. Competent social and intellectual behavior is either discouraged or encouraged by social institutions leading to individual's internalization of these expectations. Such a socialization process produces conditions and attitudes that result in a self-fulfilling depreciation of abilities and functioning (Bengston and Kuyper 1973; Labouvie-Vief 1985). If negative expectations and the lack of encouragement and affirmation for one's abilities has a negative effect, it follows that positive experiences or the encouragement of others—particularly colleagues in the field—are likely to promote self-confidence and subsequent professional development. In this way, during later adulthood one's sense of self, ability, and competence are generally enhanced by the affirmation of colleagues and the admiration of students and younger people in the field.

Based on her research, Amabile (1983, 1990) claims that external evaluation plays a negative role in creative production. Likewise, her work implies that the absence of such evaluation from the consciousness will invariably have a positive impact on one's creativity and work. Moreover, public recognition and fame is constantly discussed among critics and artists as one of the greatest possible threats to the artist's creativity and continued growth. Once artists earn a reputation and begin to sell their work, there is pressure to continue to produce work that "sells". In this way, the marketability of the work can become an inherent part (and sometimes destructive element) of the artistic process. At the same time, external evaluations, affirmation, and praise for ideas and work often leads to continued work in that area, but also to the assimilation of valued work into the larger domain. In this way there appears to be a more complex relationship between the value of intrinsic and extrinsic reward systems for creativity and eminence.

As noted earlier, the field plays a critical role in the recognition and assimilation of ideas into the domain. Our research suggests that highly eminent and creative individuals are often able to take advantage of the opportunities that come their way.

I really have a lot of ability in management. At the age of 29, I was totally unaware of it. When the war broke out I was thrown into a management position in the *Federal Communications*

Commission. Almost immediately I received very high praise for my management skills. I was totally surprised because I had no image of myself in that way [M8].

A professor at the University of Wisconsin who later became a professor at Harvard. It was through his influence that I got an appointment at the Society of Fellows at Harvard after I got my PhD [M1].

One of the biggest influences came when I was 34. I worked with men in their 50 and 60s who had held quite high responsibilities all their life. They were a remarkable group. After the war I met these individuals who lived with a sense of responsibility about what went on in the world. That had a big impact on me. They displayed a sense of social responsibility that was inspiring. They had strong good characters and a largeness of view with a deep sense of responsibility. So it's a little later than one normally thinks of having influences, but it was one of those influences that can have a big impact on you [M8].

In another ease, although one of the women scientists did not have a significant mentor during graduate school, 16 years after completing her PhD she had the opportunity to work with an older, well-established female colleague with similar interests. This relationship was particularly meaningful to her.

It was really a very remarkable year for me because, apart from actually working with (her), and doing the work that I was interested in, I really learned that she was interested in my ideas. I think it was the first time I was in a position where someone took me seriously as an astronomer [F5].

In addition to the direct influence of older colleagues, people discuss the relevance of peer feedback and affirmation for their work. Overall, among our group of eminent individuals men were more frequently affirmed for their work and accepted by professional institutions.

Of course the feedback is very strong in both (science and writing)… after you have published a book it is out in the world you get a tremendous enrichment of contacts…. The most enjoyable part of doing science or writing is the response. Telling your Mends about it and being involved with *people*. People either saying it is good or it isn't, or else just talking about the problems…. When I am writing I write for a particular person or a particular audience, not just to create something for myself [M10].

The success of the book earned me respect among colleagues as well as served to open doors for me professionally. Although my reputation was "defamed" by another prominent colleague in the field, I am proud of the fact that the book has remained popular [M12].

I think I have earned my way into the National Academy of Sciences five times over… but every time my name was proposed I was turned down because I had offended various big shots, by treading on their toes in the work I had done. Obviously I was disappointed. Most objective people agree that I have earned it… but somewhere along the road I decided I didn't really care if I was a member. What I have instead is people who say to me "you know I read your book and it changed my life." That's good too [M13].

I have accepted and welcomed criticism. It is important to not be indifferent to criticism and new information [M2].

For the most part, previous research has found that women receive less positive affirmation from the field for their interests and abilities. Professional institutions reward women less than men for comparable achievements. Women receive less pay for performing similar tasks and are promoted and honored less than men for similar accomplishments.

> There are only 10 % women in Research and Development. Most of them are in the lower positions such as scientific assistants. The management is still all male and they talk to each other. A lot of the news about what opportunities are available at the laboratory does not filter down. Two times I went to talk to the management because the pay of women was significantly less than the pay of men. They made some adjustments. But they did not admit there was a problem. They never announced to the employees that they were making this adjustment. So, a lot of women still did not know if they were making the same pay as the men. All of the managers are male and they don't pass the information down. Women are very unsure of where they stand and want some kind of feedback. They are just not told or rewarded like the men. I talked with a young woman who received an absolutely stellar evaluation from her boss, yet she did not get a raise. The evaluation process is very difficult for everyone, but it is especially bard for women because they are always talking to men. These women don't know where they stand. They don't know if there is going to be a cut back so they are very insecure. The young men may get together on the golf course and be told, "Hey you are doing a great job. I like what you are doing." Somehow a lot of women do not get any sense of how they are doing [F4].

> The biggest barrier was trying to find a place where both my husband and I could work [F6].

> I had what was called a research development award. There was a provision in that the university was supposed to make a place for me. So, one year I sent back my contract. It took 18 months before I got a reply. They wrote back and said something about not having anything against women. I wrote back and... within a week I was a member of the department. This was about 1970 [F1].

> I felt very frustrated.... That was a time when I felt there was no where to go and decided I should get out and let someone else in. As a woman I did not feel I was going to get promoted because upper management was all male [F4].

Many eminent men and women find ways to continue working in spite of the conflict their work may evoke. Some choose to pursue less contested problems whereas others choose to persevere in their current endeavors even if doing so embroils them in controversy. It does seem, however, that conflict, controversy, and competition may be more abrasive to women. It may also be that women may have more difficulty "detaching" themselves emotionally form work. As a result, they may have trouble receiving criticism about their work. Pursuing creative ideas often results in critical feedback from the field. Unless gifted men and women have the self-confidence and assurance to persevere in spite of such feedback, it is unlikely that they will be able to withstand such scrutiny. One eminent female scientist noted that controversy from the field often caused her to switch problems in order to avoid a highly visible and challenged position, and the competitive aggressive atmosphere connected with it. Because she has multiple ideas and projects of interest, she prefers to direct her research to another problem rather than wasting energy in professional debates:

> I really found it very unpleasant. I just didn't like to be in that environment. So I decided to find a problem to study that no one would bother me with and work on it by myself for a couple of years. Hopefully people would be very interested in what came out of it.... There is really both a public and a private controversy. I really found the private part of it

very unpleasant…. Getting calls and letters from people saying "I know you are wrong and you shouldn't be doing this. I know what the answer is"… I don't know, maybe I am a coward. That just made my life unpleasant. Part of the reason I was doing astronomy was because it had always been pleasant. So rather than continue to compete in this unpleasant environment, I would do something else…. Lately, in retrospect, I am sorry I have done that because there was still so much more to be learned and some of it has now been learned by just the people who made my life unpleasant… I almost feel these, people robbed me of the pleasure of continuing the problem. It was just unpleasant [F5].

Men, on the other hand, more easily disregard negative feedback. *Likewise, they are more comfortable* when confronted with professional conflict. None of the men, for example, ever considered changing their professional position or problem due to controversy engendered by work. Instead, they asserted the opposite:

I talked to a professor of organic chemistry. He decided the next course for me and I asked him whether I should take it this semester or later and he said I could take the course later on if I wanted to and if I lasted. I never forgot that conversation because it was a serious source of unhappiness *for me*. I had gone through a number of struggles including working for a while between a previous master's degree. I had saved up enough money to get to Michigan. After I struggled for many years hoping I would finally find a niche for myself I was not pleased with this statement. It didn't affect my work. If anything I was more determined than ever to succeed. But I thought it was the perfect example of how one should not deal with students [M17].

Trust (your) intuition, don't necessarily listen to others, peer pressure or other kinds of influences that have a counterbearing influence…. Overcoming obstacles that have to do with people seeing things differently is just a matter of persisting and finding ways and means around the obstacles [M14].

I always follow my own path. I always have [M13].

In any case, social selection and affirmation contribute to a greater differential in the career paths of men and women during adulthood. Invariably, attitudes and responses from the field are interpreted and constructed based on earlier experiences. Hence, the Matthew effect (Merton 1968) applies to the emergence of eminence and creativity during later life as well.

Conclusion

This chapter examines some of the ways societal expectations and influences impact the careers of eminent individuals during their lives. In particular it examines how creativity exists within a social and historical context made up of multiple interacting systems including an individual, field, domain, and culture. The following conclusions are based on preliminary analyses of the interviews:

1. Social support systems and interactions are critical throughout the life span for the emergence of creativity. Interactions with others often determine the provision of relevant academic and professional opportunities. The value of the social support received depends on the particular needs of the individual.

For some, emotional support is crucial, whereas for others professional connections or intellectual affirmation are vital for advancement in the field.

2. The nature of the social support will vary depending on one's specific
   developmental stage. During childhood, parents or teachers recognize,
   encourage, and affirm a talented young person's interests and ability. In
   addition, they provide materials and opportunities that facilitate the development of interests.

3. During adulthood relevant interactions are with people in the field such as
   teachers, mentors, or colleagues. Mentors serve as teachers, sponsors, friends,
   counselors, and role models. They advance young people by teaching specific
   skills and relevant problem finding and solving strategies. They also provide
   opportunities and challenge and encourage interests and abilities, and build
   self-confidence and protection from negative feedback.

4. Colleagues provide critical and affirmative feedback for work. In addition,
   they render professional recognition in the form of awards, exposure, and
   promotions within the field.

5. Spouses are a significant source of support for both eminent men and women.
   For men, wives offer emotional support, general encouragement and professional sacrifices. For women, husbands often provide professional opportunities and intellectual *affirmation* for career interests and ambitions.

6. The field interacts with characteristics of individuals and the needs of the
   domain to provide opportunities that contribute to the advancement of creative
   individuals. The field's perceptions of an individual's ability and potential to
   succeed influence the emergence of eminence by determining if an individual's contribution will be accepted into the domain.

7. There is a dialectic between interpersonal relationships and identity formation.
   Both are influenced by experiences, opportunities, aspirations, and achievements. Talent development is influenced by the provision of opportunities and
   positive experiences as well as restrictions from, or negative experiences with,
   educational and professional social systems.

8. Early educational opportunities and the availability of later professional
   experiences vary between groups of individuals. For the most part, people
   within a field consider students and colleagues most similar to themselves as
   more likely to be successful,

9. Men and women have different experiences and exposure to academic and
   professional communities. Although men in our culture tend to strive for
   personal and professional independence and autonomy, on the whole they are
   generally less socially isolated than eminent women during adulthood.

10. During childhood, parents and teachers affirm and promote the abilities of
    talented girls less frequently than talented boys. During young adulthood
    women have fewer relationships with mentors. During later stages of their
    careers women have less social interaction with colleagues and receive less
    social affirmation for their work.

In conclusion, recent theories have expanded previous models of creativity that tended to ignore the social context. Nevertheless, current theories lack an adequate treatment of the ways social and cultural systems transmit values, provide opportunities, encourage interests, and develop competencies and self-confidence that contribute to eminent careers. Understanding creativity and how interpersonal relationships and social norms influence the development of eminence requires a more comprehensive view of the social system's contribution to early career choices and achievements. In light of the fact that cultures impose particular expectations and reinforce attitudes that shape people's perceptions of themselves and others, different populations are selectively rewarded and discouraged from intellectual and creative endeavors.

For instance, women's chances of emerging as eminent and creative in a field are reduced because women do not have equal access to the people responsible for acknowledging their contributions. Moreover, although this chapter has not addressed the issue of discrimination faced by minorities, there is some evidence to suggest that the Jewish and African American interviewees also faced comparable limitations and barriers to professional development. Studies of creative women and minorities will do well to attend to the role of the historical context, the availability of social support systems, and differential familial and cultural expectations surrounding their lives. Definitions of creativity need to incorporate multiple definitions of success and competence which are influenced by personal and social directives that lead to lives characterized by eminence. Future inquiry might reveal that adult creativity and eminence are as much a function of the interaction between social responses to early biological determinants such as sex and race as they are a function of the motivational and intellectual characteristics on which previous theories have been based.

References

Albert, R. S. (1983). Family positions and the attainment of eminence: A study of special family positions and special family experiences. In R. J. Albert (Ed.), *Genius and eminence: The social psychology of creativity and exceptional achievement* (pp. 141–154). Pergamon: Oxford.

Albert, R. S. (1990). Identity, experience and career choice among exceptionally gifted and eminent. In R. Albert & M. Runco (Eds.), *Theories of creativity* (pp. 13–34). Newbury Park: Sage.

Albert, R. S. & Runco, M. A. (1987). The possible personality dispositions of scientists and nonscientists. In D. N. Jackson & J. P. Rushton (Eds.), *Scientific excellence: Origins and assessment* (pp. 67–97). Newbury Park: Sage.

Amabile, T. (1983). *The social psychology of creativity*. New York: Harcourt.

Amabile, T. (1990). Within you, without you the social psychology of creativity and beyond. In R. Albert & M. Runco (Eds.), *Theories of creativity* (pp. 61–91). Newbury Park: Sage.

Astin, H. (1974). Sex differences in mathematical and scientific precocity. In J. Stanley, D. Keating, & L. Fox (Eds.), *Mathematical talent: Discovery, description, and development* (pp. 70–86). Baltimore: Johns Hopkins University Press.

Bengston, V. L. (1973). *The social psychology of aging*. New York: Bobbs-Merrill.

Bloom, B. S. (1985). *Developing talent in young people*. New York: Ballantine.

Cox, C. (1926). *The early mental traits of three hundred geniuses*. Stanford: Stanford University Press.

Csikszentmihályi, M. (1988). Society, culture and person: A systems view of creativity. In R. J. Sternberg (Ed.), *The nature of creativity: Contemporary psychological perspectives* (pp. 325–339). Cambridge: Cambridge University Press.

Csikszentmihályi, M. (1990). The domain of creativity. In M. A. Runco & R. S. Albert (Eds.), *Theories of creativity* (pp. 325–339). Newbury Park: Sage.

Csikszentmihályi, M., Rathunde, K., & Whalen, S. (1993). *Talented teenagers: A longitudinal study of development*. Cambridge: Cambridge University Press.

De Groot, A. D. (1965). *Thought and choice in class*. The Hague: Mouton.

Droege, R. (1982). A psychosocial study of the formation of the middle adult life structure in women. Unpublished doctoral dissertation, California School of Professional Psychology, Berkeley, CA.

Erikson, E. (1950). *Childhood and society*. New York: Norton.

Feldman, D., & Goldsmith, L. (1986). *Nature's gambit: Child prodigies and the development of human potential*. New York: Basic Books.

Fox, L. (1977). Sex differences: Implications for program planning for the academically gifted. In J. Stanley, W. George, & C. Solano (Eds.), *The gifted and the creative: A fifty year perspective* (pp. 113–138). Baltimore: Johns Hopkins University Press.

Furst, K. (1983). Origins and evolution of women's dreams in early adulthood. Unpublished doctoral dissertation. California School of Professional Psychology, Berkeley, CA.

Galton, F. (1869). *Hereditary genius*. New York: Appleton.

Gergen, M. (1990). Finished at 40: Women's development within the patriarchy. *Psychology of Women Quarterly, 14*, 471–493.

Getzels, J., & Csikszentmihályi, M. (1976). *The creative vision*. New York: Wiley.

Goertzel, V., & Goertzel, M. (1962). *Cradles of eminence*. Boston: Little, Brown.

Gruber, H. (1980). And the bush was not consumed: The evolving systems approach to creative work. In S. Modgil & C. Modgil (Eds.), *Toward a theory of psychological development* (pp. 269–299). Windsor: NFER Press.

Gruber, H. (1981). *Darwin on man: A psychological study of scientific thinking*. Chicago: University of Chicago Press.

Gruber, H. (1982). On the hypothesized relation between giftedness and creativity. In D. H. Feldman (Ed.), *Developmental approaches to giftedness and creativity* (pp. 7–29). San Francisco: Jossey-Bass.

Gruber, H. (1986). The self-construction of the extraordinary. In R. J. Sternberg & J. Davidson (Eds.), *Conceptions of giftedness* (pp. 247–263). Cambridge: Cambridge University Press.

Gruber, H., & Davis, S. (1988). Inching our way up Mount Olympus: The evolving-systems approach to creative thinking. In R. J. Sternberg (Ed.), *The nature of creativity: Contemporary psychological perspectives* (pp. 243–270). Cambridge: Cambridge University Press.

Helson, R. (1990). Creativity in women: Outer and inner views over time. In M. Runco & R. Albert (Eds.), *Theories of creativity* (pp. 46–60). Newbury Park: Sage.

Hollinger, C. (1985). Multidimensional determinants of traditional and nontraditional career aspirations for mathematically talented female adolescents. *Journal for the Education of the Gifted, 5*(4), 245–265.

Hollinger, C. (1986). Career aspirations as a function of Holland personality type among mathematically talented female adolescents. *Journal for the Education of the Gifted, 9*(2), 133–145.

Holloway, S. (1986). The relationship of mother's beliefs to children's mathematics achievement: some effects of sex differences. *Merrill-Palmer Q, 32*(3), 231–250.

James, J. (1990). Employment patterns and midlife well-being. In H. W. Grossman & N. L. Chester (Eds.), *The experience of meaning of work in women's lives* (pp. 103–120). Hillsdale: Lawrence Erlbaum Associates.

Jerachim, J., & Shapiro, P. (1992). *Women, mentors and success*. New York: Fawcett Columbine.

Kanigel, R. (1986). *Apprentice to genius: The making of a scientific dynasty*. New York: Macmillan.

Kerr, B. (1985). *Smart girls, gifted women*. Columbus: Ohio Publishing Company.

Kram, K. (1985). *Mentoring at work*. Glenview: Scott Foresman.

Labouvie-Vief, G. (1985). Intelligence and cognition. In J. E. Birren & K. W. Schaie (Eds.), *Handbook of the psychology of aging* (2nd ed., pp. 500–530). New York: Van Nostrand Reinhold.

Levinson, D., Darrow, C., Klein, E., Levinson, M., & McKee, B. (1978). *The seasons of a man's life*. New York: Knopf.

MacKinnon, D. W. (1978). *In search of human effectiveness*. New York: Creative Education Foundation.

Merton, R. K. (1968). The Matthew effect in science. *Science, 159*, 56–63.

Mockros, C. (1993). The mentor-apprentice relationship: interpersonal influences on creative and eminent adults. Paper presented at the Esther Katz Rosen Symposium, Lawrence, KS.

Ochse, R. (1990). *Before the gates of excellence: The determinants of creative genius*. Cambridge: Cambridge University Press.

Pariser, D. (1991). Normal and unusual aspects of juvenile artistic development in Klee, Lautrec, and Picasso. *Creativity Research Journal, 4*(1), 51–65.

Roberts, P., & Newton, P. (1987). Levinsonian studies of women's adult development. *Psychology and Aging, 2*(2), 154–163.

Roe, A. (1953). *The making of a scientist*. New York: Dodd Mead.

Simonton, D. (1983). Intergenerational transfer of individual differences in hereditary monarchs: Genes, role-modeling, cohort, or sociocultural effects? *Journal of Personality and Social Psychology, 44*, 354–364.

Simonton, D. (1984). Artistic creativity and interpersonal relationships across and within generations. *Journal of Personality and Social Psychology, 46*, 1273–1286.

Simonton, D. (1986). Biographical typicality, eminence, and achievement style. *Journal of Creative Behaviour, 20*, 14–22.

Simonton, D. (1988). Creativity, leadership, and chance. In R. J. Sternberg (Ed.), *The nature of creativity* (pp. 125–147). Cambridge: Cambridge University Press.

Simonton, D. K. (1978). The eminent genius in history: the critical role of creative development. *Gifted Child Quarterly, 22*, 187–200.

Solano, C. (1983). Self-concept in mathematically gifted adolescents. *Journal of General Psychology, 108*, 33–42.

Stewart, W. (1977). A psychosocial study of the formation of the early adult life structure in' women. Unpublished doctoral dissertation, Columbia University, New York.

Tannenbaam, A. (1987). Giftedness: A psychosocial approach. In R. Sternberg & J. Davidson (Eds.), *Conceptions of giftedness* (pp. 21–52). New York: Cambridge University Press.

Terman, L., & Oden, M. (1959). *The gifted child grows up. Genetic studies of genius* (Vol. 5). Stanford: Stanford University Press.

Tomlinson-Keasey, C., & Burton, E. (1992). Gifted women's lives: Aspirations, achievements and personal adjustment. In J. Carlsohn (Ed.), *Cognition and educational practice: An international perspective* (pp. 151–176). Greenwich: JAI Press.

Valliant, G. E. (1977). *Adaptation to life*. Boston: Little, Brown.

Walters, J., & Gardner, H. (1986). The crystallizing experience: Discovering an intellectual gift. In R. J. Sternberg & J. Davidson (Eds.), *Conceptions of giftedness* (pp. 306–331). Cambridge: Cambridge University Press.

Zey, M. (1984). *The mentor connection*. Homewood: Dow Jones-Irwin.

Zuckerman, H. (1977). *Scientific elite: Nobel laureates in the United States*. New York: The Free Press.

Chapter 10
New Conceptions and Research Approaches to Creativity: Implications of a Systems Perspective for Creativity in Education

Mihaly Csikszentmihalyi and Rustin Wolfe

Introduction

At the beginning of the third millennium, the importance of creativity becomes ever more critical. Age-old problems, such as coexistence on an increasingly interdependent planet, need new solutions for our species to survive. And the unintended results of the creativity of past centuries require even more creativity to be resolved, as we must learn to cope with the aftermath of previous successes, such as increasing population density and chemical pollution.

For several millions of years young people have learned how to adapt successfully by learning practical skills from their elders. But during the last few generations, they have become dependent on schools for acquiring the information necessary to cope with their environment. Thus we might expect that creativity, inasmuch as it can be taught, would be learned and practiced in schools. Yet—with notable exceptions—schools seem to be inimical to the development of creativity. For instance, Getzels and Jackson (1962) found that students who scored high on creativity tests were generally disliked by teachers, who preferred students who were highly intelligent but less creative.

In a recent study of 91 exceptionally creative writers, musicians, businessmen, and Nobel-prize winning scientists, these individuals almost never mentioned their elementary or secondary schools as having helped them to develop the interest and

Reproduced with permission from International Handbook of Giftedness and Talent, K.A. Heller, F.J. Monks, R.J. Sternberg & R. Subotnik (Eds.), 2000, pages 81–93, Elsevier, U.K.

M. Csikszentmihalyi (✉)
Claremont Graduate University, Claremont, CA, USA

R. Wolfe
The University of Chicago, Chicago, USA

M. Csikszentmihalyi, *The Systems Model of Creativity*,
DOI: 10.1007/978-94-017-9085-7_10,
© Springer Science+Business Media Dordrecht 2014

Fig. 10.1 General model of creativity

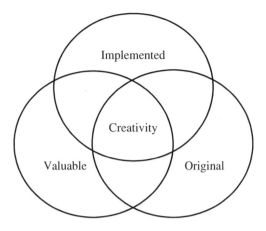

expertise that led to their later accomplishments. Almost every person could mention one or two very influential teachers, but classroom activities as such were generally remembered as boring and repressive (Csikszentmihalyi 1996). Is this a necessary feature of institutionalized mass education? Or are there ways to make schools more friendly to the development of creativity? Before attempting to deal with such questions, it will be useful to present our perspective on what creativity consists of.

A Definition of Creativity

Creativity can be defined as an idea or product that is original, valued, and implemented. Traditionally creativity has been viewed as a mental process, as the insight of an individual genius. Psychologists have assumed that creativity consists of breaking down conceptual paradigms as they are solving problems. But where do paradigms come from? Where do problems come from? On second thought, it becomes obvious that creativity cannot exist in a vacuum; new is relative to old. Without norms there can be no variation; without standards there can be no excellence. Such obvious considerations should alert us to the fact that whatever individual mental process is involved in creativity, it must be one that takes place in a context of previous cultural and social achievements, and is inseparable from them.

While originality refers to any new idea or product, creativity is a subset of originality that is also valuable (Fig. 10.1). But how do we know whether or not an original solution is worth implementing? From where do we get our internal standards? Who is to judge what is valuable? These questions point at the importance of a supportive and evaluative context beyond the individual. Most definitions of creativity also stipulate that an idea must be implemented before its success can be evaluated. Implementation, in turn, requires inputs and resources that are usually beyond the individual's control.

While individual originality clearly plays a necessary role in the creative process, it is only one part. In this chapter, we will propose that an intrapsychic approach cannot do justice to the complex phenomenon of creativity, which is as much cultural and social as it is a psychological event. To develop this perspective, we will use a 'systems' model of the creative process, that takes into account its essential features. Later, we shall consider what role educational institutions can play in fostering creativity according to the systems model.

The Systems Model of Creativity

Creativity research in recent years has been increasingly informed by a systems perspective. Starting with the observations of Morris Stein (Stein 1953, 1963), and the extensive data presented by Dean Simonton showing the influence of economic, political, and social events on the rates of creative production (Simonton 1988a, b, 1990), it has become increasingly clear that variables external to the individual must be taken into account if one wishes to explain why, when, and where new ideas or products arise from and become established in a culture (Gruber 1988; Harrington 1990). Magyari-Beck (1988) has gone so far as to suggest that because of its complexity, creativity needs a new discipline of 'creatology' in order to be thoroughly understood.

The systems approach developed here has been described before, and applied to historical and anecdotal examples, as well as to data collected to answer a variety of different questions (Csikszentmihalyi 1988b, 1990b, 1996, 1999; Csikszentmihalyi et al. 1993; Feldman et al. 1994; Csikszentmihalyi and Sawyer 1995).

Why is a Systems Approach Necessary?

When the senior author started studying creativity over 30 years ago, like most psychologists he was convinced that it consisted of a purely intrapsychic process. He assumed that one could understand creativity with reference to the thought processes, emotions, and motivations of individuals who produced novelty. But each year the task became more frustrating. In a longitudinal study of artists, for instance, it was observed that some of the potentially most creative persons stopped doing art and pursued ordinary occupations, while others who seemed to tack creative personal attributes persevered and eventually produced works of art that were hailed as important creative achievements (Getzels and Csikszentmihalyi 1976; Csikszentmihalyi and Getzels 1988; Csikszentmihalyi 1990b). To use just a single example, young women in art school showed as much, or more creative potential than their male colleagues. Yet 20 years later, not one of the cohort of women had achieved outstanding recognition, whereas several in the cohort of men did.

Psychologists have always realized that good new ideas do not automatically translate into accepted creative products. Confronted with this knowledge, one of two strategies can be adopted. The first was articulated by Abraham Maslow and involves denying the importance of public recognition (Maslow 1963). In his opinion it is not the outcome of the process that counts, but the process itself. According to this perspective a person who re-invents Einstein's formula for relativity is as creative as Einstein was. A child who sees the world with fresh eyes is creative; it is the quality of the subjective experience that determines whether a person is creative, not the judgment of the world. While we believe that the quality of subjective experience is the most important dimension of personal life, we do not believe that creativity can be assessed with reference to it. In order to be studied by the interpersonally validated tools of science, creativity must refer to a process that results in an idea or product that is recognized and adopted by others. Originality, freshness of perceptions, divergent thinking ability are all well and good in their own right, as desirable personal traits. But without some form of public recognition they do not constitute creativity. In fact, one might argue that such traits are not even necessary for creative accomplishment.

In practice, creativity research has always recognized this fact. Creativity tests, for instance, ask children to respond to divergent thinking tasks, or to produce stories, or designs with colored tiles. The results are assessed by judges or raters who weigh the originality of the responses. The underlying assumption is that an objective quality called 'creativity' is revealed in the products, and that judges and raters can recognize it. But we know that expert judges do not possess an external, objective standard by which to evaluate 'creative' responses. Their judgments rely on past experience, training, cultural biases, current trends, personal values, idiosyncratic preferences. Thus whether an idea or product is creative or not does not depend on its own qualities, but on the effect it is able to produce in others who are exposed to it. Therefore it follows that what we call creativity is a phenomenon. that is constructed through an interaction between producer and audience. Creativity is not produced by single individuals, but by social systems making judgments about individuals' products.

A second strategy that has been used to accommodate the fact that social judgments are so central to creativity is not to deny their importance, but to separate the process of *creativity* from that of *persuasion,* and then claim that both are necessary for a creative idea or product to be accepted (Simonton 1988a, b, 1991, 1994). However, this stratagem does not resolve the epistemological problem. For if you cannot persuade the world that you had a creative idea, how do we know that you actually had it? And if you do persuade others, then of course you will be recognized as creative. Therefore it is impossible to separate creativity from persuasion; the two stand or fall together. The impossibility is not only methodological, but epistemological as well, and probably ontological. In other words, if by creativity we mean *the ability to add something new to the culture*, then it is impossible to even think of it as separate from persuasion.

Of course, one might disagree with this definition of creativity. Some will prefer to define it as an intrapsychic process as an ineffable experience, as a subjective event that need not leave any objective trace. But a definition of creativity that aspires to objectivity, and therefore requires an inter-subjective dimension, will have to recognize the fact that the audience is as important to its constitution as the individual to whom it is credited.

Thus, starting from a strictly individual perspective on creativity, we were forced to adopt a view that encompasses the environment in which the individual operates. This environment has two salient aspects: A cultural, or symbolic aspect which here is called the *domain;* and a social aspect called the *field.* Creativity is a process that can be observed only at the intersection where individuals, domains, and fields interact.

An Outline of the Systems Model

In the *Origin of Species,* Charles Darwin described the process by which nature 'invents', To paraphrase:

"Nature's mechanism of invention lies in the process of natural selection. Unpacked into its details, natural selection depends on three subprocesses: (1) genetic variation; (2) selection of adaptive results via the test of survival and reproduction; (3) inheritance of the adaptive results. According to the Darwinian perspective, this trio of subprocesses, over millennia, leads to the emergence of new species" (Perkins 1988, p. 367).

Describing biological evolution may, at first, seem an odd way to present a model of creativity (Fig. 10.2), but the process of evolution at the level of species is analogous to the creativity at the level of cultural traits. Biological evolution occurs when an individual organism produces a genetic *variation* that is *selected* by the environment and *transmitted* to the next generation (see Campbell 1976; Mayr 1982; Csikszentmihalyi 1993). In biological evolution, it makes no sense to say that a beneficial step was the result of a particular genetic mutation alone, without taking into account environmental conditions. For instance, a genetic change that improved the size or taste of corn would be useless if at the same time it made the corn more vulnerable to drought, or to disease. Moreover, a genetic mutation that cannot be transmitted to the next generation is also useless from the point of view of evolution.

According to Sterman, this paradigm has now been widely accepted in the social sciences as a model of learning in general:

"John Dewey ... recognized the feedback-loop character of learning around the turn of the century when he described learning as an iterative cycle of invention [variation], observation, reflection [selection], and action [transmission] (Schon 1992). Explicit feedback accounts of behavior and learning have now permeated most of the social sciences. Learning as an explicit feedback process has even appeared in practical management tools such as Total Quality Management, where the so-called Shewhart-Deming PDCA cycle (Plan-Do-Check-Act) lies at the heart of the improvement process in TQM (Shewhart 1939; Walton 1986; Shiba et al. 1993)" (Sterman 1994, p. 293).

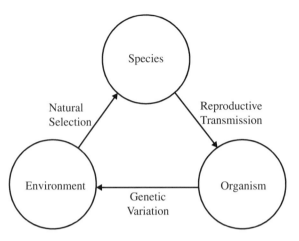

Fig. 10.2 Model of biological evolution

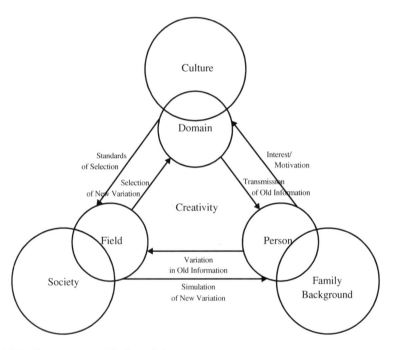

Fig. 10.3 The systems model of creativity

Creativity occurs at the interface of three subsystems: An Individual who absorbs information from the culture and changes it in a way that will be selected by the relevant Field of gatekeepers for inclusion into the Domain, from whence the novelty will be accessible to the next generation (see Fig. 10.3).

The systems model of creativity is formally analogous to the model of evolution based on natural selection. The variation which occurs at the individual level of biological evolution corresponds to the contribution that the person makes to creativity; the selection is the contribution of the field, and the transmission is the contribution of the domain to the creative process (cf. Simonton 1988a, b; Martindale 1989). Operating within a specific cultural framework, a person makes a variation on what is known, and if the change is judged to be valuable by the field, it will be incorporated into the domain, thus providing a new cultural framework for the next generation of persons (Csikszentmihalyi 1988b). Thus creativity can be seen as a special case of evolution. Creativity is to cultural evolution as the mutation, selection, and transmission of genetic variation is to biological evolution. In creativity, it makes no sense to say that a beneficial step was the result of a particular person alone, without taking into account environmental conditions. To be creative, a variation has to be adapted to its social environment, and it has to be capable of being passed on through time.

What we call creativity always involves a change in a symbolic system—a change that, in turn, will affect the thoughts and feelings of other members of the culture. A change that does not affect the way others think, feel, or act will not be creative. Thus creativity presupposes a community of people who share ways of thinking and acting, who learn from each other and imitate each other's actions. Instead of 'genes', it is useful to think about creativity as involving a change in *memes*—the units of imitation that Dawkins (1976) suggested were the building-blocks of culture. Memes are similar to genes in that they carry instructions for action. The notes of a song tell us what to sing; the recipes for a cake tells us what ingredients to mix and how long to bake, the rules of mathematics tell us how to operate with numbers. But whereas genetic instructions are transmitted in the chemical codes we inherit on our chromosomes, the instructions contained in memes are transmitted through learning. By and large we learn memes and reproduce them without change. The great majority of individuals are perfectly content to obey cultural instructions without dreaming of changing them. But occasionally some people develop the notion that they can write a new song, bake a better recipe, or develop a new equation—and then we may have creativity.

Creativity is the engine that drives cultural evolution. The notion of 'evolution' does not imply that cultural changes necessarily follow some single direction, or that cultures are getting any better as a result of the changes brought about by creativity, Following its use in biology, evolution in this context means increasing complexity over time. In turn, complexity is defined in terms of two complementary processes (Csikszentmihalyi 1993, 1996). First, it means that cultures tend to become *differentiated* over time—they develop increasingly independent and autonomous domains. Second, the domains within a culture become increasingly *integrated*; that is, related to each other and mutually supportive of each others' goals—in analogy to the differentiated organs of the physical body that help each others' functioning.

The Place of Schools in the Systems Model

If we apply this model to educational institutions, schools might be seen as consisting of the same three components; a body of knowledge to be transmitted (Domain), teachers who controls the knowledge (Field), and finally a number of individuals, the students, whose task is to learn the knowledge and who are evaluated by "teachers" in terms of their learning.

This perspective immediately makes clear why schools and creativity are inimical. In a creative process, the point is to innovate on the content of the domain in such a way that the field will deem the innovation better than what existed before. But in schools, the point is for the students to replicate the content of the domain as closely as possible, without deviations. The teachers' task is to ensure conformity with prior knowledge, without even trying to evaluate whether the students' deviations might be 'better' than what is written in the textbooks. Thus the main task of schools is to transmit knowledge with as little change as possible —a necessary task which many might argue should not be tampered with.

On the other hand, good teachers everywhere have always been alert for signs of original thinking in their students. Even though it is very rare for a young student to improve on the content of an existing discipline, the very fact of trying to invent a new poetic expression, or a more efficient mathematical calculation, is taken by some teachers to show an involvement with learning that is extremely important to encourage and nurture. From such a perspective learning can be seen as a rehearsal and preparation for later creativity, when the student has mastered the content of the domain to the point that he or she can make a genuinely valuable innovation in it.

In terms of Education as an institution, typically the individual student, teacher, or administrator submits a novel idea to the teacher, administration, or school board, respectively. This field then selects which *good* ideas are to be; respectively, added to the curriculum, passed on to a higher level of management, or implemented as policy. The cumulative sum of these decisions becomes the domain of Education.

Figure 10.4 describes the specific manifestation of creativity in the classroom. When a student produces a variation in the curriculum of a subject, a variation that the teachers feel is worthy of being preserved in some form, then we can observe an instance of creativity. Of course, the problem usually is that teachers are neither looking for innovations from their students, and even if they notice a promising one they have few mechanisms for incorporating it into the curriculum. It is for this reason that most instances of creativity in schools occur outside the classroom, such as in science fairs, artistic competitions, literary prizes, and so on.

The Individual's Contribution to Creativity

We have said that creativity occurs when a person makes a change in a domain, a change that will be transmitted through time. Some individuals are more likely to make such changes, either because of personal qualities, or because they have the good fortune to be well-positioned with respect to the domain—they have better access to it, or their social circumstances allow them more free time to experiment.

The systems model makes it possible to see the contributions of the person to the creative process in a theoretically coherent way. In the first place, it brings attention to the fact that before a person can introduce a creative variation, he or she must have access to a domain, and must want to learn to perform according to its rules. This implies that motivation is important—a topic already well understood by scholars in the field of creativity. But it also suggests a number of additional factors that are usually ignored; for instance, that cognitive and motivational factors interact with the state of the domain and the field. For instance, the domain of nuclear physics promised many interesting intellectual challenges during the first half of this century, and therefore it attracted many potentially creative young people; now the domain of molecular genetics has the same attraction.

Second, the system model reaffirms the importance of individual factors that contribute to the creative process. Persons who are likely to innovate tend to have personality traits that favor breaking rules, and early experiences that make them want to do so. Divergent thinking, problem finding, and all the other factors that psychologists have studied are relevant in this context.

Finally, the ability to convince the field about the virtue of the novelty one has produced is an important aspect of personal creativity. One must seize the opportunities to get access to the field and develop a network of contacts. The personality traits that make it possible for one to be taken seriously, the ability to express oneself in such a way as to be understood are also part of the individual traits that make it easier for someone to make a creative contribution.

Personal Qualities

Having the right background conditions is essential, but certainly not sufficient, for a person to make a creative contribution. He or she must also have the ability and inclination to introduce novelty into the domain. These are the traits that psychologists have most often studied, and it is to these that we shall now turn. Because the individual traits of creative people have been so widely studied, we shall only touch on them briefly and without being able to do them justice.

Perhaps the most salient characteristic of creative individuals is a constant curiosity, an ever renewed interest in whatever happens around them. This enthusiasm for experience is often seen as part of the 'childishness' attributed to creative individuals (Gardner 1993; Csikszentmihalyi 1996). Without this interest, a person would be unlikely to become immersed deeply enough in a domain to be able to change it.

Besides this indispensable quality of being curious and interested, the picture becomes more complicated. One view we have developed on the basis of our studies is that creative persons are characterized not so much by single traits, but rather by their ability to operate through the entire spectrum of human characteristics. So they are not just introverted, but can be both extroverted and introverted depending on the phase of the process they happen to be involved in at the moment. When gathering ideas a creative scientist is gregarious and sociable; but as soon as he starts working, he might become a secluded hermit for weeks on end, Creative individuals are sensitive and cold, arrogant and humble, masculine and feminine, as the occasion demands (Csikszentmihalyi 1996). What dictates their behavior is not a rigid inner structure, but the demands of the interaction between them and the domain in which they are working.

In order to want to introduce novelty into a domain, a person should first of all be dissatisfied with the status quo. It has been said that Einstein explained why he spent so much time on developing a new physics by saying that he could not understand the old physics. Greater sensitivity, naivete, arrogance, impatience, and higher intellectual standards have all been adduced as reasons why some people are unable to accept the *conventional wisdom* in a domain, and feel the need to break out of it.

Values also play a role in developing a creative career. There are indications that if a person holds financial and social goals in high esteem, it is less likely that he or she will continue for long to brave the insecurities involved in the production of novelty, and will tend to settle instead for a more conventional career (Getzels and Csikszentmihalyi 1976; Csikszentmihalyi et al. 1984). A person who is attracted to the solution of abstract problems (theoretical value) and to order and beauty (aesthetic value) is more likely to persevere.

Another way of describing this trait is that creative people are intrinsically motivated (Amabile 1983). They find their reward in the activity itself, without having to wait for external rewards or recognition. A recurring refrain among them goes something like this: "You could say that I worked every day of my life, or with equal justice you could say that I never did any work in my life." Such an attitude greatly helps a person to persevere during the long stretches of the creative process when no external recognition is forthcoming.

The importance of motivation for creativity has long been recognized. Cox advised that if one had to bet on who is more likely to achieve a creative breakthrough, a highly intelligent but not very motivated person, or one less intelligent but more motivated, one should always bet on the second (Cox 1926). Because introducing novelty in a system is always a risky and usually an unrewarded affair, it takes a great deal of motivation to persevere in the effort. One recent formulation of the creative person's willingness to take risks is the 'economic' model of Sternberg and Lubart (Sternberg and Lubart 1995).

Probably the most extensively studied attributes of the creative cognitive style are divergent thinking (Guilford 1967) and discovery orientation (Getzels and Csikszentmihalyi 1976). Divergent thinking—usually indexed by fluency, flexibility, and originality of mental operations—is routinely measured by psychological tests given to children, which show modest correlations with childish measures of creativity, such as the originality of stories told or pictures drawn (Runco 1991). Whether these tests also relate to creativity in 'real' adult settings is not clear, although some claims to that effect have been made (Torrance 1988; Milgram 1990). Discovery orientation, or the tendency to find and formulate problems where others have not seen any, has also been measured in selected situations, with some encouraging results (Baer 1993; Runco 1995). As Einstein and many others have observed, the solution of problems is a much simpler affair than their formulation. Anyone who is technically proficient can solve a problem that is already formulated; but it takes true originality to formulate a problem in the first place (Einstein and Infeld 1938).

Some scholars dispute the notion that problem finding and problem solving involve different thought processes; for example the Nobel-prize winning economist and psychologist Herbert Simon has claimed that all creative achievements are the result of normal problem-solving (Simon 1985; 1988). However, the evidence he presents, based on computer simulation of scientific breakthroughs, is not relevant to the claim, since the computers are fed pre-selected data, pre-selected logical algorithms, and a routine for recognizing the correct solution—all of which are absent in real historical discoveries (Csikszentmihalyi 1988a, c).

The personality of creative persons has also been exhaustively investigated (Barron 1969, 1988). Psychoanalytic theory has stressed the ability to regress into the unconscious while still maintaining conscious ego controls as one of the hallmarks of creativity (Kris 1952). The widespread use of multi-factor personality inventories suggest that creative individuals tend to be strong on certain traits such as introversion and self-reliance, and low on others such as conformity and moral certainty (Csikszentmihalyi and Getzels 1973; Getzels and Csikszentmihalyi 1976; Russ 1993).

How these patterns of cognition, personality, and motivation develop is still not clear. Some may be under heavy genetic control, while others develop under the conscious direction of the self-organizing person. In any case, the presence of such traits is likely to make a person more creative if the conjunction with the other elements of the system—the field and the domain—happen to be propitious.

Measurements Techniques

How can one appropriately measure individual creativity? By definition, the ability to develop useful products never before developed seems quite unpredictable. Nevertheless, some attempts have been made. To expand on the categories of

Davis (1983), these approaches are summarized by the following five methods: *Self-Assessment, Peer Nomination, Personality Correlates, Divergent Thinking Tests,* and *Historical Recurrence* (for greater detail see; Davis 1997; Wolfe 1997).

One method is *Self-Assessment.* This approach elicits the subject's opinion of himself. A substantial problem with such tools is the desirability effect. People like to think of themselves of possessing a positive trait such as creativity. Other people are too modest to accurately report their own strengths. Further, it is extremely difficult to lay out a standard from which the subject can judge what is *creative.* Consequently, popular stereotypes shared in the culture conflate the findings.

A second method is *Peer Nomination.* This approach allows respondents to evaluate each other. The idea is that while creativity is difficult to operationalize, people will recognize it when they see it. As with self-assessment, this measure does not require an external framework. But unlike self-assessment, with other people evaluating the subject, the desirability effect is less intrusive. Amabile (1983) and Csikszentmihalyi (1996) are among those who have used this method by asking experts in specific domains to judge each other. This approach explicitly includes a component of social evaluation.

A third method is *Personality Correlates.* This approach uses personality traits to predict creativity. Dispositions believed to be associated with creativity include confidence, risk-taking, curiosity, and tolerance for ambiguity. Davis and Rimm (1982) developed an omnibus test called the *Group inventory for Finding Interests* (GIFFI) I and II based on these assumptions. The problem with this approach is that in real life personality traits are dependent on context. What is important is whether these traits are present in a particular situation, within a particular domain. Furthermore, as previously argued the creative person is distinguished by the ability to alternate between usually fixed characteristics. For instance, he or she must be conformist enough to learn the knowledge available in the domain, and non-conformist enough to want to change it.

A fourth approach measures *Divergent Thinking.* Here creative ability is measured by the quality and quantity of responses to a series of hypothetical problems. The best known creativity tests are the Torrance Tests of Creative Thinking (TTCT) (Torrance 1966; Davis 1983, 1997). These pencil and paper tests show reasonable relationships to the preceding general creative personality traits. There is a question, however, as to how the hypothetical problems presented in divergent thinking tests translate into real life. Whether generating numerous fantastic uses for a box really predicts any sort of creative achievement is unclear. Further, divergent thinking as a general skill may not represent the reality of a domain specific world. Some support does exist for the generalizability of divergent thinking tests to creative behavior in later life as reported by Torrance (1988). An advantage of these tests is that they may pick up unrealized potential, if such a thing exists.

A fifth method is *Historical Recurrence.* This approach uses biographical data from previous creative involvement to predict future creative involvement. Simonton wrote "What distinguishes the [creative] genius is merely the cognitive

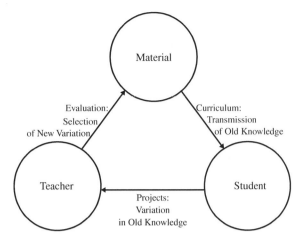

Fig. 10.4 A model of creativity in the classroom

and motivational capacity to spew forth a profusion of chance permutations pertaining to a particular problem" (1988b, p. 422). It follows that participation in a particular domain and public recognition of that participation can be measured and used as a predictive tool. Milgram (1990) designed a useful test for measuring creative activity and achievement applicable to ordinary school children. A criticism of this method is that it does not pick-up latent divergent thinking ability. But is the detached latent ability of an individual relevant? The ability to merely think in original ways may not be an appropriate predictor of creative achievement. Csikszentmihalyi (1990a) has tried to measure the mechanism through which intrinsic motivation operates. In studying the creative *experience*, he coined the term 'flow' to describe the feeling people report when skills become so second nature that everything one does seems to come naturally, and when concentration is so intense that one loses track of time. Csikszentmihalyi argued that it is this optimal feeling of flow that fuels the intrinsic motivation engine which propels creativity (Schmidt and Wolfe 1998).

Flow

People report the most positive experiences and the greatest intrinsic motivation when they are operating in a situation of high opportunities for action (Challenges) and a high capacity to act (Skills); see Fig. 10.5.

Flow experiences also play a critical role in the development of complex patterns of thought and behavior and in the successful development of talent. This theoretical assumption has received empirical support in studies of adolescents (Csikszentmihalyi et al. 1993; Adalai-Gail 1994; Hektner 1996; Heine 1996).

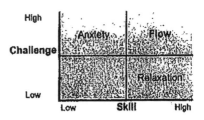

Fig. 10.5 The experience of flow

Educational Implications at the Individual Level

In applying the Systems Model to education we shall begin on familiar ground, at the level of the person. After all, the great majority of psychological research assumes that creativity is an individual trait, to be understood by studying individuals. Considering which personal characteristics promote variation in thought and behavior suggests the following implications for educational practice.

Students' Curiosity and Interest are the Main Sources of Potential Creativity

To the extent that the curriculum and the methods of instruction will stimulate and sustain students' interests, the likelihood of them being motivated to ask new questions and explore divergent solutions will be enhanced (Csikszentmihalyi 1996). Unfortunately pedagogy usually either takes students' interests for granted, or ignores them altogether. One of the most important pedagogical steps would be for teachers to acquaint themselves with each student's particular inclination and interest, so that the curricular material could be connected with it.

Potential Creativity is Enhanced by Intrinsic Motivation, and Suppressed by Excessive Reliance on Extrinsic Rewards

If students learn to enjoy the acquisition of knowledge for its own sake, they will be more likely to engage in extended exploration and experimentation (Amabile 1983). If teachers use mainly extrinsic rewards—grades, discipline, promises of conventional success—as inducements to study, it is less likely that students will be stimulated to think new thoughts. Enjoyment does not imply relaxation or laziness; the most enjoyable activities are usually those that require great effort and skill.

Activities Need to be Designed with the Conditions Necessary For Flow in Mind

To experience flow, a challenging activity must meet the skills of the student. Therefore activities must be adapted, or at least adaptable, for each student's ability. Additionally, activities need to be designed such that goals are clear and relevant feedback is not delayed. Without clear goals, students are not certain where they should be headed; and without immediate feedback, they are not sure whether or not they are successfully headed toward that goal.

Learning to Formulate Problems Should be Part of the Curriculum

Educational practice currently relies almost exclusively on teaching students how to solve problems. The ability to formulate new problems (Getzels and Csikszentmihalyi 1976)—or even to engage in divergent thinking—is seldom encouraged and even more rarely taught. Yet these are among the essential cognitive requirements for potentially creative thought.

Respecting Creative Personality Traits

Students who are potentially creative are almost by definition unusual in their attitudes, values, and demeanor. Therefore, they often come in conflict with teachers who consider their responsibility to enforce conformity and discipline. As a result, many young people who might contribute useful new ideas are intimidated into mediocrity, it is important for teachers to tolerate the idiosyncrasies of children who are otherwise curious and committed to learning.

Promoting the Internalization of Learning

A young person will be best prepared to introduce valuable novelty into a domain if he or she has identified himself with the rules and contents of a given discipline, and developed internal criteria of excellence in it. It is more important to nurture development of these internal standards than to make sure that students are able to perform according to standards set externally, as when they take tests and examinations.

The Contribution of the Domain

A new idea can be observed only against the background of already accepted ideas. These are grouped into domains that constitute the heritage of information we call a 'culture'. The purpose of education is to acquaint individuals with the contents of the most important domains. Gardner (1983) has argued that there are at least seven main classes of such domains, each based on specific neurological potentialities. These include linguistic (e.g. poetry, literature, rhetoric, drama), logical-mathematical, musical, spatial (e.g. painting, sculpture, architecture), bodily-kinesthetic (e.g. dance, athletics), interpersonal (e.g. politics) and intra-personal (e.g. philosophy, psychology) domains. Schools typically address only the content of the first two groups, and the emphasis is almost exclusively on the transmission of information, not on innovation.

As the system models suggests (cf. Fig. 10.3), in order for a creative process to begin, it is necessary that individuals become interested to assimilate the contents of a domain, and for the information contained in the domain to be transmitted to the person. These conditions suggest several issues for the enhancement of creativity in schools.

Educational Implications at the Level of the Domain

Among the issues to be considered for educational practice are the following questions.

How Attractive is the Information Presented to Students?

Regardless of the domain, if the information in it is not connected to students' interests and needs, few students will be motivated to learn beyond what is required to get good grades, and hence few will be in a position to know where the lacunae in knowledge are located, or will be moved to formulate new problems.

Given the nature of learning, it is inevitable that teachers should provide structure and goals to the curriculum, but unless students have some latitude in exploring and making decisions about the acquisition of their own knowledge, it is unlikely that they will feel enough ownership about the material to want to play with it for its own sake. The flow model also suggests that being able to match challenges with skills—in other words, to access information that is neither too difficult nor too easy—is essential for students to be attracted to learning.

How Accessible is the Information?

Often the creative process cannot start for the simple reason that the necessary information is either unavailable, or difficult to access. Textbooks and lectures are often unnecessarily abstract and mystifying, so that even motivated students often give up in frustration. It is important to encourage students to explore as many sources of information as possible, and to allow them some flexibility to do so at their own pace. Computers and the internet have a mixed record in supporting the acquisition of personalized knowledge so far, but these new information technologies have a great potential for making the contents of domains accessible.

How Integrated is the Information?

While it is important to delineate clearly the boundaries and limitations of each subject matter, it is also important for teachers to show how each subject relates to others—both differentiation and integration are essential for complex learning. Creative problems often arise at the interface of disciplines, and thus excessive compartmentalization stifles genuinely new ideas.

It is also important to help students integrate the knowledge (hey are acquiring —whether it is mathematics or history—to the issues students already know, and to what they care about. Few students care enough about purely abstract information to want to experiment with it. Courses that combine different disciplines (e.g. 'Physics for Poets') are only the first step in this direction; much more effort could be devoted to the planning of integrated curricula that while preserving the integrity of distinct domains, will attempt to show their mutual interaction.

Are There Opportunities for Mentorships and Apprenticeships?

In many domains, it is essential for a young person to be trained by experts as soon as possible, or the potential for creativity will not be fulfilled (Bloom 1985). To study physics or music long enough to be able to innovate in it depends in part on whether there are laboratories or conservatories in which one can practice and learn state-of-the-art knowledge in the particular domain. Parents have to be able to afford tutors as well as the time and expense involved in driving the child back and forth to lessons and competitions. The careers of creative individuals are often determined by chance encounters with a mentor who will open doors for them, and such encounters are more likely in places where the field is more densely represented—certain university departments, laboratories, or centers of artistic activity.

Schools can contribute to matching potentially creative young people with tutors and enhancement programs through tests for identifying talent, and the organization of mentorships.

The Contribution of the Field

Novel ideas are not recognized or adopted unless they are sanctioned by some group entitled to make decisions as to what should or should not be included in the domain. These gatekeepers are what we call here the field. The term 'field' is often used to designate an entire discipline or kind of endeavor. In the present context, however, we want to define the term in a more narrow sense, and use it to refer only to the social organization of the domain—to the teachers, critics, journal editors, museum curators, textbook writers and foundation officers who decide what belongs to a domain and what does not. In physics, the opinion of a very small number of leading university professors was enough to certify that Einstein's ideas were creative. Hundreds of millions of people accepted the judgment of this tiny field, and marveled at Einstein's creativity without understanding what it was all about. It has been said that in the United States ten thousand people in Manhattan constitute the field in modem art. They decide which new paintings or sculptures deserve to be seen, bought, included in collections—and therefore added to the domain. A society can then be defined as the sum of its interrelated fields—from architects to zookeepers, from mothers to consumers of computer peripherals.

The recognition that culture and society are as involved in the constitution of creativity certainty does not answer all the questions. In fact, it brings a host of new questions to light. New ideas often arise in the process of artistic or scientific collaboration (Dunbar 1993; Csikszentmihalyi and Sawyer 1995), and peers play an important role in supporting the creativity of individuals (Mockros and Csikszentmihalyi 2000).

Perhaps the major new question this perspective brings to light is: Who is entitled to decide what is creative? According to the individual-centered approach, this issue is not problematic. Since it assumes that creativity is located in the person and expressed in his or her works, all it takes is for some 'expert' to recognize its existence. So if some kindergarten teachers agree that a child's drawing is creative, or a group of Nobel Prize physicists judge a young scientist's theory creative, then the issue is closed, and all we need to find out is how the individual was able to produce the drawing or the theory.

But if it is true, as the systems model holds, that attribution is an integral part of the creative process, then we must ask: What does it take for a new meme to be accepted into the domain? Who has the right to decide whether a new meme is actually an improvement, or simply a mistake to be discarded? How are judgments of creativity influenced by the attributional process (Kasof 1995)?

In any case the point is that how much creativity there is at any given time is not determined just by how many original individuals are trying to change domains, but also by how receptive the fields are to innovation. It follows that if one wishes to increase the frequency of creativity, it may be more advantageous to work at the level of fields than at the level of individuals. For example, some large organizations such as Motorola, where new technological inventions are essential, spend a large quantity of resources in trying to make "engineers think more creatively. This is a good strategy as far as it goes, but it will not result in any increase in creativity unless the field—in this case, management—is able to recognize which of the new ideas are good, and has ways for implementing them—i.e. including them in the domain. Whereas engineers and managers are the field who judge the creativity of new ideas within an organization such as Motorola, the entire market for electronics becomes the field that evaluates the organization's products once these have been implemented within the organization. Thus at one level of analysis the system comprises the organization with innovators, managers, and production engineers as its parts; but at a higher level of analysis the organization becomes just one element of a broader system that includes the entire industry.

Teachers constitute a field that judges the ideas and products of students. It is they who decide which test responses, essays, or portfolios are to be considered creative. So it is true that teachers can measure creativity—as long as it is recognized that what is meant by 'creativity' is not a real objective quality, but refers only to the acceptance by teachers. Such creativity, while part of the domain of education, may have nothing to do with creativity in any other domain outside of it. At every level, from considering Nobel Prize nominations to considering the scribbles of four-year olds, fields are busy assessing new products and deciding whether or not they are creative—in other words, whether they are enough of an improvement to deserve inclusion in a particular domain. And as the biographies of creative individuals suggest, teachers are not particularly good at recognizing future creativity in their students.

Educational Implications at the Level of the Field

The Role of Funding

Other things being equal, a school that enjoys material resources is in a better position to help the creative process. A wealthier school is able to make information more readily available, allows for a greater rate of specialization and experimentation, and is better equipped to reward and implement new ideas. Subsistence schools have fewer opportunities to encourage and reward novelty, especially if is expensive to produce. Only schools with ample material reserves can afford to build great gymnasiums, great auditoriums, great scientific laboratories.

How Open are Teachers to New Ideas?

It is important that teachers enjoy students' explorations beyond the boundaries of textbooks and lesson plans, instead of feeling threatened by them. Teachers who allow deviation from the curriculum, who encourage students to ask questions, to explore alternative paths to solve problems, are more likely to see novelty produced by their students.

Do Teachers Stimulate Students' Curiosity and Interest?

Given the importance of problem formulation in the creative process, it seems important for teachers to stimulate students to find and frame problems of their own, problems that they care about. Every field sooner or later develops self-serving tendencies, so that the effort of its members goes towards making life easier for themselves instead of serving the social purposes for which they are paid.

For teachers the danger is to teach with the least effort, relaying on familiar formulae and texts, without regard for the needs and interests of students. Teachers can stimulate creativity by keeping their lessons and outlines fresh, by exposing students to extracurricular opportunities to learn, by getting to know the interests and strengths of their students.

Can Teachers Distinguish Good New Ideas from Bad Ones?

As the evolutionary model makes clear, most variations are not an improvement on existing knowledge. Teachers who praise every novelty without discrimination do not help students develop the essential internalized criteria that will eventually allow them to make informed evaluations of their own ideas.

Like good parenting, good teaching requires both support and challenge, appreciation and evaluation, freedom and discipline (Csikszentmihalyi et al. 1993). Here again extracurricular opportunities could help classroom activities: science fairs, writing contests, athletic tournaments expose students to accepted criteria of evaluation, helping them to internalize standards.

Are There Ways of Implementing Student Creativity in the School?

Recognizing a valuable novelty is the first step of the process, but bringing it to fruition is equally important. Schools can help through the production of plays, compositions, math competitions, science fairs, Similarly, it is important to pass the novel product on to others. Publication in a school paper or literary magazine, or a publicly viewed art exhibit, play, or science fair allow novelty to spread beyond the classroom.

Conclusion

It is perhaps unrealistic to expect schools to become a major force in the development of creativity. After all, the major function of formal education is to pass on knowledge to young people as accurately as possible, without losing much of the hard-earned knowledge of previous generations in the process. Yet, as we have argued, the future will require individuals who are able to formulate new problems, come up with new solutions, and adapt readily to the new ideas of others. Much of this training for a flexible, creative approach to information should be the responsibility of schools.

Traditionally, education has been focused on transmitting the knowledge of major socially sanctioned domains (i.e. Science, Mathematics, Literature), at the expense of encouraging the evolution of those domains which might lead to individual variation through challenging questions and original answers. The Systems Model suggests an important issue: To foster creativity, education needs to do more than transfer information from teacher to student. So, without sacrificing the domain's information *transmission,* how can educators add to the field's value *selection* and the student's product *variation?*

Creativity in the past has been viewed as a mental process, as the product of individual genius. But new ideas come from existing domains of knowledge; problems arise and standards are internalized from them. And we know whether or not an original solution is worth implementing because of the evaluation of an expert field. It is certain that psychologists interested in the phenomenon of creativity will continue to focus on the individual and his or her thought processes. After all, the unique qualities of creative geniuses are so attractive that we cannot curb our curiosity about them.

What the present chapter seeks to accomplish, however, is to point out that creativity cannot be recognized except as it operates within a system of cultural rules, and it cannot bring forth anything new unless it can enlist the support of experts. If these conclusions are valid, then it follows that the occurrence of creativity in schools is not simply a function of how many gifted students there are, but also of how accessible is the information they need, and how responsive teachers are to novel ideas. Instead of focusing exclusively on students, it makes more sense to focus on educational institutions that may or may not nurture novelty. For in the last analysis creativity in schools is a joint result of well-presented knowledge, interested students, and stimulating teachers.

References

Adalai-Gail, W. S. (1994). *Exploring the autotelic personality.* Unpublished doctoral dissertation. The University of Chicago.

Amabile, T. M. (1983). *The social psychology of creativity.* New York: Springer.

Baer, J. (1993). *Creativity and divergent thinking.* Hillsdale, NJ: Lawrence Erlbaum.

Barron, F. (1969). *Creative person and creative process.* New York: Holt, Rinehart and Winston.

Barron, F. (1988). Putting creativity to work. In: R. J. Sternberg (Ed.), *The Nature of Creativity* (pp. 76–98). Cambridge, UK: Cambridge University Press.

Bloom, B. (1985). *Developing talent in young people.* New York: Ballantine Books.

Campbell, D. T. (1976). Evolutionary epistemology. In D. A. Schlipp (Ed.), *The library of living philosophers: Karl Popper.* La Salle: Open Court.

Cox, C. (1926). *The early mental traits of three hundred geniuses.* Stanford, CA: Stanford University Press.

Csikszentmihalyi, M. (1988a). Motivation and creativity: Toward a synthesis of structural and energistic approaches to cognition. *New Ideas in Psychology, 6*(2), 159–176.

Csikszentmihalyi, M. (1988b). Society, culture, person: a systems view of creativity. In: R. J. Sternberg (Ed.), *The Nature of Creativity* (pp. 325–339). New York: Cambridge University Press.

Csikszentmihalyi, M. (1988c). Solving a problem is not finding a new one: A reply to Simon. *New Ideas in Psychology, 6*(2), 183–186.

Csikszentmihalyi, M. (1990a). *Flow: The psychology of optimal experience.* New York: Harper and Row.

Csikszentmihalyi, M. (1990b). The domain of creativity In: M. A. Runco & R. S. Albert (Eds), *Theories of Creativity* (pp. 190–212). Newbury Park, CA: Sage.

Csikszentmihalyi, M. (1993). *The evolving self: A psychology for the third millennium.* New York: HarperCollins.

Csikszentmihalyi, M. (1996). *Creativity: Flow and the psychology of discovery and invention.* New York: HarperCollins.

Csikszentmihalyi, M. (1999). Implications of a systems perspective for the study of creativity. In: R. J. Sternberg (Ed.), *The Handbook of Human Creativity* (pp. 313–338). New York: Cambridge University Press.

Csikszentmihalyi, M., & Getzels, J. W. (1973). The personality of young artists: An empirical and theoretical exploration. *British Journal of Psychology, 64*(1), 91–104.

Csikszentmihalyi, M., & Getzels, J. W. (1988). Creativity and problem finding. In: F, 0. Farley & N, R. W, (Eds), *The Foundations of Aesthetics, Art, and Art Education* (pp. 91–106). New York: Praeger.

Csikszentmihalyi, M., Getzels, J. W., & Kahn, S. P. (1984). *Talent and achievement: A longitudinal study of artists.* [A report to the Spencer Foundation.] Chicago: The University of Chicago.

Csikszentmihalyi, M., Rathunde, K., & Whalen, S. (1993). *Talented teenagers: The roots of success and failure.* New York: Cambridge University Press.

Csikszentmihalyi, M. & Sawyer, K. (1995). Shifting the focus from individual to organizational creativity. In: C. M. Ford & D. A. Gloia (Eds.), *Creative Action in Organization* (pp. 167–172). Thousand Oaks, CA: Sage Publications.

Davis, G. A. (1983) Creativity is forever. Hunt Publishing Company, Kendall.

Davis, G. A. (1997). Identifying Creative Students and Measuring Creativity. In: N. Colangelo & Davis (Eds.), *Handbook of Gifted Education* (2nd ed., pp. 269—281). Boston: Allyn and Bacon.

Davis, G. A. & Rimm, S. (1982). Group inventory for finding interests (GIFFI) I and II: Instruments for Identifying creative potential in the junior and senior high school. *Journal of Creative Behavior, 16,* 50–57.

Dawkins, R. (1976). *The selfish gene*. Oxford: Oxford University Press.

Dunbar, K. (1993). Scientific reasoning strategies for concept discovery in a complex domain. *Cogn Sci, 17*, 397–434.

Einstein, A. & Infeld, L. (1938). *The evolution of physics*. New York: Simon & Schuster.

Feldman, D., Csikszentmihalyi, M. & Gardner, H. (1994). *Changing the world: A framework for the study of creativity*. Westport, CT: Praeger.

Gardner, H. (1983). *Frames of mind: The theory of multiple intelligences*. New York: Basic Books.

Gardner, H. (1993). *Creating minds*. New York: Basic Books.

Getzels, J. W., & Csikszentmihalyi, M. (1976). *The creative vision: A longitudinal study of problem finding in art*. New York: Wiley.

Getzels, J. W., & Jackson, P.W. (1962). *Creativity and Intelligence*. New York: Wiley

Gruber, H. (1988). The evolving systems approach to creative work. *Creativity Res J, 1*(1), 27–51.

Guilford, J. P. (1967). *The nature of human intelligence*. New York: McGraw-Hill.

Harrington, D. M. (1990). The ecology of human creativity: a psychological perspective. In M. A. Runco & R. S. Albert (Eds.), *Theories of creativity* (pp. 143–169). Newbury Park: Sage.

Hektner, J. (1996). *Exploring optimal personality development: A longitudinal study of adolescents*. Unpublished doctoral dissertation. The University of Chicago.

Heine, C. (1996). *Flow and achievement in mathematics*. Unpublished doctoral dissertation, Chicago.

Kasof, J. (1995). Explaining creativity: The attributional perspective. *Creativity Res J, 8*(4), 311–366.

Kris, E. (1952). *Psychoanalytic explorations in art*. New York: International Universities Press.

Magyari-Beck, I. (1988). New concepts about personal creativity. *Creativity and Innovation Yearbook, 1* (pp. 121–126), Manchester, UK: Manchester Business School.

Martindale, C. (1989). Personality, situation, and creativity. In: R. R. J. Glover & C. R. Reynolds (Eds.), *Handbook of creativity* (pp. 211–232). New York: Plenum.

Maslow, A. H. (1963). The creative attitude. *The Structuralist, 3*, 4–10.

Mayr, E. (1982). *The growth of biological thought*. Cambridge: Belknap Press.

Milgram, R. M. (1990). Creativity: an idea whose time has come and gone? In M. A. Runco & R. S. Albert (Eds), *Theories of Creativity* (pp. 215–233). Newbury Park, CA: Sage Publications.

Mockros, C. & Csikszentmihalyi, M. (2000). The social construction of creative lives. In R. Purser & A. Montuori (Eds.), *Social creativity* (pp. 175–182). Creskill, NY: Hampton Press.

Perkins, D. N. (1988). The Possibility of invention. In R, J. Sternberg (Ed.), *The Nature of Creativity* (pp. 362–385). New York: Cambridge University Press.

Runco, M. A. (1991). *Divergent thinking*. Norwood: Ablex.

Runco, M. A. (Ed.). (1995). *Problem finding*. Norwood: Ablex.

Russ, S. W. (1993). *Affect and creativity*. Hillsdale: Lawrence Erlbaum.

Schmidt, J. A. & R. N. Wolfe. (1998) *Preparing for Careers* in *Technology: course-taking, time allocation, and daily experience of American adolescents*. Unpublished paper presented at the 6th Biennial Conference for the European Association for Research on Adolescence, June 1998. Budapest, Hungary.

Simon, H. A. (1985). *Psychology of scientific discovery*. Keynote presentation at the 93rd Annual Meeting of the American Psychological Association. Los Angeles, CA.

Simon, H. A. (1988). Creativity and motivation: a response to Csikszentmihalyi. *New Ideas in Psychology, 6*(2), 177–181.

Simonton, D. K. (1988a). *Scientific genius*. Cambridge: Cambridge University Press.

Simonton, D. K. (1988b). Creativity, leadership, and chance. In *R. J. Sternberg* (Ed.), *The Nature of Creativity* (pp. 386–426). New York: Cambridge University Press.

Simonton, D. K. (1990), Political pathology and societal creativity. *Creativity Research Journal, 3*(2), 85–99.

Simonton, D. K. (1991). Personality correlates of exceptional personal influence. *Creativity Research Journal, 4*, 67–68.

Simonton, D, K. (1994). *Greatness: Who makes history and why*. New York: Guilford.

Stein, M. L. (1953). Creativity and culture. *Journal of Psychology, 36*, 311–322.

Stein, M. I. (1963). A transactional approach to creativity. In C. W. Taylor & F. Barron (Eds.), *Scientific creativity* (pp. 217–227). New York: Wiley.

Sterman, J. D. (1994). Teaming in and about complex systems. *System Dynamics Review, 10*(2–3), 291–330.

Sternberg, R. J., & Lubart, T. I. (1995). *Defying the crowd: Cultivating creativity in a culture of conformity*. New York: The Free Press.

Torrance, E. P. (1966). *Torrance tests of creative thinking*. Bensenvillo: Scholastic Testing Service.

Torrance, E. P. (1988). The nature of creativity as manifest in its testing. In R. J. Sternberg (Ed.), *The nature of creativity* (pp. 43–75). Cambridge: Cambridge University Press.

Wolfe, R. N. (1997). *Creative involvement, task motivation, and future orientation in adolescence*. Unpublished masters thesis. The University of Chicago.

Chapter 11
Catalytic Creativity

The Case of Linus Pauling

Mihaly Csikszentmihalyi and Jeanne Nakamura

This article illustrates how creativity is constituted by forces beyond the innovating individual, drawing examples from the career of the eminent chemist Linus Pauling. From a systems perspective, a scientific theory or other product is creative only if the innovation gains the acceptance of a field of experts and so transforms the culture. In addition to this crucial selective function vis-à-vis the completed work, the social field can play a catalytic role, fostering productive interactions between person and domain throughout a career. Pauling's case yields examples of how variously the social field contributes to creativity, shaping the individual's standards of judgment and providing opportunities, incentives, and critical evaluation. A formidable set of strengths suited Pauling for his scientific achievements, but examination of his career qualifies the notion of a lone genius whose brilliance carries the day.

Editor's note. Robert J. Sternberg and Nancy K. Dess developed this section on creativity.

Author's note. Jeanne Nakamura, Committee on Human Development, University of Chicago, and Quality of Life Research Center, Peler F. Drucker Graduate School of Management, Claremont Graduate University; Mihaly Csikszentmihalyi, Quality of Life Research Center, Peter F. Drucker Graduate School of Management, Claremont Graduate University.

The Creativity in Later Life Project was generously supported by the Spencer Foundation.

Correspondence concerning this article should be addressed to Jeanne Nakamura Quality of Life Research Center, Peter F. Drucker Graduate School of Management, Claremont Graduate University, 1021 North Dartmouth Avenue, Claremont, CA 91711. Electronic mail may be sent to Jeanne.nakarniira@cgu.edu.

M. Csikszentmihalyi (✉) · J. Nakamura
Quality of Life Research Centre, Claremont Graduate University,
1021 North Dartmouth Avenue, Claremont, CA 91711, USA

J. Nakamura
Commitee on Human Development, University of Chicago, Chicago, IL, USA

M. Csikszentmihalyi, *The Systems Model of Creativity*,
DOI: 10.1007/978-94-017-9085-7_11,
© Springer Science+Business Media Dordrecht 2014

Many people today associate the chemist Linus Pauling (1901–1994) with the two campaigns that preoccupied him during the second half of his long life: the advocacy of nuclear disarmament, which earned him the Nobel peace prize in 1963, and the subsequent controversial advocacy of Vitamin C for fighting cancer and the common cold. A full appreciation of Pauling's accomplishments is impossible without discussion of his efforts on behalf of peace; however, this article focuses on the first half of Pauling's life, when his attention was trained single-mindedly on research and the creativity of his output was indisputable. His scientific contributions during those years were acknowledged with the 1954 Nobel prize in chemistry.

Like some others in psychology (e.g., Amabile 1983, 1996; Gardner 1993; Kasof 1995; Simonton 1984; Sternberg and Lubart 1991) and like many sociologists of knowledge (for a recent example, see Collins 1998), we do not think of creativity as a quality or product of exclusively intrapsychic processes. Instead, we view it as the transformation of a cultural system (e.g., chemistry, medicine, poetry)—the incorporation of novelty into the culture (see Csikszentmihalyi 1988, 1996, 1999; Feldman et al. 1994, for fuller discussions of this topic). We contend that a creative contribution is jointly constituted by the interaction of three components of a system: (a) the innovating *person*; (b) the symbolic *domain* that the individual absorbs, works with, and contributes to; and (c) the social *field* of gatekeepers and practitioners who solicit, discourage, respond to, judge, and reward contributions. It is a model of cultural evolution, with individuals as the generators of variation; the field as the mechanism of selection, determining what gets preserved; and the domain as the mechanism by which innovations are retained and transmitted to the next generation.

In the space of this brief article, our goal is to make more concrete, through a case example, the constitutive role played in creativity by forces beyond the individual (see also Csikszentmihalyi and Sawyer 1995; Mockros and Csikszentmihalyi 2000). To do so, we narrow our focus to the positive role of the field in creativity, a topic that to date has received limited treatment by psychologists. We draw on a 1990 interview with Linus Pauling from the Creativity in Later Life Project (CLL 1990; see Csikszentmihalyi 1996, for a description of the study) and published writings about Pauling's life and work (e.g., Goertzel and Goertzel 1995; Hager 1995; Marinacci 1995; Pauling 1965, 1970, 1986, 1992; Servos 1990).

Linus Pauling

We have selected for this analysis a hard case from the standpoint of illustrating the contribution of the social field to creativity. Linus Pauling's Nobel prize in chemistry was unshared (as was his later peace prize), and his scientific persona was larger than life. To his contemporaries, he must have seemed predestined for both scientific greatness in general and for his groundbreaking work in theoretical structural chemistry in particular (CLL 1990; Goertzel and Goertzel 1995; Hager 1995; Marinacci 1995). Pauling had the intense curiosity and abiding love of science needed to fuel long, hard work. Moreover, he had both a quick, fertile, playful mind suited to theorizing and a prodigious memory that enabled him to amass a vast store of chemical knowledge to draw on in theorizing. He had an exceptional capacity for visualization, equipping him to analyze three-dimensional structures, and the strong mathematical ability needed for absorbing and applying quantum physics. He had an inclination toward the big picture and was comfortable with approximation and conjecture. Pauling exemplified the productive fit between "a remarkable individual's mind and a domain's most challenging problems" (Feldman 1999, p. 178). In recent years, some creativity research has moved away from the notion of creativity as an abstract attribute, toward this notion of person-domain fit.

These personal qualities contributed to Pauling's accomplishments by enabling effective interactions with the domain. Other qualities enabled Pauling to shape, or benefit from, his interactions with the field. He had infectious enthusiasm; ample self-confidence; and, especially important (Simonton 1984), a legendary ability to clearly, simply, and convincingly communicate complex ideas. These qualities helped him persuade the field to accept his ideas. Reciprocally, he showed responsiveness to stimulation from the field that made varied interactions fruitful. As a student, he readily absorbed lessons, guidance, and ideas; throughout his career, he was capable of drawing motivation from competition and skepticism that he encountered rather than being paralyzed (Goertzel and Goertzel 1995; Hager 1995; Marinacci 1995). Given how well this set of strengths suited him for the discoveries he made at chemistry's borders with physics, biology, and medicine, it is tempting to begin and end an analysis of Pauling's creative efforts here. How did the social field play a significant role in the creative accomplishments of such a force of nature (Hager 1995)?

The Role of the Field

From the systems perspective, the person, domain, and field jointly determine a contribution's creativity. The field's most obvious role is in judging would-be additions to the domain. In fact, however, (the field touches the creative process, broadly defined, at many points. At each point, it may have a positive effect on creativity, even though it also can discourage or deform it. Beyond the sheer preserving of the works selected for retention, the field's positive role is catalytic; it actively fosters productive interactions between person and domain (the act of selection can also be catalytic, of course; e.g., by affirming and invigorating). Pauling's case illustrates all of the following impacts: (a) the formative influence of the field on the individual's relationship to the domain; (b) the constructive role of concentric circles of evaluation in the problem-solving process; (c) the contribution of field characteristics to the acceptance of a given work; (d) (the positive impact of extrinsic motivation on the evolution of the individual's research program; and, to shift frames, (e) the creator's catalyzing influence, as part of the field, on others' creative efforts.

The Formative Role of the Field

The field profoundly influences the future of the domain not only by deciding the fate of current contributions but also by determining what is learned by newcomers. In the course of training, students internalize a particular version of the domain and field, which then informs the work that they do. The former encompasses a body of knowledge, skills, and practices. The latter encompasses criteria of evaluation and opinions about worth: a sense of what constitutes an important and interesting problem, where the frontier is, what comprises a good versus bad idea, and when a solution is complete (Pauling 1970). The field as a set of formative environments is heterogeneous, and the lessons learned depend on where they are learned, with the best place being among the field's elite (Zuckerman 1977). Pauling was fortunate to do his learning in the program directed by the distinguished chemist A. A. Noyes at Caltech, an institution on the discipline's leading edge, and at Arnold Somerfield's institute in Munich, Germany, a major center of quantum physics. By Pauling's account, these formative experiences were crucial catalysts of his creative achievements, including his proudest accomplishment, his 1931 paper applying quantum mechanics to the understanding of chemical bonds (CLL 1990).

In the 1920s, Caltech was small but ambitious. Pauling pursued research on the structure of crystals using X-ray diffraction; he later called this focus "just about the most fortunate accident that 1 have experienced in my life" (Pauling 1992, p. 5). The orientation was determinedly interdisciplinary; leading quantum physicists visited from Europe, and the chemists attended their lectures. Pauling studied the new physics and was animated by the vision of a quantum mechanical understanding of chemical phenomena. Then, in Munich, he was exposed to critical ideas in quantum theory just as these were being articulated, and he absorbed Somerfield's "practical, flexible" style of mathematics, which would serve him well in his work at the intersection of quantum physics and chemistry (Hager 1995, p. 126).

Pauling's accounts of this period acknowledge the training that uniquely suited him for interdisciplinary success by shaping his interests, expertise, and standards of quality; it was the "greatest good luck" that brought him to Caltech (Pauling 1965, p. 348). A further aspect of the field's positive impact, obscured by Pauling's reference to luck, was Noyes's guiding influence. Noyes's goal was the integration of chemistry and physics, and at Caltech he made training his primary tool: He shaped the domain by actively shaping the field. He was "capable of identifying and nurturing exceptional talent, of matching that talent with important and timely opportunities in his science, and of securing the resources necessary to realize these opportunities" (Servos 1990, p. 298). Pauling was his "greatest discovery" (Servos 1990, p. 275). In fact, Noyes probed Pauling's interests and aptitudes, steered him toward X-ray work on the structure of crystals, counseled him to study the new physics abroad, and kept his focus on chemistry after his enthusiasm for quantum theory was ignited.

Concentric Circles of Evaluation

Pauling returned from Munich to a faculty position at Caltech, where those around him continued to positively influence his work. He had a large lab with outstanding students. Colleagues in neighboring disciplines, such as the eminent biologists Max Delbrück and George Beadle, provided stimulation. In the Rockefeller Foundation's head, Warren Weaver, he had an enthusiastic patron. Noyes, who had brought Pauling to Caltech as a student, remained a powerful sponsor, protecting his demanding, sometimes arrogant young star from critics within the institution and promoting Pauling's reputation in (the wider field (Goertzel and Goertzel 1995; Hager 1995; Marinacci 1995).

Pauling's way of working had an important social dimension (Csikszentmihalyi and Sawyer 1995), It is easy to think about the evaluation of contributions purely in terms of (a) self-evaluation by the individual during the creative process and (b) acceptance or rejection of the eventual contribution by the field's gatekeepers. The actuality is more differentiated, with concentric circles of critics varying in their distance from the creative process. These intermediate sources of evaluation played a crucial role in Pauling's accomplishments.

We have seen that the individual internalizes a version of the field's evaluative criteria and brings these to bear in the course of work. Pauling liked to say that the route to creativity was having a lot of ideas and discarding the bad ones. He maintained that he had developed "pretty good judgment about what are good ideas and what are bad ideas" (CLL 1990). Furthermore, like other scientists, his internalization of the field's standards sometimes convinced him to postpone, even for years, presentation of ideas that he deemed good while he sought more convincing support (CLL 1990; Hager 1995).

However, Pauling was a theorist, and his inclinations were speculative, optimistic, and self-confident. Consequently, sources of evaluation intermediate between his internal standards and the field's formal gatekeepers played a particularly important role for him in screening out bad ideas (Goertzel and Goertzel 1995; Hager 1995). During his career, he benefited most from the circle of students and collaborators who were both participants in the creative process (cf. Csikszentmihalyi and Sawyer 1995) and representatives of the wider field, critically reacting to the ideas he generated. In particular, he collaborated for decades with the crystallographer Robert Corey, whose experimental skill, precision, and persistence effectively complemented Pauling's strengths—and his weaknesses—as a researcher. For Pauling, colleagues and correspondents provided another, somewhat more distant, sounding board. When this evaluative process was short-circuited—for example, by Pauling's impatience—bad ideas could reach print. His incorrect DNA structure is the best-known example.

The Receptiveness of the Field as a Contributor to Creativity

A discipline's gatekeepers judge the worth of a work and its fate; this is the most obvious way in which the field determines creativity. In doing so, the field may accept contributions for unexpected reasons, for example, because of its own limitations. Everyone is familiar with the case of a creative idea being ignored because the knowledge of the field lags behind that of the creator. This lag sometimes helps a creative contribution that is ahead of, but not a great deal above, the common knowledge shared by the field. Pauling's valence-bond theory transformed chemistry and enabled him to generate a remarkable set of insights into the nature of the chemical bond in the early 1930s (Goertzel and Goertzel 1995; Hager 1995). The approach represented a creative breakthrough even though it was ultimately supplanted by Robert Mulliken's molecular orbital approach. Its early success over this alternative theory was due in large part to limitations on the field's capacity to absorb new knowledge.

Acceptance of Pauling's ideas about the chemical bond occurred in two phases. Scientists working at the border of physical chemistry and quantum theory had shaped his integrative aspirations, multidisciplinary skills, and scientific judgment; they heralded his paper as a major achievement. However, this community was small. In the early 1930s, most chemists were neither interested nor expert enough in math and physics to absorb the new chemistry. The ignorance extended to the field's gatekeepers; Pauling's 1931 paper reportedly was published in the *Journal of the American Chemical Society* without review because the editor could think of no one qualified to evaluate it (Hager 1995).

The widespread acceptance of Pauling's theory over Mulliken's was abetted by this state of ignorance in the field. Pauling's approach was less mathematical, was simpler, and made greater intuitive sense to chemists. In addition, he was the vastly superior communicator, both in the classroom and on the written page. The two theories were ultimately found to be equivalent at a deep level. The valence-bond approach was adopted in large part because it was more accessible to chemists who were unaccustomed to theoretical chemistry, physics, and math; it better matched the field's capacities (Hager 1995). Chemists "could use his ideas with the assurance that they were grounded in the new physics, but they did not have to learn the physics" (Hager 1995, p. 326).

The influence of the field later turned negative. As subsequent generations of chemists emerged, trained in quantum mechanics and math as a consequence of Pauling's impact on the field, "they were hungry for a more quantitative, less intuitive approach" (Hager 1995, p. 327). The valence-bond theory's acceptance by the field thus led—through transformation of the field—to its own supplanting. The history of Pauling's approach illustrates a kind of bootstrapping process in the evolution of culture.

The Shift to Molecular Biology: The Funder's Role

Definition of a research problem or direction is a key point at which the field can influence creativity. A decisive instance of the field's catalytic role in Pauling's success was in effecting his shift during the late 1930s from inorganic to organic chemistry. His fruitful but reluctant change of research focus came as a pragmatic response to urgings from his patron, the Rockefeller Foundation's Warren Weaver. Weaver envisioned a new domain that he called molecular biology and wielded the foundation's funding to foster it. In the 1930s he began pressing Pauling to shift his research focus. Pauling was engrossed in Rockefeller-funded mineralogical and other studies at the time, had been "repelled" by organic chemistry as a student (Marinacci 1995), and had no background in biology, but he had a large lab and growing staff to support. It became clear that Rockefeller funding would continue only if he "became interested in chemistry in relation to biology"; he "followed the money" (Hager 1995, p. 188). Pauling acknowledged the field's role in shaping his research program and the domain, observing that "granting agencies can influence the progress of science" (as quoted in Hager 1995, p. 189).

The outcome of Weaver's intervention confirms that extrinsic motivation does not universally undermine interest and creativity (Amabile 1996). It is undoubtedly critical that here the external influence did not extend its reach into the creative process itself. However, in a clear instance of the functional autonomy of motives (Crutchfield 1962), once Pauling's attention had been redirected, he threw himself wholeheartedly into the study of the far more complex and challenging biological molecules. Energized by his own growing interest, the initial push from outside led to a second period of wide-ranging creative achievement for Pauling. He is viewed today as one of the founders of molecular biology (Crick 1992; Goertzel and Goertzel 1995). This example suggests that the field can play a significant and sometimes fruitful role by instigating deviations from an ongoing line of enterprise.

Pauling's Role as a Catalytic Influence on Others

Thus far, we have focused on the role of the field in fostering Pauling's creativity, but Pauling himself was a powerful catalytic influence on other chemists' work. His most pervasive influence was felt through his 1939 text-book: "For the first time, the science was presented not as a collection of empirical facts tied together by practical formulae but as a field unified by an underlying chemical theory" (Hager 1995, p. 217). The theory it transmitted was Pauling's own quantum-mechanical view. He was already a leader in the field by 1939; through the text-book—written in a "somewhat pontifical style," according to a reviewer (Hager 1995, p. 218)—he presented his own ideas as canonical. Instantly successful and ultimately one of the most heavily cited of all scientific works, the text reshaped the field. Like the 1931 paper, its clear and intuitive exposition made the new science accessible to chemists without Pauling's training in physics and math, enabling them to use valence-bond theory in the solution of chemical structures.

The most visible example of the latter impact was, without a doubt. Crick and Watson's discovery of the double helix in 1953. In late 1952, Pauling himself had rushed to publish what proved to be a notoriously incorrect solution, a triple helix (Goertzel and Goertzel 1995; Hager 1995). From a systems view of creativity, however, it would be inaccurate to say that Pauling did not contribute to deter-mining the structure of DNA. If one relinquishes a strictly individualist account of creativity, the role played by Pauling is evident. He was both a central player in the field and the scientist whose ideas and approaches at the time shaped and domi-nated the domain.

We have more in mind here than the notion that all innovation necessarily builds on the domain of existing knowledge constituted from the contributions of earlier, frequently anonymous creators. Just as Pauling's contributions did not spring from his prodigious intellect operating in isolation, neither did Crick and Watson's double helix. Each had met Pauling, knew his reputation, and was in awe; he was the scientist who by all logic should have solved the structure of DNA. The pair's basic plan for solving the DNA structure was simple: "Imitate Linus Pauling and beat him at his own game" (Watson 1968, p. 48). Trained in biology and physics, both learned their chemistry largely from Pauling's classic text and believed that they would find within it the key to the structure of DNA (Crick 1992; Watson 1968). Moreover, they emulated Pauling's use of three-dimensional models and his philosophy of first considering the simple solution, despite the skepticism of British colleagues. They painstakingly studied his papers on protein structure, noting even the way he had written up the papers (Watson 1968). Insofar as they internalized the field of structural chemistry, it was in the form of Pauling. When the double helix was unveiled, the victory was capped for Crick and Watson by Pauling's gracious acknowledgment that they had gotten it right.

Pauling also made inadvertent contributions to their progress in the roles of rival and former teacher. Watson (1968) vividly recalled racing against the distant rival. The two monitored his efforts through mutual acquaintances, including Pauling's son Peter, who—along with one of Pauling's former lab members, Jerry Donohue—improbably shared a work space with Watson and Crick. Furthermore, Donohue, a crystallographer, proved directly instrumental to their success—as if they had brought Pauling himself into their circle. He drew on a deep knowledge of chemical structure, gained during his years in Pauling's Caltech tab, to supply crucial infor-mation and to correct key errors in the pair's theorizing (Hager 1995; Pauling 1986; Watson 1968). Watson observed that "but for Jerry, only Pauling would have been likely to make the right choice and stick by its consequences" (p. 209); Pauling would later suggest that Donohue should have shared the Nobel prize.

Conclusion

Drawing on events across the course of Linus Pauling's career, we have illustrated the formative influence of the field on an individual's relationship to the domain, the positive impact of concentric circles of evaluation, the implicating of field characteristics in the widespread acceptance of a work, and the constructive influence of the field on the evolving network of enterprise. In addition, we have suggested that Pauling played a role in the successful solution of the DNA puzzle, despite his own erroneous proposal of a triple helix.

The systems approach recognizes the individual innovator's role in creativity. Given Pauling's formidable set of strengths, it may seem he was predestined for the pivotal role that he played in the history of science (Feldman 1999). However, the individual is only the most salient (Kasof 1995) among a set of interacting forces that jointly transform the culture. Throughout his career, Pauling's achievements were ascribable to multiple influences rather than to his intellectual and personal qualities alone, Pauling was not shy about accepting credit for the accomplishments that streamed from his Caltech lab. Nevertheless, he himself in fact offered more complex accounts for his success than personal qualities alone (CLL 1990), ascribing even his proudest creative achievement to context as well as to his own doing.

Thus, Pauling's case illustrates well what is true of creativity in general. The phenomena we agree to call "creative" cannot be observed, measured, evaluated, or reported independently of the judgments of a field of experts whose opinion has currency in a particular society at a specific point in time. The field not only constitutes a given phenomenon as "creative" by giving it legitimacy but also helps to bring it about by setting the agenda for the creative individual and by providing the necessary knowledge, incentives, and critical evaluation. The creative individual, in turn, as a member of the field helps peers and the next generation of practitioners to actualize their own creative potential.

References

Amabile, T. (1983). *The social psychology of creativity*. New York: Springer.

Amabile, T. (1996). *Creativity in context*. Boulder: Westview Press.

Collins, R. (1998). *The sociology of philosophies: a global theory of intellectual change*. Cambridge: Harvard University Press.

Creativity in Later Life Project. (1990). Unpublished interview with Linus Pauling conducted on 20 Nov 1991.

Crick, F. (1992). The impact of Linus Pauling on molecular biology: A reminiscence. In A. Zewail (Ed.), *The chemical bond: structure and dynamics* (pp. 87–98). New York: Academic Press.

Crutchfield, R. (1962). Conformity and creative thinking. In H. Gruber, G. Terrell, & M. Wertheimer (Eds.), *Contemporary approaches to creative thinking* (pp. 120–140). New York: Atherton.

Csikszentmihalyi, M. (1988). Society, culture, and person: a systems view of creativity. In R. J. Sternberg (Ed.), *The nature of creativity* (pp. 325–339). New York: Cambridge University Press.

Csikszentmihalyi, M. (1996). *Creativity: flow and the psychology of discovery and invention*. New York: Harper Collins.

Csikszentmihalyi, M. (1999). Implications of a systems perspective for the study of creativity. In R. J. Sternberg (Ed.), *Handbook of creativity* (pp. 313–335). Cambridge, England: Cambridge University Press.

Csikszentmihalyi, M., & Sawyer, K. (1995). Creative insight: the social dimension of a solitary moment. In R. J. Sternberg (Ed.), *The nature of insight* (pp. 329–363). Cambridge: MIT Press.

Feldman, D. (1999). The development of creativity. In R. J. Sternberg (Ed.), *Handbook of creativity* (pp. 169–186). Cambridge, England: Cambridge University Press.

Feldman, D., Csikszentmihalyi, M., & Gardner, H. (1994). *Changing the world: A framework for the study of creativity*. Westport: Praeger.

Gardner, H. (1993). *Creating minds*. New York: Basic Books.

Goertzel, T., & Goertzel, B. (1995). *Linus Pauling: A life in science and politics*. New York: Basic Books.

Hager, T. (1995). *Force of nature: the life of Linus Pauling*. New York: Simon & Schuster.

Kasof, J. (1995). Explaining creativity: the attributional perspective. *Creativity Research Journal 8*, 311–366.

Marinacci, B. (Ed.). (1995). *Linus Pauling in his own words*. New York: Simon & Schuster.

Mockros, C., & Csikszentmihalyi, M. (2000). The social construction of creative lives. In A. Montouri & R. Purser (Eds.), *Social creativity* (Vol. 1, pp. 175–218). Creskill: Hampton Press.

Pauling, L. (1965). Fifty years of physical chemistry in the California institute of technology. In G. H. Bishop et al. (eds.) The excitement and fascination of science: a collection of autobiographical and philosophical essays (pp. 346–360). Palo Alto: Annual Reviews.

Pauling, L. (1970). Fifty years of progress in structural chemistry and molecular biology. In G. Holton (Ed.), *The twentieth-century sciences: Studies in the biography of ideas* (pp. 281–307). New York: Norton.

Pauling, L. (1986). Early days of molecular biology in the California institute of technology. *Annual Review of Biophysics and Biophysical Chemistry, 15*, 1–9.

Pauling, L. (1992). X-ray crystallography and the nature of the chemical bond. In A. Zewail (Ed.), *The chemical bond: structure and dynamics* (pp. 3–16). New York: Academic Press.

Servos, J. W. (1990). *Physical chemistry from Ostwald to Pauling: The making of a science in America*. Princeton: Princeton University Press.

Simonton, D. K. (1984). *Genius, creativity, and leadership*. Cambridge: Harvard University Press.

Sternberg, R. J., & Lubart, T. (1991). An investment theory of creativity and its development. *Human Development, 34*, 1–31.

Watson, J. D. (1968). *The double helix: A personal account of the discovery of the structure of DNA*. New York: Atheneum.

Zuckerman, H. (1977). *Scientific elite: Nobel laureates in the United States*. New Brunswick: Transaction.

Chapter 12
The Motivational Sources of Creativity as Viewed from the Paradigm of Positive Psychology

Jeanne Nakamura and Mihaly Csikszentmihalyi

Appearing at the dawn of a new paradigm, this volume affords a chance to reflect about the goals of the emerging psychology of strengths, its promise, and its limits. With Seligman, Csikszentmihalyi elsewhere has discussed psychology's long neglect of positive functioning and identified some of the key problems that a positive psychology ought to address in the coming years (Seligman and Csikszentmihalyi 2000). In the present chapter, we draw on work on optimal experience and development, in particular work on creativity, to illustrate the promise of a strengths approach.

Positive psychology extends an umbrella over multiple existing, emerging, and envisioned programs of research. Its current core consists in the study of particular strengths or dimensions of positive functioning: optimism, hope, resilience, wisdom, happiness—in our case, creativity, intrinsic motivation, flow. But beyond specific research directions, the emerging paradigm enriches the discipline by foregrounding a different perspective from the one most psychologists are in the habit of using.

The topic of creativity's motivational underpinnings provides an excellent example of such a shift in perspective. From Freud's earliest writings on the subject, it has been tacitly accepted that the single-minded dedication of such geniuses as Leonardo or Michelangelo must be the result of the displacement of repressed needs. For creativity, as in most areas of human behavior, a deficit was the prime mover, and everything that needed to be explained had to be reduced and assimilated to it. The deficit model of creativity has added necessary depth to the conventional view of behavior and has helped illuminate human motivations with greater complexity. At the same time, as the sole paradigm it runs the risk of

Reference: "The Motivational Sources of Creativity as Viewed from the Paradigm of Positive Psychology" by Jeanne Nakamura and Mihaly Csikszentmihalyi in L.G. Aspinwall and U.M. Staudinger (Eds.) A Psychology of Human Strengths. Washington, DC: American Psychology Association, pages 257–280.

The Creativity in Later Life study was generously supported by the Spencer Foundation.

M. Csikszentmihalyi, *The Systems Model of Creativity*,
DOI: 10.1007/978-94-017-9085-7_12,
© Springer Science+Business Media Dordrecht 2014

flattening the field's perspective once again, substituting a one-dimensional explanatory framework based on deficit for the earlier and equally one-dimensional Victorian view of complacent rationalism.

Creativity, or the process by which new ideas, objects, or processes are introduced into the evolution of culture (Csikszentmihalyi 1992, 1996; Simonton 1984), is in large part a function of a specific kind of motivation. Even more than particular cognitive abilities, a set of motivational attributes—childlike curiosity, intrinsic interest, perseverance bordering on obsession—seem to set individuals who change the culture apart from the rest of humankind. Already in one of the earliest studies of creative geniuses, Cox (1926) concluded that in predicting which of two young people would make a creative contribution, one who was intellectually brilliant but not very motivated and another who was less brilliant but more motivated, the better bet would be on the latter person. But what are the sources of this motivation? It is in answering this question that positive psychology can provide a different and complementary account from traditional interpretations, which often stress the morbidly pathological sources of the motivation that leads to creativity.

To illustrate what difference it makes to use one or the other paradigm, it may be useful to apply the deficit and strengths perspectives to a recent biographical account of a creative individual. This is not intended to be a weighing of the two perspectives' relative merits; rather, we are interested in juxtaposing them in order to understand the phenomenon of creativity better. The particulars may be of interest to researchers studying creativity or intrinsic motivation; more generally, however, it serves as an exploration into whether, and how, the strengths perspective on a phenomenon broadens understanding as a whole.

The analysis was stimulated by a recent article in *The Atlantic Monthly* entitled "Fame: The Power and Cost of a Fantasy" by psychotherapist Bloland (1999). She is the late Erik Erikson's daughter and, like her father, a gifted writer. The article is an eloquent, personal discussion of the costs of celebrity, which was inspired by and describes the case of her father on the one hand and those around him on the other. In an account embraced by others (e.g., Eckersley 2000), Bloland analyzed the phenomenon of fame and the idealization of the famous in deficit terms, as pathologies of narcissism. As the child of a celebrity, she discussed with particular clarity the collateral damage to family members of individuals caught up in the pursuit of fame.

Briefly, Bloland argued that the pursuit of fame is "a defense against shame" (1999, p. 55). It is an attempt to overcome "a sense that the self is deeply flawed or deficient" through the particular means—destined to fail—of gaining from others the admiring attention that the parents did not adequately or appropriately provide (p. 55). An individual's full development of significant talent is "always" energized by this drive to become famous.

Bloland (1999) viewed others' idealization and pursuit of the celebrated individual through the lens of deficit as well: "The purpose of setting up figures who seem superpowerful, infinitely wise or infinitely kind, larger than life itself, is to make us feel safe" (p. 62). Other people's relationships to a celebrated individual are energized by their need to find a hero and thereby deny death and helplessness (Becker 1973).

Bloland's analysis of her father's pursuit of fame consistently located motive force in deficit and in human relationships. Relationships with others are the cause of deficits (in Erikson's case, abandonment by the father and narcissistic needs of the mother), the place where the costs of these deficits are felt (for Erikson, in his relationships with Bloland and his other children), the arena in which one tries to overcome them (by winning attention and admiration), and the only sphere where true repair of self-esteem can occur (by revealing feelings of shame and inadequacy to another person and finding that one can still be accepted).

Creative Accomplishment and Its Motivation

Deficit-Based Motivations

Bloland's (1999) article, with its emphasis on deficit and human relationships, remains almost entirely silent about the interest in and enjoyment of the cultural and natural worlds, which are such powerful motives in any creative process. It is likely that the single-minded pursuit of fame has a basis in narcissistic deficit. In addition, we defer to Bloland's insight into her father's inner life when she ascribes to him a lack of self-confidence and, rooted in that deficit, a profound hunger for recognition. Human motivation is complex, however it is rarely an either-or proposition. Research on accomplished creators (Csikszentmihalyi 1996) leads us to question her analysis of Erikson's motivations, and more importantly her generalization beyond them, on two points: (a) her downplaying of his enjoyment of the work process and (b) her silence about the content of his work, meaning the specific questions with which he grappled throughout his lifetime as a psychologist.

In her one passing allusion to Erikson's subjective experience of the work itself, Bloland (1999) observed that the exercise of skills at a high level is a source of joy. A large body of research has documented the intense enjoyment found in demanding activities and has shown that it is intrinsically motivating—no other reason is needed to engage in activities that produce it (Csikszentmihalyi, 1975/2000; Deci 1975). Through the lens of deficit, however, this is viewed as merely a gratifying by-product of the pursuit of fame and is quickly passed by in Bloland's analysis:

> Of course, there is enormous gratification in exercising one's talents for their own sake—a joy in one's mastery of any highly skilled activity. But I would suggest that *extraordinary talent is characteristically fueled by a desperate longing for human connection*, (Bloland 1999, p. 58, italics added).

Thus, Erikson's work is reduced to a defense, a futile effort at repairing early deficits. This reductionism characterizes an established tradition within the study of creativity (for a discussion, see Ochse 1990). The tradition is often but not exclusively identified with psychoanalytic psychology, where it reaches back to Freud's pathographies. It describes a troubled individual whose motivation for creative work is fundamentally negative and for whom the work lacks transformative power. It ignores the psychoanalytic notion of healthy narcissism that exists within the very paradigm drawn on by Bloland.

It is particularly problematic to pathologize creative accomplishment in general, as Bloland does when she extends the argument beyond the specific case of her father:

> Family friends learned to treat with good humor his disappearances from picnics, or parties to find a quiet place where he could read or write. His brilliance was coupled with an overwhelming need to achieve. *I suspect that the full realization of great talent is always fueled by such an intense need. And what, exactly, is the source of this drive? An early experience of shame* so overwhelming to the sense of self that to become someone extraordinary seems the only way to defend against it. (Bloland 1999, p. 55, italics added).

Passion for the Work

Erikson's behavior at family gatherings sounds strikingly similar to stories we heard many times in interviews with eminent older creators. Such behavior, however, can be interpreted very differently in the context of those accomplished individuals' lives. The emphasis in such accounts was on the passion for the work itself, one of two positive motivations that are evident from a strengths perspective on creativity. For example, the 83-year-old inventor Jack Rabinow invents because it's "a lot of fun" and selects problems because they "move" him. He struggled to answer our question about how he has balanced work and family life:

> I remember once at one of our parties here, we had a big party and Gladys [his wife] said that Jack sometimes walks to a different drummer. In other words, he's so involved in an idea he's working on, he's so carried away, that he is all by himself. He's not listening to what anybody says. This sometimes happens. That you're so—you've got a new idea and you feel that it's very good, and you're so involved that you're not paying attention to anybody. And you tend to drift away from people…. I'm social, I like people, I like to tell jokes, I like to go to theater. But it's probably true that there are times when Gladys would have liked me to pay more attention to her and to the family than I do…. I love Gladys and I love my children. But it could be that I sometimes am in a different world … there's not much you can do about it. I'm sure this is true of most people who love their job. That they can be carried away. (Creativity in Later Life Project 1993).

Another example involves the tumor biologist George Klein. Once he described the feeling he gets when working at the bench in his lab as "the happiness of a deer running through a meadow". But he violently dislikes small talk, parties, and idle social encounters. One evening in the early 1970s, everyone in the lab at the Karolinska Institute in Stockholm went to a traditional celebration of Midsummer's Eve, involving a party that lasts till dawn. Horrified at the thought of having to waste all that time, Klein excused himself by telling his colleagues that a shipment of Burkett's lymphoma cultures had just arrived by plane from South Africa, and he had to process them before they spoiled. So he stayed in the laboratory alone to carry out the delicate procedures that previously had been performed by his assistants. He found that he was completely inept at this task and ruined all the specimens. This is how he described the conclusion of that day:

> I remained into the wee hours studying tube after tube and could only confirm that everything was spoiled, At four in the morning I admitted total defeat and gave up. I was in a total state of euphoria. While driving home that bright Midsummer's morning, I wondered how I could be so happy after having destroyed the excellent samples. The answer was obvious: I had been excused from participating in the Midsummer's dance (Klein 1990, p. 154).

Should we consider the attitude decried by Bloland, and exemplified by many creative individuals, "antisocial," "selfish," and "defensive"? Why do we ascribe a higher moral purpose to being bored than to being happy? And are the fruits of creativity to be accounted for less than satisfying the emotional needs of others?

Focusing on narcissistic pathology can create a susceptibility to interpreting as deficit-based and extrinsically motivated an undertaking that instead arises from intrinsic interest and coexists with positive human relationships. Within psycho-analytic psychology, White (1959) and others—including Erik Erikson himself—have written in this vein about ego processes, and Kohut (1966) has analyzed creativity as a positive transformation of narcissism. Research on flow, interest, and intrinsic motivation has addressed the creator's enjoyable absorption in the work itself (Collins and Amabile 1999; Csikszentmihalyi 1996). Put more generally, the strengths perspective perceives the creator's strivings in terms of proactive, constructivist tendencies of the organism (cf. Brandstädter 1998) rather than reaction, coping, and repair.

Meaningful Purpose

A meaningful purpose is a second possible positive motivation for engaging a domain. Lifelong vocations are often based on goals formulated to make sense of an experienced threat or stress (Csikszentmihalyi and Beattie 1979). A pressing existential problem encountered early in life (e.g., poverty, marginality, social injustice) inspires first a process of meaning construction, and then the channeling of energy into a sphere that is construed as addressing the problem. Frequently, the motivation for engaging the domain becomes functionally autonomous of its origins as a transformational response to threat, evolving into intrinsic interest in the work itself. A young person who has lost a family member to illness thus might frame the problem as one of inadequate medical knowledge and therefore decide to become a medical researcher. Along the way, the individual might discover that the process of scientific discovery is inherently enjoyable.

Despite the superficial resemblance to the narcissistic deficit model invoked by Bloland, the differences are critical. In the latter, creative accomplishment is traced to one kind of problem only: a sense of personal inadequacy. Only one solution to the problem is identified: securing fame. The work is pursued as a means of undoing a deep sense of inadequacy by garnering attention; the work's specific content is unimportant. In other words, the deficit model leaves out the role of meaning-making in motivating action. Erikson never knew the father who abandoned him—indeed, his mother refused even to reveal the father's identity. Erikson was haunted by this throughout his life. His daughter contends that his life's work was a tool to secure the attention he never got from his father.

The strengths model is more general in the sense that any problem is possible and any solution might be conceived. It is also more specific:

The solution chosen is organically rooted in the nature of the particular problem, as formulated by the individual, and in the particular resources that the person deploys to solve it. Further, it is possible for the individual to generalize the personal problem and try to solve it in more universal terms. Rather than simply being a bid for attention, it may have been in this manner that Erikson's lifelong intellectual exploration of identity crisis and identity development was animated by his early loss.

Integrating the Deficit and Strengths Perspectives: The Systems Model

To see more clearly the different implications of the strengths and deficit perspectives, it may help to introduce at this juncture a model of creativity that encompasses both the interpersonal sphere on which the deficit view focuses and the work activity on which the strengths view focuses. The systems model (Csikszentmihalyi 1988, 1999) depicts creativity not as an exclusively intrapsychic process, but as the outcome of interactions among three components of a system: (a) the innovating individual, whose motivation is the focus of this chapter; (b) the domain of knowledge about the empirical world, or ways of shaping it, to which the individual contributes (e.g., psychology, science, art); and (c) the social field of teachers, gatekeepers, and practitioners who respond to and judge the individual's contributions to the domain (i.e., praising, rejecting, ignoring, or embracing them). A given contribution is creative insofar as it gains the acceptance of the field and becomes part of the corresponding domain of knowledge by extending or transforming it.

Within this framework, the medium of *attention* (Csikszentmihalyi 1978) bridges the deficit and strengths perspectives. Investment of attention provides the basis for exchange between the individual and the environment, including the interpersonal environment (the social field, in the systems model) and the symbolic sphere that mediates understanding of the world (the cultural domain, in the systems model). Both perspectives ascribe a key role to attentional processes. Figure 12.1 shows the creator's investment of attention from the two perspectives. Arrows represent flows of attention within the system, Solid lines represent the creator's investment of attention in a sphere for its own sake, whereas broken lines represent the investment of attention in a sphere instrumentally in the service of other goals. The thickness of a line suggests the amount of attention invested.

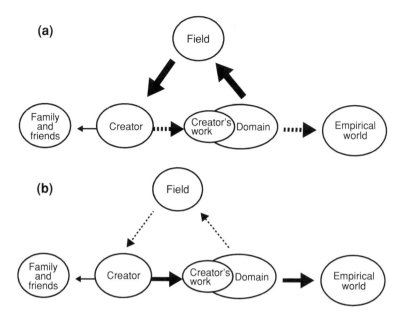

Fig. 12.1 The creator's investment of attention in deficit and strengths models of creativity. *Arrows* represent the flow of attention, *Solid lines* represent investment of attention in something for its own sake. *Broken lines* represent investment of attention instrumentally in the service of other goals. *Thickness of a line* represents amount of attention invested, **a** In a (narcissistic) deficit model, attention is heavily invested in the sphere of creativity (vs. other possible life spheres). Although attention is invested in using the domain to understand the empirical world, this activity is instrumental to eliciting feedback from the field (hopefully, acclaim). **b** In a strengths model, attention is heavily invested in the sphere of creativity (vs. other possible life spheres). Attention is invested in understanding the empirical world, through use of the domain, as an end in itself. Feedback from the field is attended to secondarily and instrumentally as one source of information about the adequacy of current understanding

Attention might be considered the essential commodity in the psychology of narcissism. In the narcissistic deficit model, receiving inadequate or inappropriate attention from parents results in a lasting hunger for attention from others, a channeling of energy into its pursuit, and a sense of gratification or despair depending on the success in attracting it. From a deficit perspective (Fig. 12.1a), the creator's attention is heavily invested in using the domain to understand or shape the empirical world; however, this activity is in the service of winning favorable attention from the various audiences that constitute the field. From a strengths perspective (Fig. 12.1b), the creator's attention is again heavily invested in understanding or shaping the empirical world through use of the domain. From this perspective, however, the activity is an end in itself. Attention to the domain, motivated by interest, is eager and undivided. When the activity goes well, attention becomes focused and effortless and the creator may enter a state of complete involvement, or *flow* (Csikszentmihalyi 1996, 1997); this is what Bloland (1999) referred to in passing as the joy accompanying the mastery of highly skilled activities.

What are the implications of adopting one perspective rather than the other? We briefly identify three illustrative points of divergence. First, the two perspectives differ with respect to the creator's use of feedback to guide activity. From the deficit perspective, the creator pays close attention to the field, seen as a potential source of affirmation. Lack of affirmation, whether this means being rejected or ignored, might discourage persistence even if there has been promising feedback from the work itself. On the other hand, a positive reception by the field might lead the creator to persist in a line of work even if interest or enjoyment wanes or the work stagnates, because the creator's fundamental need for attention continues to be met. The underlying principle is that the creator is motivated to adjust involvement in the domain in the ways that maximize others' admiring attention.

From a strengths perspective, creators attend to the field's reception of their work instrumentally, as a form of feedback about their work's progress (cf. Collins and Amabile 1999). The negative as well as the positive reactions from the field are therefore valued as sources of information. The more primary and more immediate source of feedback is the progress of the work itself, however (e.g., Is the medium expressing the artist's intentions? Is the theory fitting the empirical data?). Focusing on feedback from the activity itself might lead the creator to persist when things are going well despite receiving negative or no attention from the field.

A second point of divergence concerns the creator's relationship to other people. Bloland (1999) discussed the costs of fame for the people around an accomplished individual, particularly the immediate circle of family and friends. Creators devote enormous amounts of attention to their work (Ochse 1990; Roe 1952). Because attention is a finite resource (Csikszentmihalyi 1978), individuals who choose to invest a great deal of attention in work necessarily have less attention to devote to other commitments, including family and friends (see Fig. 12.1). This is true regardless of whether the accomplished creator's work life is viewed from a deficit perspective or a strengths one.

The differences emerge when other relationships are considered, as in the accomplished individual's relationship to students or followers. Both perspectives might suggest that the creator's attention is focused elsewhere (on the wider field, in the case of deficits; on the work itself, in that of strengths) more than on education of students. Beyond this, however, they differ. From the narcissistic deficit perspective, creators may view students as another potential source of affirmation and may actively seek students' admiration rather than directing their attention to the domain. Furthermore, regardless of the creator's intentions, the student motivated by the need for a hero may independently fix idealizing attention on the creator rather than focusing on the domain. Other ways of relating to accomplished individuals may be obscured when limited to a deficit perspective like Bloland's.

An alternative reading of teacher-student interactions, from the strengths perspective, is that the creative individual invests attention in the domain for its own sake, and so does the student. The motivation of the student, like the teacher, lies in curiosity, interest, and enjoyment of the activity. Rather than feeling neglected because of the creator's absorption in the work, the student relishes their joint involvement in the domain based on shared interest. Furthermore, students eager to learn an approach may do so regardless of the teacher's attentiveness to them by investing their own attention well in becoming keen observers of how the teacher approaches the domain.

Finally, deficit and strengths perspectives on the motivational underpinnings of creativity imply divergent therapeutic models. From the first perspective, the creator's absorption in work is motivated by deficit and signals a need for therapeutic treatment; in the latter, the creator's absorption illustrates what therapeutic treatment might seek to make possible. To return to the systems model, from the narcissistic deficit perspective, the individual's involvement with the domain represents a futile attempt to bolster self-worth through direct pursuit of affirmation (i.e., winning the regard of the field). The origin of the person's sense of inadequacy is relational, and treatment correspondingly must occur within an affirming therapeutic relationship. Activity in the domain is a barometer of the pathological need for attention; however, the relationship with the therapist is the medium of cure.

An alternative therapeutic model is associated with the strengths perspective. In it, involvement with a domain of activity is viewed as a route to engagement and a legitimate pathway to an increased sense of self-worth. Massimini and colleagues developed therapeutic interventions guided by flow principles (Delle Fave and Massimini 1992; Inghilleri 1999; Massimini et al. 1987). They sought to identify activities that a person enjoys and oriented therapy toward building on those interests and strengths, taking advantage of the growth of skill and confidence that attends flow experience (Csikszentmihalyi 1997), and enabling the individual to reduce dysphoric experience as a by-product of this growth. The therapist serves as a source of feedback and a guide in reflecting on experience; however, involvement in the domain is the key medium of cure. The continuity between this therapeutic course and naturally occurring developmental processes is illustrated by Erikson's (1968) own notion of "self-chosen therapies", in which a person's identification and mastery of meaningful challenges leads them out of an identity crisis. His work is consistent with the view that people are capable of showing considerable initiative and ingenuity in fostering their own development.

The systems model helps put the deficit and strengths perspectives in contact with one another. In each of the illustrative areas identified in this chapter—the creator's use of feedback, the creator-student relationship, the approach to therapy—the implications of the two approaches largely diverge. Considering both perspectives yields a fuller, potentially more generative picture of the complex dynamics of creativity.

Conclusion

A paradigm based on deficit assumptions alone can give only a limited view of creativity. It cannot explain why some persons dedicate their energies to the pursuit of activities that bring them no external recognition, yet provide great joy. On the broader canvas of human evolution, the deficit perspective cannot adequately explain why people run risks to defy tradition and convention in order to experiment with new ways of seeing, describing, or understanding the world. Positive psychology assumes that the rewards of creativity—and more generally, of any behavior that stretches and enlarges the self—are as genuine and as primary as those homeostatic rewards that reduce discomfort and disease.

Within psychology's own field of creativity, those adopting deficit and strengths views rarely talk to each other, with a resultant loss to each in terms of stimulation and context for their research. Either focus, in isolation, runs the risk of finding only what it is looking for. As one example of the fruitfulness of an open stance, King (2001) brought a strengths perspective to bear on the literature concerning the benefits of self-disclosure writing. As long as subjects were asked only to write about past trauma, the health benefits of writing could be plausibly explained by catharsis, a deficit account. Because King questioned the completeness of this analysis, she proceeded to ask whether writing about positive events also carries health benefits. The finding that health improved after writing about either positive futures or negative pasts led her to frame a higher-order account in terms of writing's effect on self-understanding.

Those who pursue a psychology of strengths need not place borders around it and fix attention on strengths, in a rigid way. There are clear examples of evolving research programs in which the study of strengths was stimulated by or grew out of the study of deficit. These include Bandura's. transition from a concern with social learning of aggression to an interest in self-efficacy (Bandura 1973, 1997); Seligman and colleagues' move from the study of helplessness and depression to the study of optimism and hope (Peterson 2000; Seligman 1990); and Haidt's (2000) passage from research on disgust to research on elevation, the response to witnessing moral acts. In each case, the established line of research suggested the study of strengths. Clearly, human behavior includes both positive and negative aspects, and what is important is to be open to the reality of both.

Through a psychology of strengths, the field hopes to overcome reductionist treatments of positive functioning, such as the reading of all creative accomplishment as a bid for attention (discussed in this chapter) or the interpretation of optimism as a form of denial (discussed in Aspinwall and Brunhart 2000). At the same time, a psychology that denies the existence and dynamics of deficit, in practice even if not by design, would be equally reductionistic. In the case we have sketched, we found it helpful to identify a conceptual tool (the systems model) that bridges the deficit and strengths perspectives and thereby affords the possibility of ultimately integrating the two perspectives in a more encompassing model.

References

Aspinwall, L. G., & Brunhart, S. M. (2000). What I do know won't hurt me: Optimism, attention to negative information, coping, and health. In: J. Gill-ham (Ed.), *The science of optimism and hope: Research essays in honor of Martin Seligman EP* (pp. 163–200). Philadelphia: Templeton Foundation Press.

Bandura, A. (1973). *Aggression: A social learning analysis.* Englewood Cliffs: Prentice Hall.

Bandura, A. (1997). *Self-efficacy: The exercise of control.* New York: Freeman.

Becker, E. (1973). *The denial of death.* New York: Free Press.

Bloland, S. E. (1999, November). *Fame: The power and cost of a fantasy* (pp. 51–62). The Atlantic Monthly.

Brantdstädter, J. (1998). Action perspectives in human development. In R. M. Lerner (Ed.), *Handbook of child psychology* (Vol. 1, pp. 807–863)., Theoretical models of human development New York: Wiley.

Collins, M. A., & Amabile, T. (1999). Motivation and creativity. In R. J. Sternberg (Ed.), *Handbook of creativity* (pp. 297–312). Cambridge: Cambridge University Press.

Cox, C. (1926). *The early mental traits of three hundred geniuses.* Stanford: Stanford University Press.

Creativity in Later Life Project (1993) [Interview]. Unpublished interview.

Csikszentmihalyi, M. (1978). Attention and the holistic approach to behavior. In K. S. Pope, & J, L. Singer (Eds.), *The stream of consciousness: Scientific investigations into the flow of human experience* (pp. 335–358). New York: Plenum.

Csikszentmihalyi, M. (1988). Society, culture, and person: A systems view of creativity. In R. J. Sternberg (Ed.), *The nature of creativity* (pp. 325–339). New York: Cambridge University Press.

Csikszentmihalyi, M. (1992). Motivation and creativity. In R. S. Albert (Ed.), *Genius and eminence* (pp. 19–34). Oxford: Pergamon.

Csikszentmihalyi, M. (1996). *Creativity: Flow and the psychology of discovery and invention.* New York: HarperCollins.

Csikszentmihalyi, M. (1997). *Finding flow.* New York: Basic Books.

Csikszentmihalyi, M. (1999). Implications of a systems perspective for the study of creativity. In R. J. Sternberg (Ed.), *Handbook of creativity* (pp. 313–335). New York: Cambridge University Press.

Csikszentmihalyi, M. (2000). *Beyond boredom and anxiety: The experience of play in work and games.* San Francisco: Jossey-Bass. (Original work published 1975).

Csikszentmihalyi, M., & Beattie, O. (1979). Life themes: A theoretical and empirical exploration of their origins and effects. *Journal of Humanistic Psychology, 19,* 45–63.

Deci, E. (1975). *Intrinsic motivation.* New York: Plenum Press.

Delle Fave, A., &. Massimini, F. (1992). The ESM and the measurement of clinical change: A case of anxiety disorder. In M. de. Vries (Ed.) The *experience of psychopathology* (pp. 280–289). Cambridge, England: Cambridge University Press.

Eckersley, R. (2000). The mixed blessings of material progress: Diminishing returns in the pursuit of happiness. *Journal of Happiness Studies, 1,* 267–292.

Erikson, E. (1968). *Identity: Youth and crisis.* New York: Norton.

Haidt, J. (2000). The positive emotion of elevation. *Prevention and Treatment,* vol 3. http://journals.apa.org/prevention/volume3/pre0030003c.html. Accessed 15 August 2002.

Inghilleri, P. (1999). *From subjective experience to cultural change.* Cambridge: Cambridge University Press.

King, L. (2001). The health benefits of writing about life goals. *Personality and Social Psychology Bulletin, 27,* 798–807.

Klein, G. (1990). *The atheist and the holy city: Encounters and reflections.* Cambridge: MIT Press.

Kohut, H. (1966). Forms and transformations of narcissism. *Journal of the American Psychoanalytic Association, 14,* 243–272.

Massimini, F., Csikszentmihalyi, M., & Carli, M. (1987). The monitoring of optimal experience: A tool for psychiatric rehabilitation. *Journal of Nervous and Mental Disease, 175,* 545–549.

Ochse, R. (1990). *Before the gates of excellence: The determinants of creative genius.* Cambridge: Cambridge University Press.

Peterson, C. (2000). The future of optimism. *American Psychologist, 55,* 44–55.

Roe, A. (1952). *The making of a scientist.* New York: Dodd, Mead.

Seligman, M. (1990). *Learned optimism*. New York: Knopf.
Seligman, M., & Csikszentmihalyi, M. (2000). Positive psychology: An introduction. *American Psychologist, 55*, 5–14.
Simonton, D. K. (1984). *Genius, creativity, and leadership*. Cambridge: Harvard University Press.
White, R. (1959). Motivation reconsidered: The concept of competence. *Psychological Review, 66*, 297–333.

Chapter 13
The Group as Mentor

Social Capital and the Systems Model
of Creativity

Charles Hooker, Jeanne Nakamura and Mihaly Csikszentmihalyi

In recent years, several significant studies of creativity have highlighted the importance of apprenticeship experiences in shaping the potential of young scientists, artists, thinkers, performers, and entrepreneurs. Walberg et al. (1980) found that at least two-thirds of their sample of eminent personalities had been exposed to people of distinction in their field during early life experiences. Simonton (1984, 1988) showed that role models, whether impersonal paragons or personal mentors, played an irreplaceable role in the lives of most creative individuals. Feldman (1999) echoed the same point, and Gardner (1993), after reviewing the lives of Freud, Picasso, Einstein, Stravinsky, T. S. Eliot, Martha Graham, and Gandhi, found it inconceivable to envision any mature expert or creator devoid of competent mentoring.

Csikszentmihalyi's (1996) interviews with over 90 creative individuals in later life confirmed once again the crucial importance of master-apprentice relationships in fashioning careers of significant contribution and productivity. At the same time, however, some of the themes from these interviews raised questions that had been previously unaddressed: what are the practices of good mentors? How are knowledge and skills effectively transmitted from one generation to the next? How are guiding values attached to the instrumental knowledge bequeathed by mentors?

A particularly salient example from the creativity in later life sample (Csikszentmihalyi 1996) will help illustrate the genesis of our present research. As part of the 1996 study, we interviewed three physicists about 80 years of age who had worked with Niels Bohr at some point in their career. Each of them had won some of the most prestigious awards in their field, short of the Nobel prize, and all three mentioned Bohr as a seminal influence in the development of their respective vocations—a mentor from whom they learned important insights about physics as well as how to lead a good life. During their interviews, all three emphasized Bohr's

P. Paulus and M. Nijstad (Eds.), Group Creativity, 2003, pages 225-244.

M. Csikszentmihalyi, *The Systems Model of Creativity*,
DOI: 10.1007/978-94-017-9085-7_13,
© Springer Science+Business Media Dordrecht 2014

importance in terms of the broad discussions they had with him about important life issues (both concerning and beyond the scope of physics). They recounted times they shared with him eating meals, taking walks, and doing other everyday life activities, and they reflected on the general way he cared about them as persons as much as scientists. For each of them, Bohr had a "special way of teaching" that incorporated a holistic purview and a caring touch and that served to model not only scientific excellence but also civic integrity and humane responsibility. One of Bohr's students explained, "I lived as a member of his family... he had a great feel for people, their careers, and their problems." Another said, "He was always living with or among us... although he was much better than us, he was accessible.... He was interested to talk to us not only about physics, but also about philosophy, politics, and art. We went together to the movies." A third added, "As he walked around the table in his office talking about some of the great questions, you would have the feeling that you could understand how people such as Buddha or Confucius really existed.... He took his role as citizen and scientist very seriously... he had a great feeling of responsibility and citizenship."

From this example and others like it in the sample, we became intrigued with the notion that mentors such as Bohr, who embody such estimable ways of being in addition to excellence in their field, have an especially profound and lasting effect on their students, both as professionals and as people. From what we know of wider society, however, such mentoring unfortunately appears to be quite rare. The brilliance of teachers and mentors such as Bohr is not well understood and thus probably rarely practiced. Thus, we took the questions of good mentoring and the transmission of knowledge, skills, and values as our research agenda.

Surprisingly, many of our findings point to group dynamics and social networks as integral components of optimal mentoring practices. In this chapter, we first frame our research in the context of past research on mentoring. We then introduce the systems model of creativity and the concepts of social and cultural capital as helpful theoretical frameworks and vocabulary for our analysis of mentoring to follow. Next, we briefly recount our method and sample and provide a case study from our recent research illustrating, among other things, the importance of group dynamics in mentoring. We then further discuss group dynamics in mentoring and give broader perspective to the interaction we have observed between social capital and the systems model of creativity. Finally, we offer suggestions for extending our conventional conceptions of optimal mentoring.

Conceptions of Mentoring

Historically, social scientists have painted a picture of mentoring that looks very much like the image of Niels Bohr depicted by his intellectual offspring. Levinson (1978), for instance, described a mentor as someone who serves as advisor, sponsor, host, exemplar, and guide for a young person moving from dependence and naivete into independence and sophistication in terms of vocational identity.

The mentor's role, according to Levinson, is to welcome the initiate into a new work-related world; to acquaint him or her with its values, customs, resources, and key players; to provide a model that the protégé can admire and seek to emulate; and to offer counsel and moral support in times of stress. Most important, the "true mentor" will support and facilitate the realization of a dream of the young person, bestowing responsibility and trust on the burgeoning young novice.

Levinson (1978) also noted the complexity and variation inherent in mentoring relationships in general. They are not, as he said, "simple or an all-or-none matter" (p. 100). Rather, they may be only partially beneficial to a young person or seriously flawed and destructive, depending on the motives, capabilities, and disposition of the mentor (and of the apprentice). It is also possible for a mentoring relationship to be very limited and yet highly valuable to a young person's development. For example, some people have purely symbolic mentors whom they have never met, such as an inspiring figure from the past, but who nonetheless may have taught them a great deal about the nature and standards of a domain of interest. In all, theorists such as Levinson, Erikson (1959) and Vaillant (1977) have asserted that "good enough" mentoring relationships provide young people with sustained feelings of support, admiration, respect, appreciation, and gratitude that outweigh, but may not completely prevent, the opposite feelings of resentment, inferiority, and intimidation.

In addition to identifying mentors as basic sources of support and nurturance, the literature in both psychology and sociology has advanced the idea that a young person's prospects can be dramatically increased by apprenticing under a highly successful practitioner from a preceding generation, especially in the field of science (Crane 1965; Kanigel 1986; Simonton 1988; Zuckerman 1977). Zucker-man's study of Nobelists in science revealed this trend perhaps most interestingly. She found that apprentices who became successful scientists themselves reported scientific knowledge as the least important advantage bestowed on them by the laureates who trained them. Far more significant were other influences, such as professional connections and exemplary work standards. As students of the elite, Zuckerman's participants reported unparalleled access to resources (both physical and human), high visibility within their field, and the development of a self-image as one to whom the mantle of excellence and distinction was being passed. Because of these contributions, apprentices said they were able to develop exceptionally high levels of self-confidence. Concordantly, students attributed to the master scientists' example their own high standards of work, along with their ability to intuit important and feasible research problems and elegant solutions— forms of tacit knowledge crucial to creative scientific work and best learned through apprenticeship.

Thus, over the years, social science has documented the many positive (and negative) outcomes of apprenticeship. In so doing, it has also constructed, both implicitly and overtly, an ideal image of the mentor-apprentice relationship, which looks a great deal like the supportive, nurturing connection described by Bohr's students. It has also been shown, at least in the sciences, that training under eminence leads to eminence. Thus, the established ideal proffers elite practitioners supporting promising young novices with emotional, financial, and physical resources in addition to intangible assets such as high visibility, increased self-confidence, and domain-specific intuition. Although this is a helpful map to the process of mentoring and apprenticeship, it is nevertheless incomplete. What is left to be identified and articulated are the specific mechanisms involved in training those who become the best in their given field. We begin this process by examining the training structures and practices used by a highly successful lab in space science. We will see that there are other mechanisms that contribute to the overall effectiveness of training and mentorship. One such mechanism, which is explored in depth, is the role of a group of peers and colleagues in the apprenticeship process. However, before entering that discussion, it will be helpful to first introduce the systems model of creativity to provide a more precise vocabulary and a way of locating our investigation within the broader scope of research on creativity.

The Systems Model of Creativity

In contradistinction to other approaches to understanding creativity, Csikszentmihalyi (1988) introduced the systems model of creativity as an attempt to more fully acknowledge and explain the interaction between the individual and social and cultural factors involved in the creative process. Extended by Feldman et al. (1994), Csikszentmihalyi (1996, 1999), the systems perspective (see Fig. 13.1) views creativity not as the product of an isolated individual's aptitude or quirkiness, but as an interaction occurring among a talented individual, a domain of knowledge or practice, and a field of experts. Csikszentmihalyi (1988, 1996, 1999), Nakamura and Csikszentmihalyi (2002) and Feldman et al. have fully articulated and defined the components of this model. Put briefly, the model begins with an individual who is dissatisfied with the existing state of affairs and wants to change a domain. To accomplish something creative, however, the newcomer must first apprehend an existing body of knowledge, develop a set of skills and abilities, and internalize key standards of quality, values, and beliefs. Having sufficiently mastered the rules, symbols, skills, values, and practices of a domain, the individual may then transform its content in a meaningful way (e.g., by developing a new process, proposing a new theory, finding, or tool), which may then be labeled *creative* only if the associated field of experts deem it so. Gardner (1993) has pointed out that, averaged across domains, this process of acquisition, internalization, and incubation (preceding an initial creative contribution to a domain) generally takes a person about 10 years.

Let *us* briefly unpack this process and provide a brief example. The first step for an aspiring creator rests in adequately mastering what the systems model refers to as the *domain*: some already existing set of objects, rules, representations, or notations. It is simply the content the individual intends to work with or alter. The domain must be included as a component of the creative process because creativity

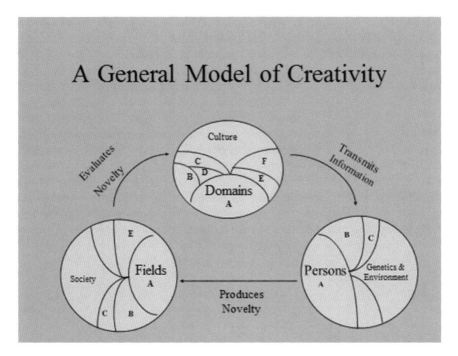

Fig. 13.1 The systems model of creativity. For creativity to occur, a set of rules and practices must be transmitted from the domain to the individual. The individual must then produce a novel variation in the content of the domain. The new variation must then be selected by a field of experts for inclusion in the domain. In this chapter, we focus on the relationship between the field and the individual who aspires to add creatively to the domain. It is here that social capital is generated through mentoring and peer relationships

does not exist in a vacuum (Csikszentmihalyi 1999). It is impossible to introduce something "new" without reference to that which has preceded it: the "old," the already existing patterns or representations of knowledge.

Simply introducing novelty does not, of course, constitute an act of creativity. Many new ideas are generated every day and are quickly forgotten or ignored. To be creative, a variation must somehow be endorsed by *the field*: a group of experts entitled through their own accomplishments or position to decide what should or should not be included in the domain. The field is the social organization of the domain. It consists of gatekeepers—teachers, critics, editors, museum curators, agency directors, and foundation officers—whose role is to decide what should and should not be added to the existing set of knowledge and passed on to subsequent generations.

Let's take a brief example from the visual arts. An aspiring artist must first come to know the relevant domain. She must learn as much as possible about past works of art, historical movements, ideas, and leading figures in sculpture, painting, and drawing. She must develop abilities to expressively manipulate some medium—paint, pencil, paper, stone, metal, or clay. Perhaps most important, she must sufficiently internalize the standards and values of the field by paying attention to the things expressed by the teachers, experts, peers, and critics surrounding her, who ultimately will decide the merits of her work. In some cases, the field may not immediately open itself to a creator's ideas for change. In such cases, the successfully creative person must, for a time, create an entirely new field. This is what the Impressionist painters had to do in Paris in the late 19th century; when the field of academic art spurned their works, the Impressionists enlisted peers, collectors, critics, and galleries to generate enough energy to bring their cause to center stage. Having suitably mastered enough of the knowledge, symbols, and skills of the domain and having internalized the values and practices of the field, the budding artist may contribute to the content of the domain by developing new forms of representation or new techniques, by coming up with a new style, or perhaps by shifting aesthetic criteria in some meaningful way that is accepted and promulgated by the field.

Creativity involves social judgment. The systems model, therefore, seeks to move the concept of creativity from the plane of purely individual (subjective) recognition to a social (intersubjective) arena, wherein the full complexity of creativity can be recognized. Furthermore, it locates creativity within the larger process of cultural evolution, that is, creativity as analogous to the biological process of evolution. Evolution occurs when an individual organism produces a variation that is selected by the environment and transmitted to subsequent generations. So too, in cultural evolution, individuals create variation that is selected by the environment and passed on to future generations. What the systems model calls the field corresponds to the environment; the domain is analogous to the evolutionary genome. As such, creativity is the engine that drives cultural evolution.

Dawkins (1976) introduced the term "meme" to denote the building blocks of culture. Analogous to the role of genes in biological evolution, memes also carry instructions for action (e.g., the laws of physics, the principles of an artistic style, the recipe for baking a cake). However simple or complex, memes make up culture and provide blueprints for individuals, groups, and societal action. Memes make up domains. Domains in turn are subsets of culture.

Whereas genetic instructions are transmitted in sequences of nucleic acids, the instructions contained in memes are conveyed through learning. In this chapter, we are concerned with the process by which aspiring creators are taught the knowledge and skills of a domain and are socialized into the values and standards of the field. In other words, we are concerned with the transmission of memes. It is mainly in this capacity that the mentor-apprentice relationship impacts the development of a nascent individual creator; from our perspective this may be the crucial point at which guiding values and practices are instilled in individuals who will go on to control the field and domain and thereby direct a portion of our society and culture. From this perspective, a mentor is a gatekeeper to a domain who furthers a novice's access to a field, or, as we will come to discover, a mentor serves to increase a novitiate's social capital.

In what follows, we present and expand on a case study to demonstrate key mentoring mechanisms and techniques that, based on our observations, we believe to account for a significant amount of success and creative output in scientific lineages as well as in other fields. Central to all of the mechanisms we discuss is the idea of social capital. Indeed, we see the linking of social capital to mentorship and creativity as a key contribution of this chapter, and so let us turn now to introduce and discuss the concept.

Social Capital

A growing consensus among sociologists has come to define social capital as "the ability of actors to secure benefits by virtue of membership in social networks or other social structures" (Portes 1998, p. 6); Bourdieu (1985), a French sociologist, first introduced the concept decades ago in his work with educational systems in Europe. He defined the term more specifically as "the aggregate of the actual or potential resources which are linked to possession of a durable network of more or less institutionalized relationships of mutual acquaintance or recognition" (p. 248). Bourdieu was interested in the way that social status and power interact with educational systems to directly affect children's educational outcomes and eventual social status as adults. In short, he documented ways in which the social status of a child affected his or her eventual level of educational attainment and position in society. By and large, Bourdieu and his colleagues argued that children from higher social classes retained their position in these ranks of society through relationships they formed, or were given access to, by virtue of their family's position in society (Bourdieu and Passeron 1977). Bourdieu developed the concepts of social and cultural capital to provide a vocabulary for these processes. Social capital, for Bourdieu, is the relationships with other adults (parents, etc.) and peers that avail children access to resources (economic and human) and cultural information that help ensure the child's eventual success in schooling and in attaining status in society. Cultural capital, for Bourdieu, is embodied cultural information. This can be in the form of other people, such as teachers, experts, or peers who internalize areas of cultural information, or it can be found in materials such as books, computers, museums, or other cultural artifacts. For Bourdieu, social capital generally increases a person's access to cultural capital and thereby augments that person's own cultural capital (Portes 1998). This boost in cultural knowledge, when coupled with the accompanying social networks and opportunities, helps pave the way for high achievement.

Coleman (1990) popularized the idea of social capital in the United States. Borrowing from Loury (1987), he defined the term as "the set of resources that inhere in family relations and in community social organization and that are useful for the cognitive or social development of a child or young person" (Coleman 1990, p. 302). Like Bourdieu, Coleman was interested in the intangible factors that contribute strongly to children's educational achievement and career success. Coleman's work was less of a critique and more practical in orientation than Bourdieu's, and so he broadened the definition of social capital somewhat, identifying it by its function of "making possible the achievement of certain ends that would not be attainable in its absence" (p. 304). In other words, we can use social capital to mean the social resources and relationships that assist an individual in the developing vocational and career opportunities that would otherwise not exist.

Having clarified relevant concepts, vocabulary, and perspective, let us now turn to our recent research in hopes that it will allow us to meaningfully relate social capital and the systems model and, in so doing, forge new ideas about apprenticeship and the importance of the group in mentoring and in creativity.

Sample and Method

The sample we used came from a larger ongoing study of apprenticeship across multiple professional domains, including medical genetics, journalism, business, modern dance, martial arts, and coaching. In both the case to follow and the overall project, the sampling strategy was "lab-" or "shop-focused." That is, through expert recommendations and our own research, leading figures were identified within a given field as individuals who led creative careers and who became known for training high-caliber successors who remained in the field and contributed significantly to the domain.

The case examined in this chapter came from a space science lab at a major Midwestern research university. We interviewed five scientists: the generation one (G1) lab head/mentor and four generation two (G2) students. All were White males (which was representative of this field), ranging in age from the G1, who was 81 years old, to the youngest G2, who was in his forties. The participants were dispersed across several regions of the United States, including the Midwest, the South, and the East and West Coasts.

The primary source of data was in-depth, semistructured interviews, which were designed to take approximately two and a half hours and covered broad as well as specific topics, including initial interest in the field; formative experiences; apprenticeship experiences; valued goals, practices, and beliefs; obstacles, pressures, and rewards; training the next generation; and larger vocational vision or purpose. The interviews were recorded and transcribed and then analyzed using a simple coding scheme.

Exploring Apprenticeship and Creativity in a Space Science Lab

With even a cursory review of his career, one must categorize G1 as a supremely successful scientist and mentor. "My theme is to get out of the classroom and into the world of discovery and exploration of new frontiers—and the earlier the better. That's my advice to students." As much as this was his pedagogy, it was also a direct reflection of the kind of life and career led by G1. A giant in the world of space science, G1 wasted no time delving into his own life's work. Immediately after completing his doctoral degree he was recruited to the Manhattan Project, where he joined the team that achieved the first self-sustaining nuclear reaction on the floor of a squash court turned makeshift laboratory. On the day after the United States dropped the atomic bomb on Hiroshima, G1 and a group of conscientious colleagues organized an aggressive campaign to bring nuclear power under civilian control to ensure its peaceful future use. The public concern and leadership evident in this effort proved indicative of G1's entire, lengthy career.

Soon after the Manhattan Project, G1 was appointed to the faculty of a major Midwestern university, where he remained for his entire career, continuing throughout to publicly promote his values in relation to science. During his tenure, G1 received numerous teaching awards and many of the most prestigious scientific awards, short of the Nobel. He supervised the construction and operation of some 35 space experiments and sponsored the work of 34 doctoral students, many of whom are among today's most eminent leaders in space science. One of G1's early apprentices explained, "He was a towering figure in 20th-century science. A large number of his students are research faculty members around the country. His impact has been extremely broad." In fact, G1's teaching and mentoring produced elite scientists who have headed major space science and space exploration laboratories around the country and who continue his concern for science and public policy.

Although one would have to characterize G1 as a supremely successful scientist, public figure, and mentor, his mentoring principles and practices ran surprisingly counter to the predominant conception of effective mentoring espoused by previous research and exemplified in the earlier example of Niels Bohr. First, we were struck by a consistent expression among G2 respondents of what we have come to call "benign neglect." Although G1 was decidedly not hostile and for the most part not inhibitive for his students, both he and his students described a remote, hands-off, management-style approach to teaching, mentoring, and running a lab. Second, despite the paucity of one-on-one contact with their mentor, G2s came away from their training with a shared set of core memes and approaches to research and managing creative groups. Third, as foreshadowed, we were surprised by the significance that G2 respondents assigned to peers, postdocs, and lab culture as components of their training that were equal to or more important than the one-on-one interactions they had with their mentor. Finally, throughout all the interviews, respondents emphasized the way in which trust and endowing apprentices with important responsibilities had a profound effect on motivation, performance (both individual and group projects), and the absorption of the memes being conveyed by the mentor.

Although none of the G2s used the term "benign neglect" to describe the remote mentoring style of G1, all of them discussed this aspect of their training experience in his lab. They described him as "distant," "not intimate," or "off on his own lily pad," and yet, at the same time, they discussed their training experience as "excellent," "high quality," and "highly supportive." Here is the way one G2 recounted his apprenticeship experience:

> [G1 's] style of doing research was all by sort of management. I would consider [G1] "science management." He wouldn't describe himself that way. He would be horrified. But basically he would meet with research people.... He'd be building several projects at a time.... And he'd have a meeting with the students every week. We'd get together for tea and cookies for an hour or two every week. And the students would give a report or something like that. In terms of one-on-one meetings, there were very few, especially with the students. My Ph.D. thesis, I think I spent a total of 15 min discussing it with him. He was basically just unavailable. And that was typical... because [G1] was just sort of infinitely busy and he would be on the phone or in meetings, and then he'd disappear, or he didn't want to be disturbed, or something like that. So that was the way he interacted.

When asked how much time he spent with G1, another G2 responded:

> Directly, probably not a lot, maybe a few minutes every week or couple of weeks, something like that. There was an infrastructure that he had with various other staff who were working on the daily analysis and that's where I, from these guys, where I really learned most of the techniques.

Another described his interaction with G1 this way: "Well, it was less of a personal thing because he was hard to see, and a very busy person.... But he created the lab that had the kind of environment in terms of other people that helped students a lot."

From G1's perspective, there was a system to training creative space scientists who could go on to survive the vicissitudes of a competitive and rapidly changing field. Mainly, G1's approach seemed to incorporate two central principles: have multiple, overlapping projects running simultaneously, and bestow on his students high levels of trust and real responsibility. By having a whole sequence of research projects, or missions, running simultaneously, G1 was able to (1) expedite students' progress toward their Ph.D.; (2) provide students with valuable experience in various stages of different kinds of projects; and (3) increase the overall productivity of the lab and its constituent members. G1 was interested in his students' timely progression through graduate training mainly because he did not want them to become demoralized or discouraged by an overly prolonged period of arduous graduate research. "I'm a great believer in trying to keep the shortest possible time until they get their degree.... That's what alarms me about some of the other fields. I see students are up to six, seven, maybe 8 years before they get a degree. This is devastating in my mind, in terms of doing creative work." After so many years of drudgery G1 believed students lost their zeal for science and research. So, to keep their time in apprenticeship to a minimum, G1 required his students to design a mission or write a grant that would become a future project and then use an existing mission as the basis for their thesis research. By this system, each student participated in every stage of research from conception to write-up, they were exposed to multiple projects, and they short-circuited the all too often hyper-elongated process of attaining a Ph.D.

In case it appears G1 let his students off the hook too easily, let us point out the sizable responsibilities and expectations bestowed on those training in his lab. During his interview, G1 summed up the regimen:

> As I mentioned earlier, the student will help design with me a mission and if we get it... he will then have the opportunity to take data from a previous mission and find some new results and have that as a thesis. And I have a golden rule that the thesis has to be not only original, but it has to be in a refereed journal and I refuse to be a coauthor; that a student has to publish alone. It has to be a single authored student thesis.... Well, this is great because you see the reaction of some students when they suddenly get very fearful of... they're exposed to the world, no help, no support. You see, that's good. And then usually if we can... have them stay on [as a post-doc]... after they get their degree or as they're getting their degree they get their referee's reports and that can obviously be devastating... not necessarily right. But... in every field you get people who are trying to put others down, and so students who face that situation then, it's good to have them here. To be able to sort of hold their hand and say, "Look, don't worry. Let me show you one of the... referee reports I got."

This account shows clearly how G1 helped students very early to internalize the expectations of the field and thus avoid the rejection of their novel ideas and findings, or, if rejected, not to give up as a result. Of course, he himself held high expectations of his students and initiated them in a stepwise fashion into the full set of responsibilities of a tenured member of the field, at the same time maintaining a nurturing environment that would assuage the discouraging obstacles inevitably encountered by any fledgling professional.

It was not only through work on their own grant proposals and thesis publication that G1's students got a taste of real responsibility. It also came through the trust he showered on them in working on existing projects. Apprentices in G1's lab performed most, if not all, of the functions of conceptualizing research questions, writing research proposals, and designing, building, and launching exploratory instruments. Usually they did these things before they thought they were ready. One G2 recalls:

> I remember, my first hint that this was different than anything I'd ever done before was shortly after I was there. We came across a way of improving some of the detectors that we had.... This required making some calculations, and then these detectors would be constructed by cutting them out of crystals, and it would cost a lot of money to get it done. Okay. Fine. So, we were building an instrument, and so I did the calculations to find out how these detectors—what shape they should have to go on the instrument. And so I took my results to [G1], fully expecting him to pull out a pencil and paper and check my calculation. But he just ordered them. I thought, "Oh my God!" So I went back and checked them again. I was expecting a sort of tutorial. And that's just not the way things worked. I think that's fun. This was graduate school. But it was very interesting—I was horrified. It also showed he was trusting me. He was in essence saying, "Fine. We're going to go off and have these things built at the factory to your specs."

In this way G1 embodied the pedagogy he espoused of "getting out of the class-room and into the world of discovery and exploration of new frontiers—and the earlier the better." Quite consciously, it seems, he pushed his students into and beyond what Vygotsky (1978) calls "the zone of proximal development," and in so doing provided them with experiences that built tremendous self-confidence and an identity as a scientist capable of exceeding their own and others' expectations. Throughout the rest of this chapter, we emphasize the importance of other mechanisms in the training process (especially the roles of peers and networks of colleagues), but without this deep sense of trust, responsibility, and respect con-ferred by G1 on his students, none of these other mechanisms would have taken on sufficient vitality to forge such successful young scientists. It would be hard, in our estimation, to overstate the importance of this practice of trust and the willingness, on the part of G1, to delegate real responsibility to his apprentices. Without this, it seems unlikely that apprentices in his lab would have been able to safely inter-nalize the high standards and tacit expectations of the field that have guided their contributions and creative successes since striking out on their own.

Although G1 endowed apprentices with ample physical resources and provided opportunities to take on new challenges and important responsibilities, it does not seem likely, from what has been described so far, that the apprentices from G1's lab would have received memes in any consistent or uniform fashion. That is, given the paucity of contact with G1 and the manner in which G2 s were left to learn on their own and from one another, one might expect a highly heterogeneous, haphazard transmission of memes. To a small extent this was true. There were differences in the sets of memes received by different G2 s, which seemed to stem mainly from the timing of G2 s' apprenticeships with G1. As G1's career and interests evolved, it appears that the emphasis of the work and of the students and staff in the lab shifted slightly, which in turn altered the kinds of memes afloat in the lab environment.

Overall, however, there was a common set of memes about how to do creative work shared by all of G1's apprentices, which more than likely set them apart from apprentices who trained under a different mentor. To begin with, all of the G2s we interviewed (as well as most of those we did not) were still conducting research in the basic scientific area they had pursued under G1's tutelage. It was also the case that all of the apprentices reported an especially hard-nosed commitment to "high quality" and "discovering truth." These are certainly universal scientific memes (as we have observed in our research in other domains, such as medical genetics), but G1's descendants appeared to hold these values especially dear. Finally, there was abundant evidence indicating that more specific practices and approaches to science, to public life, and to teaching were conveyed to and internalized by G1's apprentices.

All of the G2s indicated a serious commitment to fulfilling the public role of a scientist that they saw modeled by their mentor. One student said, "You could see that [G1] obviously took those kinds of responsibilities seriously. So, certainly… there has been a role model there to emulate." Another elaborated more fully:

[G1] felt that he owed something more than just his own research, that he really often made an effort to make a wider contribution to science and society. And I think that the fact that he felt very strongly about that meant that he was not just a scientist. I don't want to make this sound negative, but there are some scientists who really focus totally on their science, and don't feel any wider responsibility.... [G1] was never that way. He was focused on his science, but at the same time he felt a broader responsibility.... So I think that was something which was an important style which I observed and which has continued even long since I've been a graduate student.

This G2 discussed at length his own continuing commitment to "communicate about science to the public" and to "engage the public in the scientific process." Others expressed these same commitments and also attributed them to the influence of their mentor as something that set their training in his lab apart from others.

Another distinguishing characteristic and meme of G1's lab appears to be the very methods he used to systematically manage his lab and its resources (human and otherwise). Although each of the G2 s said they consciously attempted to spend more time with their own students because they would have liked to have received more individual attention from G1, they also reported learning important skills and strategies for managing a lab. One G2 discussed his internalization of this meme as follows:

Space research is something that requires teams of people. It requires leading those teams, formulating direction for the teams. It requires writing proposals and dealing with people who will fund it, and gaining their interest in what you're doing... So I think what I learned from [G1] was kind of research strategy in terms of how to... pick the problem, how to sort of have a bigger picture of where things were headed. Because each thing you do is usually a step. And he always had a larger view of the program.... Similarly, my style tends to be one where I encourage students I am supervising and post-docs working with me to learn and not just follow my direction.

This G2 went on to discuss how, in his first posting as director of his own lab, he attempted to set up a "miniature version" of his mentor's lab. Another G2 said he learned these group management and research strategy skills after he completed his Ph.D. but was still working with G1. Other G2s internalized these memes to greater or lesser degrees, and all acknowledged the strong presence of these memes in G1's lab.

It has been portended and discussed throughout our analysis thus far that perhaps the most striking trend in our data was the overwhelming importance of peers, post-docs, and lab culture in the apprenticeship experience. Resoundingly, apprentices described this as the primary way through which they learned the basic skills and abilities they needed to become successful in space science, and they highlighted it as one of the most important components of G1's lab that allowed them to become successful scientists. One G2 recounted:

My advisor was a very busy person, but in his lab, there were people who were really my day-to-day mentors in a way. I learned a lot from them.... . [G1] created a lab that had the kind of environment in terms of other people that helped students a lot.... I worked very closely with [a post-doc in the lab] as a graduate student, for my whole graduate career. He taught me really all the skills that you need to know—from the analysis of data and looking at problems, to the experiments themselves. He, as I said, was a great teacher in a sense by just having me work with him.... It was the kinds of hands-on stuff you don't learn in books.

Another G2 responded to the question "How did you learn things in the lab?" this way: "Well, very easy, because there were research associates working for [G1], there were other students, there were all these engineers. And that's how you worked. You were in this environment and you learned things." Another G2 added, "[G1] was managing a very good group of people, and he's a very good scientist. So the result is good stuff came out." Still another remarked, "The other graduate students were certainly—I learned a lot from them.... That was an important part of the opportunity too, was to have more senior graduate students that you could learn from. In fact, the first thing I worked on was another student's thesis experiment. That was a wonderful learning experience,"

By both G1's and the apprentices' accounts, G1 understood his role as lab head as one who provided students with a rich learning environment in which they could "get excited about creativity and discovery in science." Other mentors, such as Bohr, have approached this basic task by nurturing students with large amounts of personal attention and acting as a constant source of support and guidance. As we have seen, the literature on mentoring has well documented this approach, and in many ways idealized it, but it has not accounted for other approaches such as the one we have described here. Our aim is not to discredit mentoring approaches that resemble Bohr's and that have been celebrated in the research literature; nor is it to draw comparisons. Instead, our goals are (1) to point out the plurality of effective mentoring methods; (2) to demonstrate the importance of the largely overlooked component of mentoring that involves the group of peers and colleagues surrounding a young apprentice; and (3) to enumerate additional ideal or optimal conditions for effective mentoring. It is to the latter two points that we now turn our attention.

The Group as Mentor

It has been emphasized throughout that peers and colleagues play an integral role in the training and mentoring process of young novices. The role of peer influence is not new to the literature on creativity. Feldman (1999) and Gardner (1993) both discussed the influence of small groups of peers on a creator, especially when working on a new style, theory, or paradigm. Often, creative forms of work and creative ideas are forged within a small group of colleagues (Feldman 1999). Each of Gardner's seven exemplars benefited professionally from peer relationships. Similarly, Woodman et al. (1993) discussed the benefits of peer interaction in creative efforts. But none of these findings have been made in the context of apprenticeship or training processes. In fact, Feldman and Gardner mainly discuss the importance of these relationships after the process of formal training has already taken place. Although this is consistent with our findings, these relationships often begin and become significant during a person's apprenticeship to a particular mentor.

Recalling the concepts of social and cultural capital introduced earlier, we can more clearly articulate some of the mechanisms at play and the reasons we believe it's important to look at apprenticeship to gain a complete understanding of the role of peers and social capital in a person's career. To begin with, it appears that joining an elite lab is analogous to being born into a family of high social status, just as Bourdieu (1985) showed that access to cultural information and important social networks are conferred on children of elite community members, apprentices of eminent mentors reap similar benefits. In this way, perhaps social capital explains Zuckerman's (1977) finding that scientists who studied under Nobelists tended to become highly successful also. But how does this occur? How does social capital bestowed on a young apprentice continue to have effects years later?

It appears this works in several ways. First, novices who train under reputable mentors are given their mentor's stamp of approval and association, which facilitates their way past subsequent "gatekeepers" in the field. Certainly this was the case with students from G1's lab, and we have found it to be true in most other professional fields as well. In some cases, a mentor may even use his or her eminence to prevail on behalf of the novice. In a recent journalism interview, for example, a now prominent editor of a major national newspaper recounted a story of his mentor's weighing in on his behalf when, as a sapling reporter, his press pass was revoked in Vietnam for publishing a story the military did not yet want released. Without his press badge his career could soon be over. Realizing this, and the tenuous case the military had against him, this reporter's mentor rallied journalists from around the country and mustered enough pressure to quickly have the press pass reissued. Needless to say, this now prominent editor could not have made it to the station in life he now occupies without his mentor's placing such a substantial social investment in him. This is but one dramatic case. Sometimes mentors actively go to bat for their apprentices in this way; more often, their association alone is sufficient to open necessary doors.

A second and similar way social capital serves to promote the careers of apprentices is by raising the novice's visibility within the field. That is to say, a mentor, along with the group of peers and colleagues from the mentor's lab, together help amplify the novice's presence within the field. Through collaborations with them, aspiring novices gain greater visibility beyond the lab, in the field, by having greater opportunities to publish, present, and make known their work. In our small sample alone, most of the G2 s explicitly cited relationships they had formed while training under G1 as playing a significant role in attaining their first job. Such is the way it works in academic fields. Beyond academia, this type of social capital benefit occurs in much the same way. In the field of coaching, for example, training with a top coach and his or her staff affords a novice access to relationships with other excellent coaches and athletic staff. Several coaches we interviewed have stressed the importance of the visibility they were given as apprentices by being involved in conference meetings with other coaches, by being assistant coaches on successful teams that received mass media attention, and by developing a network of peers through their mentor. One can easily imagine how this same process works in other fields such as business management, journalism, law, and the arts.

Third, and perhaps most significant, the social capital of a mentor continues to positively affect the apprentice's career years later because apprentices often persist in working with colleagues and peers whom they have met through their mentor. In our case from the space science lab, almost all of the G2s continued collaborative relationships they had begun while under G1's tutelage, either with peers from within G1's lab or with colleagues they worked with beyond his lab. These same enduring collaborative bonds occur in other fields as well. Returning to coaching and journalism for further examples, in each of these fields, many, if not most, of our respondents reported continuing collegial relationships with peers forged during their time of training long after their apprenticeships were over. In fact, in both coaching and journalism, trust in one's colleagues appears to be so, important that these relationships often continue to be primary throughout one's career. Journalists at times move en masse from one newspaper to another because these relationships are so crucial. Similarly, entire coaching staffs often change when a new head coach is appointed. People in these fields tend to hire people they have previously worked with or people recommended by colleagues they know they can trust.

There is another dimension to this last social capital benefit. The importance of the relationships with peers and colleagues formed during a person's training extends beyond trust. Put differently, there is a *creative* benefit that stems from this trust, namely, that it allows for a milieu to develop wherein creative ideas can incubate. It is said that Leonardo da Vinci learned as much from his fellow apprentices, such as Lorenzo di Credi, as he did from the workshop master Verrocchio, and Michelangelo learned from his fellow pupils in Ghlrlandaio's atelier and from the other young men who assembled at the court of the Medici to discuss art and philosophy. In much the same way, many of our respondents said that their creativity was augmented as much by their peers and colleagues as by their mentor, and that the creative milieu did not cease when their time with the mentor ended. Instead, colleagues who share a deep sense of trust and safe feeling forged during their years of mutual apprenticeship often continue to draw on one another's insights, ideas, support, and reflection and, in so doing, find their creativity continuously enhanced.

Extending Our Conception of Optimal Mentoring

In light of our findings regarding the importance of social capital in apprenticeship, a new set of optimal mentoring conditions emerges. First, based on our observations, granting trust and real responsibility to the young apprentice appears crucial to the development of expertise and self-confidence. Through trust and real responsibility apprentices gain a palpable and contagiously exciting sense that their work really matters. It gives their training a new weight, without which their ideas would remain groundless, abstract, and casual. Only by experiencing real responsibility through the trust of the mentor do apprentices begin to gain a sense for what it must be like to be a practitioner in their selected domain. Only through this experience, and the awareness it brings, do they begin to value and internalize the standards and practices of the field.

Second, our research shows that a degree of psychological and social distance from the mentor is beneficial. Some might consider G1 from our case study an extreme example of this. His style of mentoring, which we at times termed benign neglect, was indeed especially hands-off. However, his heavy reliance on the milieu and networking of his lab both for day-to-day teaching of apprentices and for aiding them with career opportunities once they completed their time in training was in many ways exemplary. As such an extreme yet effective example, G1's lab points out mechanisms of mentorship that for the most part have been overlooked but, once discovered, can be seen at work in other lineages in other fields such as coaching and journalism. Mentors must provide support, nurturance, and guidance, but close one-on-one relationships are but one way of accomplishing this, and they alone may not be most effective.

This leads to and works hand in hand with our third and final suggested optimal mentoring condition: providing a systematized group of peers and professional colleagues within and beyond the lab or place of training. Within the lab, peers serve as sources of emotional support and expertise; they provide one another knowledge and intellectual inspiration; they model effective skills and behavior, and thereby supplement many of the roles traditionally thought to belong to mentors alone. Equally important, optimal mentors avail students a new network of colleagues in the larger field, beyond the mere confines of the place of training. From these colleagues, a novice gains not only new ideas and memes and different perspectives on the domain and the field; he or she also gains a new set of trusted collaborative partners. As we discussed earlier, all of the G2s in our sample reported other students and post-docs in G1's lab as being crucial to their training. But the importance of these relationships did not stop with the mastery of scientific principles or techniques, or even with the value of brainstorming and sharing ideas. All of the G2s extended the relationships they built in G1's lab to create important networks, which eventually made significant impacts on their career paths and professional affiliations. In most cases, a contact developed through their mentor played a direct role in securing their first job. Most G2s also continued to collaborate with colleagues from G1's lab, and in all cases they used one another as continuing sources of support and reflection for new ideas and projects. From this perspective, we can see that in addition to impacting students through modeling behavior and embodying values, an important function of mentors is to provide apprentices with state-of-the-art specialized information (cultural capital) and to help them navigate the social networks of the field (social capital).

In this way, understanding social capital enriches the definition of effective mentoring and helps to articulate more clearly a part of the systems model of creativity, namely, the role of the field (i.e., the mentor and an apprentice's peers and colleagues) in educating and socializing aspiring young people (see Fig. 13.1). To be creative in any domain, a person must be able to build the appropriate cultural and social capital—to gain access to the knowledge and the institutions that will allow his or her novel ideas to be expressed. In this process, mentors, who act as gatekeepers to the domain, can either facilitate or terminate a novice's creative aspirations. Good mentors are those who can transmit enthusiasm and knowledge while also introducing the novice to the social realities of the relevant field. As we have seen, this process of building the cultural and social capital, which is requisite for creativity, does not necessarily involve one-on-one tutoring on the part of the mentor. It can take place instead in a studio or lab rich with peers and colleagues whom the mentor makes available and who act as incubators for new ideas.

If creativity is in short supply at a particular moment in time, this may not be due to the lack of young people with good ideas and serious motivation. It may be due instead to the lack of mentors who can provide the needed cultural and social capital and thus create the necessary conditions for the flowering of novel ideas.

Note

The Transmission of Excellence Study was generously supported by the Spencer Foundation.

References

Bourdieu, P. (1985). The forms of social capital. In J.G. Richardson (Ed.), *Handbook of theory and research for the sociology of education* (pp. 241–258). New York: Greenwood.

Bourdieu, P., & Passeron, J.C. (1977). *Reproduction in education, society and culture.* (R. Nice, Trans.). London: Sage.

Coleman, J. (1990). Social capital. In J. Coleman (Ed.), *Foundations of social theory* (pp. 300–324). Cambridge, MA: Belknap Press of Harvard University Press.

Crane, D. (1965). Scientists at major and minor universities: A study of productivity and recognition. *American Sociological Review, 30,* 699–714.

Csikszentmihalyi, M. (1988). Society, culture, and person: A systems view of creativity. In R. J. Sternberg (Ed.) *The nature of creativity* (pp. 325–339). New York: Cambridge University Press.

Csikszentmihalyi, M. (1996). *Creativity.* New York: HarperCollins.

Csikszentmihalyi, M. (1999). Implications of a systems perspective for the study of creativity. In R. J. Sternberg (Ed.) *Handbook of creativity* (pp. 313–335). Cambridge, UK: Cambridge University Press.

Dawkins, R. (1976). *The selfish gene.* New York: Oxford University Press.

Erikson, E. (1959). *Identity and the life cycle.* New York: Norton.

Feldman, D. H. (1999). The development of creativity. In R. J. Sternberg (Ed.), *Handbook of creativity* (pp. 169–186). Cambridge, UK: Cambridge University Press.

Feldman, D. H., Csikszentmihalyi, M., & Gardner, H. (1994). A framework for the study of creativity. In D. H. Feldman, M. Csikszentmihalyi, & H. Gardner (Eds.), *Changing the world: A framework for the study of creativity* (pp. 1–45). Westport, CT: Praeger.

Gardner, H. (1993). *Creating minds*. New York: HarperCollins.

Kanigel, R. (1986). *Apprentice to genius*. New York: Macmillan.

Levinson, D. J. (1978). *The seasons of a man's life*. New York: Knopf.

Loury, G. (1987). Why should we care about group inequality? *Social Philosophy and Policy, 5*, 249–271.

Nakamura, J., & Csikszentmihalyi, M. (2002). The motivational sources of creativity as viewed from the paradigm of positive psychology. In L. G. Aspinwall & V. M. Staudinger (Eds.), *A Psychology of human strengths: Perspectives on an emerging field* (pp. 257–269). Washington: American Psychological Association Books.

Portes, A. (1998). Social capital: Its origins and applications in modern sociology. *Annual Review of Sociology, 24*, 1–24.

Simonton, D. K. (1984). Artistic creativity and interpersonal relationships across and within generations. *Journal of Personality and Social Psychology, 46*, 1273–1286.

Simonton, D. K. (1988). Developmental antecedents. In D. K. Simonton (Ed.), *Scientific genius: A psychology of science* (pp. 107–134). Cambridge, MA: Cambridge University Press.

Vaillant, G. E. (1977). *Adaptation to life*. Boston: Little, Brown.

Vygotsky, L. S. (1978). *Mind in society*. Cambridge, MA: Harvard University Press.

Walberg, H. J., Rasher, S. P., & Parkerson, J. (1980). Childhood and eminence. *Journal of Creative Behavior, 13*, 225–231.

Woodman, R. W., Sawyer, J. E., & Griffin, R. W. (1993). Toward a theory of organizational creativity. *Academy of Management Review, 18*(2), 293–321.

Zuckerman, H. (1977). *Scientific elite*. New York: Free Press.

Chapter 14
The Artistic Personality: A Systems Perspective

Sami Abuhamdeh and Mihaly Csikszentmihalyi

> Why do people think artists are special? It's just another job.
> —Andy Wathol (1975, p. 178)

When considering the relationship between personality and a given occupation or vocation, we usually assume the relationship remains invariant over time. One might assume, for instance, that the temperament and traits that distinguished military leaders in the 5th century BCE would be the same traits as those belonging to warriors in the Middle Ages, or in our own times. Yet the changes throughout history in the social and economic status of soldiers, and in the technology of warfare, suggest that the personalities of men (or women) attracted to a military career will be quite different in each period.

This variability is very obvious in the case of artists. Until the end of the 15th century in Europe, when even the greatest artists were considered to be merely craftsmen and when works of art required the collaboration of several individuals, the typical artist did not display the eccentric, fiercely independent qualities of the "artistic personality" that we now take for granted. In the words of an eminent sociologist of art, "The artist's studio in the early Renaissance is still dominated by the communal spirit of the mason's lodge and the guild workshop; the work of art is not yet the expression of an independent personality" (Hauser 1951, pp. 54–55).

By the middle of the 16th century, however, several artists had become celebrities, in part, because now that painting in oils on canvas was the favorite medium of expression they could work alone, and also because their status had been elevated by such stars as Michelangelo, Leonardo, and Raphael. Thus, Vasari, who in 1550 published the biographies of the "most eminent artists" in Italy, complained that

S. Abuhamdeh · M. Csikszentmihalyi (✉)
Claremont Graduate University, Claremont, CA, USA
e-mail: Mihaly.Csikszentmihalyi@cgu.edu

M. Csikszentmihalyi, *The Systems Model of Creativity*,
DOI: 10.1007/978-94-017-9085-7_14,
© Springer Science+Business Media Dordrecht 2014

nature had given the artists of his time "a certain element of savagery and madness, which, besides making them strange and eccentric… revealed in them the obscure darkness of vice rather than the brightness and splendor of those virtues that make men immortal" (Vasari 1550/1959, p. 22).

The popular idea of artistic temperament embodied in Vasari's view went through several transformations in the past five centuries, but many of its basic traits have endured. One of the most prominent American painters of the past generation, Jackson Pollock, is a good illustration of that "savagery and madness" Vasari complained about. He spent most of his 44 years battling alcoholism, depression, and self-doubt (Solomon 1987), and his stormy marriage to artist Lee Krasner was a source of unrelenting torment. When Pollock painted, he did it with a passion bordering on madness, hurling paint across the canvas in an all-out blitzkrieg of emotion, determined to give life to his singular vision.

Psychological studies suggest that artists are emotional (Barron 1972), sensitive, independent, impulsive, and socially aloof (Csikszentmihalyi and Getzels 1973; Walker et al. 1995), introverted (Storr 1988), and nonconforming (Barton and Cattell 1972). But how pervasive are these traits among successful artists—the personalities who actually shape the domain of art? Is there really such a thing as a timeless, constitutional artistic personality?

In this chapter we propose that the notion of the "artistic personality" is more myth than fact. Although it describes some of the traits that distinguish aspiring artists at certain times under certain conditions, these traits are in no sense required to create valuable art at all times, in all places. We argue that artistic creativity is as much a social and cultural phenomenon as it is an intrapsychic one. And because the social and cultural constraints on the artistic process vary significantly across time and place, the nature of the artistic personality will vary accordingly. When the predominant style or styles of a period change—from Abstract Expressionism to Op Art, Conceptual Art, Photorealism, let us say—so will the personalities of the artists.

We begin with an overview of the theoretical framework that guides this chapter—the systems model of creativity.

The Systems Model of Creativity

Creativity has traditionally been viewed as a mental process, as the insight of an individual. The majority of past psychological research on creativity, accordingly, has concentrated on the thought processes, emotions, and motivations of individuals who produce novelty: the "creative personality". However, beginning with the observations of Morris Stein (Stein 1953, 1963) and continuing with the extensive data presented by Dean Simonton (1988, 1990) showing the influence of economic, political, and social events on the rates of creative production, it has become increasingly clear that variables external to the individual must be considered if one wishes to explain why, when, and from where new ideas or products arise and become established in a culture (Gruber 1988; Harrington 1990).

The systems model proposes that creativity can be observed only in the interrelations of a system made up of three main elements. The first of these is the *domain,* which consists of information—a set of rules, procedures, and instructions for action. To do anything creative, one must operate within a domain. Art is a domain, and the various styles and movements within art can be considered subdomains.

The second component of a system is the *field,* which includes all the individuals who act as gatekeepers to the domain. It is their job to decide whether a new idea or product should be added to the domain. In the world of art, the field consists of the art critics and art historians, the art dealers and art collectors, and the artists themselves. Collectively, this group selects the art products that become recognized as legitimate art.

The final component of the system is the *individual.* In the systems model, creativity occurs when a person makes a change in the information contained in a domain, a change that will be selected by the field for inclusion in the domain.

As this overview of the systems model suggests, the nature of the creative individual—and therefore the artistic personality–is dependent on the nature of the domain and field in which the individual operates. Therefore, to gain a meaningful assessment of the artistic personality, we must pay attention to these other two components of the system. We begin with the domain.

The Domain of Art

During the premodern era, the domain of art was relatively homogeneous in its vocabulary. It consisted almost entirely of figurative works recalling images of religious, philosophical, or historical significance that were widely shared by most members of society. With the arrival of modernism, however, an explosion of artistic styles and movements broadened the boundaries of art considerably. This "de-definition of art" (Rosenberg 1972) has continued during the postmodern era, at warp speed, rendering all tidy definitions of art obsolete.

To illustrate the relationship between the content of artwork and the personality of the artist, we use a classification scheme based on two dimensions of stylistic content, *representational versus abstract* and linear versus *painterly* (see Fig. 14.1).[1] These two dimensions are among a set of five critical dimensions of stylistic content first proposed by the art historian Wölfflin (1929), and later validated by empirical research (e.g., Cupchik 1974; Loomis and Saltz 1984) as important for differentiating artistic styles. The first dimension, *representational versus abstract,* refers to the degree to which a particular artwork imitates an external reference; the second dimension, *linear versus painterly,* represents the degree to which the content of an artwork is characterized by precisely controlled

---

[1] For practical reasons, we limit out discussion of the domain of art to Western painting.

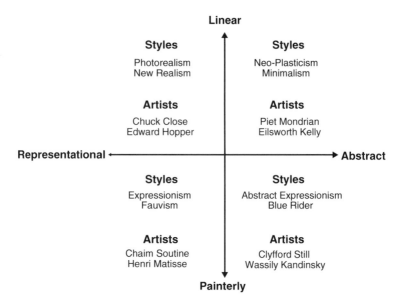

Fig. 14.1 The domain of modern and contemporary painting can be described by two continuous dimensions, *representational–abstract* and *linear–painterly*. Examples of artists and styles for each of the quadrants are given

line and distinct figures (i.e., linear) as opposed to loosely handled paint and relatively undefined form (i.e., painterly).[2]

The diversity of stylistic content represented by the two dimensions within the domain of painting are the outward manifestations of a corresponding diversity in artistic processes and artistic experience. First, let us consider the representational-abstract dimension. Artists painting in a predominantly representational manner have clear external references toward which they can direct their artistic activity—a person, an object, a scene, or any and all combinations. Artists are able to accurately monitor their progress by comparing their work with these external references. Indeed, the success of the work is highly dependent on the artist making such comparisons repeatedly and skillfully.

For those artists working in a nonrepresentational manner, the creative process differs considerably. There is little or no objective referent toward which artists can guide their activity, no clear challenges and goals to pursue.

Whereas the artistic process for the representational artist is highly structured, driven by constraints imposed by the task of representation, abstract artists must actively impose structure on the artistic process, relying on feelings or concepts to guide the process. Susan Rothenberg, who works in a predominantly abstract style, commented on this formidable challenge: "I struggle with it all the time, and a

---

[2] Clearly, the two dimensions of the classification system are not completely independent. The more "painterly" a style is, for example, the less "representational" it is likely to be.

straightforward portrait would be a kind of anchor. I envy Lucian Freud and Chuck Close (two artists with highly representational styles), waking up every morning and knowing what they're going to do" (Kimmelman 1998, p. 178).

The linear-painterly dimension is also associated with significant variety in artistic process and experience. For the artist who paints in a linear style, the artistic process must be exact and focused. Attentional resources are necessarily directed outward, away from the self, toward the technical demands of the task. Because of this, the process tends to be associated with secondary-process cognition (Fromm 1978)—rational and reality-oriented—and devoid of strong emotion. In contrast, the artist who paints using the looser brushstrokes of painterly styles is not bound by the rigid stylistic constraints of the linear style, and is therefore able to allow primary-process cognition—free-associative, irrational, and often emotional—to drive the process. As a result, the creative process is often more improvisational in nature.

The significant relationship among style and experience is exemplified by comparing the following two accounts of the artistic process. The first account is by Clyfford Still, one of the original Abstract Expressionists, and the second is by Chuck Close, a Photo Realist famous for his mural-sized, eerily lifelike portraits.

> A great free joy surges through me when I work… with tense slashes and a few thrusts the beautiful white fields receive their color and the work is finished in a few minutes (Like Belmonte [the bullfighter] weaving the pattern of his being by twisting the powerful bulls around him, I seem to achieve a comparable ecstasy in bringing forth the flaming life through these large areas of canvas. And as the blues or reds or blacks leap and quiver in their tenuous ambience or rise in austere thrusts to carry their power infinitely beyond the bounds of the limiting field, I move with them and find a resurrection from the moribund oppressions that held me only hours ago). Only they are complete too soon, and I must quickly move on to another to keep the spirit alive and unburdened by the labor my Puritan reflexes tell me must be the cost of my joy (Lucie-Smith 1999, p. 184).

Clearly, the artistic process for Clyfford Still was an expressive, intensely personal experience. Contrast this with the artistic process of Chuck Close, as described by his biographers, Lisa Lyons and Robert Storr (1987):

> Propped on an easel to his left are the griddled photographs he refers to as he paints; a shelf on the right carries a telephone and two other important pieces of equipment: a television and a radio/cassette deck. The background noise they provide helps him to maintain that subtle degree of detachment he needs from the tedious activity of building an image, part by part, with machine-like precision. In the past, Close listened to (but did not watch) television almost constantly while working, becoming in the process a connoisseur of morning game shows and afternoon soap operas. Their slow-paced soundtracks ate "of such a mundane nature that you don't really get engaged", he once said. "It's like having a dumb friend in the room. It just chatters away and you don't have to respond to it".

Personality Implications

That significantly different artistic processes exist within the domain of art has significant implications for attempts to define the nature of the artistic personality. More specifically, it suggests that the kinds of traits optimally suited to the creation of art will be dependent on the specific kind of art being created. For example, an artist who is extroverted, sociable, and moved by external norms would not be well-suited to create introspective work, as it requires a special sensitivity to private inner events. Conversely, an introverted artist would have a hard time being noticed if the prevailing style of the domain consisted in polished representations of the objective world.

Although past research on the relationship between artistic style and personality has been relatively sparse, the results of these studies support the idea of a significant relationship between the personality of the artist and the type of art he or she produces. Dudek and Marchand (1983) found a strong correspondence between artists' painting styles and the degree to which they exhibited cognitive defenses and controls. Artists who had lower cognitive defenses and controls (assessed using the Rorschach test) tended to paint in a loosely controlled, painterly manner, whereas artists who were more rigid in their psychological defenses painted in a more formal, linear style. In a study that examined the relationship between personality and the representational-abstract dimension, Loomis and Saltz (1984) found that "rational cognitive styles" were associated with representational artistic styles, whereas "irrational cognitive styles" were associated with abstract styles. Furthermore, extroverts tended to have representational styles, whereas introverts tended to have more abstract styles.

Perhaps the most compelling empirical support for a significant relationship between the personality of an artist and his artistic style comes from a study by Ludwig (1998). He compared the lifetime rates of mental disorder among artists whose work was primarily *formal* (emphasizing structural, compositional, or decorative elements) with rates of mental disorder among artists whose work was primarily emotive (emphasizing self-expression).[3] Results were dramatic: the incidence of lifetime mental disorder among the artists in the emotive category was more than three times the incidence of mental disorder among artists in the format category—22 versus 75 %, respectively ($p < 0.001$).

These results point to a significant relationship between the personality of the artist and the stylistic content of the art he or she produces. Next, we examine the field's role in shaping the personality traits that are characteristic of recognized artists.

The Field of Art

"We are not the masters of what we produce. It is imposed upon us".

—Henri Matisse (Seuphor 1961, p. 16).

---

[3] In the study, Ludwig also classified the works of certain artists as "symbolic". Because we do not use this classification category in the present chapter, Ludwig's findings relating to symbolic styles are not discussed here.

Artists have traditionally been perceived as individuals working in relative isolation, free to follow their creative urges. "Like most geniuses" wrote Ambrose Vollard, friend and biographer of Degas, "[Degas] was essentially independent of events, persons, and places, refusing to be limited by time and disregarding as unimportant everything which did not include and enrich his work" (Vollard 1986, p. 5).

A consideration of the forces at work suggests a less romantic image. One does not become an artist simply by making art. To earn a living and develop a self-concept as a bona fide artist distinct from a dilettante, one must be legitimated by the appropriate art institutions. Only when the artist's work has been recognized by the *field* of art—the critics, historians, dealers, collectors, curators, and fellow artists—can the artist continue to focus his or her energies on creating art.

So what does the art world look for? An artwork will only be accepted as significant if it provides a meaningful extension (aesthetic, political, moral, etc.) to the catalogue of past artistic achievements, the so-called "grand narrative" of art. The greater the contribution to the story, the more significant the work is judged to be. "The imperative to make abstract art comes from history", wrote the famous critic Clement Greenberg in 1940, when Abstract Expressionism was just beginning to take hold of the art world, "and the artist is held in a vise from which at the present moment he can escape only by surrendering his ambition and returning to a stale past" (Greenberg 1940, p. 310).

If an artist creates artwork that does not fulfill the needs of the field, that artist will be dismissed or ignored. Leon Golub, who like so many other artists spent a significant amount of his career living and working in New York, commented on the pressures often felt by artists and created by the field pursuing its rigid agenda:

> The critics were angry about my art. New York seemed impenetrable. I was devastated by some of the reactions, so we (Golub and his wife, artist Nancy Spero) decided to leave because, frankly, we didn't have what-ever it took to fight New York and the atmosphere of that time. There was, and still is, a force in New York, you see, that pushes art in certain directions—ideologically, rhetorically, and rather strongly (Kimmelman 1998, p. 178).

Because of the field's perpetual need for novelty, the field's aesthetic preference is guaranteed to change constantly. Within a given artistic style, this change is characterized by, among other things, an increase in complexity and unpredictability (Martindale 1990). These changes maintain the field's interest in a given style, warding off habituation and boredom. When the style has exhausted its potential for interest, the field will be actively looking for works that hold promise for ushering in a new paradigm.

Consider the emergence of Pop Art in the late 1950s. The first Pop Art paintings appeared at a time when interest and faith in Abstract Expressionism was on the wane. Warhol's mass-produced paintings were not only novel in concept, they also provided a meaningful contrast to the highly expressive paintings of Pollock, de Kooning, and other leading Abstract Expressionists. In other words, Abstract Expressionism created the opportunity for Pop Art to emerge. It is unlikely that Pop Art would have appeared at another point in the history of art.

The nature of the art field's selection process has two important implications for the current topic under consideration, the artistic personality. The first is that, at any given point in time, there will be a constellation of personality traits that are optimally suited to create the kind of art the field will recognize as significant. The nature of these traits will be strongly determined by the nature of the domain. For example, if an abstract, painterly style such as Abstract Expressionism is reigning in the art world, emotional, introverted artists will have the advantage; if a realistic, linear style such as Social Realism is in vogue, more extroverted, unemotional dispositions will be favored. It is important to note, however, that the stylistic qualities of movements often change significantly during a movement's life span, so that different personality traits will be adaptive depending on the developmental stage of the movement (Kubler 1962). For example, original, nonconforming types will flourish more during the early stages of a movement, when the task is to lay new foundations, rather than the later stages, when the task is to elaborate and refine already existing symbols and themes.

The second implication of the field's selection process, already suggested by the first, is that the artistic personality is not a stable, timeless personality type. As the field's taste for art changes, so too will the types of personalities creating the art that will be accepted as significant. Though it may have been adaptive at one point in history for artists to possess the traits associated with the archetypal "artistic personality"—introverted, nonconforming, socially aloof, and so forth—there is no reason to believe that these traits will continue to be adaptive, or even that they are adaptive in today's art world.

Indeed, a longitudinal study conducted by Getzels and Csikszentmihalyi (1976) suggests many of these traits are a recipe for failure in the contemporary art world.

A Longitudinal Study of Artistic Development and Artistic Success

The study involved 281 students at the prestigious Art Institute of Chicago. During the first phase of the study, the artists completed several personality questionnaires and engaged in problem-finding and problem-solving tasks designed to assess various dimensions of creativity. Twenty years later, 64 of the original 281 students were contacted. The primary focus of this second phase of the study was to identify and understand the factors that were most predictive of artistic success.

The picture that emerged was unexpected. Out of the handful of artists that did achieve some artistic success, the traits that distinguished them from their unrecognized peers were more characteristic of Wall Street marketing executives than what we have come to associate with artists. Compared with their less successful peers, these artists were more sociable, practical, and career-driven (Csikszentmihalyi et al. 1984). "Unless you are a social beast", said one of the artists, "it is naïve to think you are going to make it". They also demonstrated a willingness to sacrifice personal expressivity in the service of artistic recognition.

Instead of ignoring the business aspects of the art world, or pretending that they did not exist, the successful artists acknowledged, accommodated, and even embraced them. One artist put it this way: "Usually you can judge somebody's career orientation and ability in building a career by how good their career is. It has nothing to do with their art, it has everything to do with how they can build a career and who they know" (Freeman 1993, p. 115).

Consider Jim, the most successful artist of the sample. Like the handful of other successful artists in the group, Jim had an acute understanding of how the business side of the art world worked. He tailored his art to accommodate it. "You need to have a monotheistic thing on the surface for business reasons," he pointed out. "This is not Versace. This is Robert Hall. It's on the racks, like small, medium, and large. These are made to order." Jim held no illusions about where his art fit into the system: "[Art] exists as a vehicle for criticism and writing" (Freeman 1993, p. 193).

In art school, students whose traits resembled that of the archetypal artistic personality tended to be viewed by their teachers as very original and creative. But when students left school, those who lacked the extroversion, aggressiveness, and a knack for promoting themselves that attracted the attention of critics, gallery owners, and media tended to disappear from the art scene, never to be heard of again. Simpson (1981) went so far as to suggest that the "artistic mystique" has been perpetuated more by unsuccessful artists than successful artists, as a defense against artistic failure.

So we see that many of the traits traditionally associated with the artistic personality—nonconforming, socially aloof, impulsive—are incompatible with artistic success in the contemporary art world. The loft, the exhibition channels, the galleries, the New York art scene are all necessary steps a serious artist must be able and willing to negotiate. Yet these steps to success run counter to a large array of values and traits young artists hold dear and were encouraged to believe in. Today's art world is extremely inhospitable to the romantic image of the artist.

Conclusion

The systems perspective of the artistic personality admits that individual traits may be necessary for a person to be recognized as creative, but that these cannot be predicted a priori. The specific individual traits associated with the artistic personality will depend on characteristics of the other two subsystems, the domain of art and the field of art. A person who becomes a painter in a period when Abstract Expressionism is the reigning style will be more likely to be recognized if he or she possesses the emotional, imaginative, and introverted qualities that are well-suited for the creation of abstract, expressionistic art. Likewise, in a period when Photo Realism is in vogue, a cool, rational, and outward-oriented person will be more likely to make a contribution to the domain. Given the constantly evolving nature of both the domain of art and the field of art, the idea of the artistic personality as a timeless, constitutional personality type is therefore an improbable proposition.

The preceding analysis suggests that a construct as broad as the artistic *personality* may be of limited value if addressing questions related to individual differences in artistic creativity. Consider, for example, the relationship between psychopathology and artistic creativity. Though it seems reasonable to suggest a link between the psychological torment of artists like Frida Kahlo, James Ensor, and Vincent Van Gogh and their heavily affect-laden art, such a relationship in areas that allow for less self-expression (e.g., Photo-Realism, Minimalism, etc.) is highly questionable. Indeed, it is hard to imagine how psychopathology would be anything but a distraction.

It is important to keep in mind that our analysis has focused on one area of art, painting. In the highly diversified, "radical pluralism" (Danto 1998)[4] of today's postmodern art world, painting constitutes just one of many media available to artists, ranging from audio and video installations to the human body to the natural landscape. Given that each of these media involves unique artistic processes, we should expect the range of traits found among artists today to be even greater than our analysis in this chapter suggests.

Finally, it should be clear from all we have said that the same argument holds for any other profession or occupation. A biologist like Friedrich von Humboldt was an explorer, adventurer, and naturalist; a century and a half later, E. O. Wilson complains that the hegemony of molecular biology has transformed the domain into an abstract laboratory discipline (Csikszentmihalyi 1996). It is unlikely that the personality of individuals attracted to biology in Humboldt's time would be the same as those who join the field now. The links between a domain and the personality of those who work in it are not rigidly forged but change organically as the domain itself changes with time.

References

Barron, F. (1972). *Artists in the making*. New York: Seminar Press.
Barton, K., & Cattell, H. (1972). Personality characteristics of female psychology, science and art majors. *Psychological Reports, 31*, 807–813.
Csikszentmihalyi, M. (1996). *Creativity*. New York: HarperCollins.
Csikszentmihalyi, M., & Getzels, J. W. (1973). The personality of young artists: an empirical and theoretical exploration. *British Journal of Psychology, 64*(1), 91–104.
Csikszentmihalyi, M., Getzels, J. W., & Kahn, S. P. (1984). *Talent and achievement (Report)*. Chicago: Spencer and MacArthur Foundations.
Cupchik, G. C. (1974). An experimental investigation of perceptual and stylistic dimensions of paintings suggested by art history. In D. E. Berlyne (Ed.), *Studies in the new experimental aesthetics* (pp. 235–257). New York: Wiley.

---

[4] Also referred to, less favorably, as the "post-Warholian nightmare".

Danto, A. (1998). *After the end of art: Contemporary art and the pale of history.* Princeton: Princeton University Press.

Dudek, S. Z., & Marchand, P. (1983). Artistic style and personality in creative painters. *Journal of Personality Assessment, 47*(2), 139–142.

Freeman, M. (1993). *Finding the muse.* Cambridge: Cambridge University Press.

Fromm, E. (1978). Primary and secondary process in waking and in altered states of consciousness. *Journal of Altered States of Consciousness, 4,* 115–128.

Getzels, U. J. W., & Csikszentmihalyi, M. (1976). *The creative vision: A longitudinal study of problem finding in art.* New York: Wiley.

Greenberg, C. (1940). Towards a newer Laocoon. *Partisan Review, 3,* 296–310.

Gruber, H. (1988). The evolving systems approach to creative work. *Creativity Research Journal, 1*(1), 27–51.

Harrington, D. M. (1990). The ecology of human creativity: a psychological perspective. In M. A. Runco & R. S. Albert (Eds.), *Theories of creativity* (pp. 143–169). Newbury Park: Sage.

Hauser, A. (1951). *The social history of art.* New York: Vintage.

Kimmelman, M. (1998). *Portraits: talking with artists at the met, the modern, the louvre, and elsewhere.* New York: Random House.

Kubler, G. (1962). *The shape of time.* New Haven: Yale University Press.

Loomis, M., & Saltz, E. (1984). Cognitive styles as predictors of artistic styles. *Journal of Personality, 52*(1), 22–35.

Lucie-Smith, E. (1999). *Lives of the great twentieth century artists.* London: Thames and Hudson.

Ludwig, A. (1998). Method and madness in the arts and sciences. *Creativity Research Journal, 11*(2), 93–101.

Lyons, L., & Storr, R. (1987). *Chuck close.* New York: Rizzoli.

Martindale, C. (1990). *The clockwork muse.* New York: Basic Boob.

Rosenberg, H. (1972). *The de-definition of art.* Chicago: University of Chicago Press.

Seuphor, M. (1961). *Abstract painting: 50 years of accomplishment, from Kandinsky to the present* (Chevalier H, Trans.). New York: Harry Abrams.

Simonton, D. K. (1988). Age and outstanding achievement: what do we know after a century of research? *Psychological Bulletin, 104,* 163–180.

Simonton, D. K. (1990). Political pathology and societal creativity. *Creativity Research Journal, 3*(2), 85–99.

Simpson, C. R. (1981). *SoHo: the artist in the city.* Chicago: University of Chicago Press.

Solomon, D. (1987). *Jackson Pollock: A biography.* New York: Simon and Schuster.

Stein, M. I. (1953). Creativity and culture. *J Psychol, 36,* 311–322.

Stein, M. I. (1963). A transactional approach to creativity. In C. W. Taylor &. F. Barron (Eds.), *Scientific creativity* (pp. 217–227). New York: Wiley.

Storr, A. (1988). *Solitude: A return to the self.* New York: Free Press.

Vasari, G. (1959). *Lives of the artists,* Oxford, England: Oxford University Press, (Original work published 1550).

Vollard, A. (1986). *Degas, an intimate portrait.* New York: Dover.

Walker, A. M., Koestner, R., & Hum, A. (1995). Personality correlates of depressive style in autobiographies of creative achievers. *Journal of Creative Behavior, 29*(2), 75–94.

Wolrffin, H. (1929). *Principles of art history: The problem of the development of style in later art* (7th rev ed.). New York: Dover.

Chapter 15
Creativity Through the Life Span from an Evolutionary Systems Perspective

Mihaly Csikszentmihalyi and Jeanne Nakamura

What is Creativity?

Creativity has become such a commonly used term in the past few decades that everyone has formed an opinion about what it means, and there is no need to define it further. In this chapter, however, we are going to use the word in specific ways, so a few words of explanation may be useful to orient the reader. There are three main dichotomies we use, and if these are not clear, what follows might be confusing.

The first dichotomy is that between creativity with a capital C and with a lowercase *c*. Big C, or cultural creativity, refers to ideas or products that are original, are valued by society or some influential segment thereof, and are brought to completion (Csikszentmihalyi 1999; MacKinnon 1963; White 1968). This form of creativity changes the way we see, understand, and interact with the reality that surrounds us. It is the energy that propels cultural evolution. Most of this chapter deals with cultural creativity, both because it is a clearly important feature of human life and because it is the one about which most is known.

But one could argue that small c or personal creativity is just as important, if not more so. Personal creativity refers to the novel ideas or experiences that any person can have and that do not need to leave a trace anywhere else but in the consciousness of the person who has had them. A new hairdo, a shortcut in servicing one's car engine, a clever conversation may qualify. Although this form of creativity does not change the culture, it does make a vast difference to the quality of one's life—without it, existence would be intolerably drab.

These two meanings of the concept are usually thought of as being on the same continuum, the small c slowly growing into the big C. However, there are good

M. Csikszentmihalyi, *The Systems Model of Creativity*,
DOI: 10.1007/978-94-017-9085-7_15,
© Springer Science+Business Media Dordrecht 2014

reasons to consider them as relatively independent, orthogonal processes that are more different than similar, and this is how we treat the concepts here.

The second dichotomy pertains only to cultural creativity and concerns the dialectic between producers and audience. It is commonly assumed that big C creative ideas are self-sufficient, and thus creativity includes only what happens in the creative person's mind. Our approach assumes instead that without a receptive audience, the creative process is not unlike the sound of one hand clapping the Zen koan refers to. In other words, what we call creativity is co-constituted by an individual who comes up with a novelty and a social milieu that evaluates it (Brannigan 1981; Csikszentmihalyi 1988; Kasof 1995). At the very least, it should be obvious that creativity is always an attribution, and that it cannot be "seen" except when it has been so identified by some group (teachers, critics, historians) that has credibility in the eyes of society. The same is not true of personal creativity. For personal creativity, no external evaluation is necessary; only the subjective experience matters.

Finally, the third dichotomy refers to that between the distal and proximal accounts of why some people bother being creative. Distal explanations present the creative drive as motivated by the desire for fame and wealth—or, in light of the broader scope of evolutionary theory, by the selective forces of survival pressures. Although distal explanations account in part for creative behavior, they ignore the momentary experience of the creative person, which motivates the search for novelty even when wealth and fame are extremely unlikely. Distal explanations tend to be extrinsic, pointing to an external goal that is usually objective and concrete, like money, a promotion, or a prize. Proximal explanations tend to be intrinsic, subjective in nature. In the case of creativity, the intrinsic rewards include the excitement of discovery, the satisfaction of solving a problem, and the joy of shaping sounds, words, or colors into new forms.

With these preliminary distinctions in hand, we proceed to examine some of the ways that moving through the life span affects creativity. We do this first by considering the implications of evolutionary theory for aging and creativity.

Creativity and Life Span Development from an Evolutionary Perspective

According to evolutionary psychology, currently a leading paradigm concerning human behavior, one might conclude that learning—and certainly creativity—are of little use in the second half of life; being useless, that they should eventually disappear from the human behavioral repertoire as wasteful of energy, to be replaced by concerns more conducive to reproductive fitness—such as taking care of one's offspring and of their descendants. Certainly there is a great amount of evidence to the effect that among all sorts of animals, including humans, the amount of spontaneous learning and some of the behaviors underlying creativity, such as curiosity and playfulness, decrease precipitously with age (Fagan 1981).

Play, exploration, curiosity, and innovation are linked behaviors in all species. Studies of animal play show a great interspecies variability in the age at which individuals start and stop playing. Wildebeest and caribou infants start prancing playfully a few hours after birth, apparently to discourage predators from attacking them (Estes 1976). In general, however, play ceases around the time an individual first reproduces "because play at successively later ages yields successively fewer cumulative benefits and because resources devoted to reproduction are more effective for producing surviving offspring than are resources devoted to adult play" (Fagan 1981, p. 378).

Creativity has not been directly studied in nonhuman species with reference to age. Anecdotal evidence suggests that behavioral flexibility and innovation are much more likely to be shown by younger individuals. For example, Japanese macaques were observed to have trouble eating the fruits placed for them on the ground, where they were immediately covered with sand. After some time, a young female accidentally dropped a sweet potato in the water, and when she retrieved it, the fruit emerged nice and clean. After this the juvenile went on washing its fruit, and presently her mother and siblings began to imitate her (Kawai 1965). There seems to be no evidence that older males caught on to the new practice. Before one immediately jumps to conclusions about the effects of the Y chromosome on creativity, it is useful to consider the fact that Japanese macaque females, although not the dominant sex, take more of the responsibility for the maintenance of social order than males (see, e.g., Altmann 1980). This in turn suggests that the diffusion of innovation may be linked to concern for the well-being of the social network. Adult individuals who fill certain roles in the group may be more able to notice innovations and be more likely to adopt them and diffuse them than others.

In this respect it is important to recognize that the adoption of useful new ideas or practices is as important for creativity as the creative act itself. Psychologists have long accepted the popular assumption that "genius will out," meaning that a creative act will prevail and impose itself on the culture regardless of opposition. A more likely scenario is that original ideas become creative only when a critical mass of the audience recognizes them as worthy of attention. According to this systems model, creativity is co-constituted by an individual who introduces a novelty that is selected, preserved, and transmitted over time by a field of experts, or in the case of items of mass culture such as soft drinks or movies, by the market as a whole (Csikszentmihalyi 1996, 1998; Csikszentmihalyi and Wolfe 2000).

According to this model, then, the relation between creativity and age is not restricted to the individual who initiates the creative process but extends to the audience as well. The recent interest in "cultural creatives" (Anderson and Ray 2001) and in a "creative class" (Florida 2002) can be more appropriately seen as referring to audiences that are susceptible to the adoption of new ideas or products, rather than to those who are actually producing creatively. Thus one might ask: Are older adults more or less likely to recognize and adopt new ideas, practices, or artifacts than teenagers or younger adults?

Before reviewing the empirical evidence for the link between creativity and age among humans, it may be useful to consider the theoretical implications of the evolutionary perspective. To what extent is it true that among us "resources devoted to adult play [or to creativity]" are less effective than resources devoted directly to reproduction? The peculiar survival strategy of *Homo sapiens* has always rested on the use of the cortex, on the processing and abstracting of complex information. This is becoming increasingly true as we enter what has been called a "knowledge economy" or an "information age" (Drucker 1985, 1999). With useful information and new knowledge constantly coming on line, for many thousands of years now it has been advantageous for individual men and women to retain some of their exploratory curiosity, some of their playfulness and creativity. Even from a purely sociobiological standpoint, to invest energy in new learning may often be a more effective strategy for the propagation and survival of one's genes than investing energy in more conservative, traditional ways of accruing resources.

Some evolutionary psychologists are beginning to reevaluate the role of creativity in the transmission of genes. For example, Miller (2000) argued that creative individuals, especially those working in artistic domains, are more likely to be attractive to the opposite sex and thus reproduce relatively more often. Genius is a "fitness indicator" in that it is rare, valued, and takes time to develop; it is also an "ornament that appeals to the senses," thereby attracting potential mates (Miller 2000). A similar argument has been advanced by Blackmore (1999).

Two observations are appropriate in considering these extensions of the theory of sexual selection to creativity. In the first place, the reproductive advantage of creativity presumably extends to adulthood but not to old age—yet many great creative accomplishments come late in life. Second, evolutionary explanations of behavior are always distal; that is, they account for why a given behavior survives over time, as the cumulative effects of that behavior over many generations of individuals have a chance to be selected in competition with the behaviors of other individuals who do not engage in that behavior. But evolutionary explanations have little or nothing to say about proximal causes—the ones that actually motivate the individual in his or her lifetime.

Play behavior, for example, is explained by the evolutionary perspective in terms of the advantages that an adult will have if he or she played as a child. Compared to other adults who did not play extensively early in life, such a person may be slightly more savvy at interpersonal relations, better controlled, better able to compete within a clear set of rules, and so on. These are all distal reasons, however. Children do not play because they expect to become more successful adults. They play because it's fun. The proximal reason for playing is that the experience is enjoyable. A similar distinction between distal and proximal explanation holds for creativity as well. Whatever the long-term advantages it confers, the reason people involve themselves in the processes of discovery and invention is that nothing in "normal" life compares with the experience (Csikszentmihalyi 1996).

But with human beings there is perhaps an even more important difference for expecting creativity and learning to continue throughout life. As a species we are dependent on the social milieu to teach us the accumulated experience of innumerable ancestral generations. Other social organisms—such as ants, termites, or coyotes—also depend on the group to which they belong, but not for learning—what they will ever know is already programmed in their genes. Even though experience within the group is necessary to unlock most of this programmed knowledge, there is little or no evidence of unprecedented behaviors arising in such groups, unless as a result of genetic mutation. As humans we inherit not only our ancestral genes but also the memes (Csikszentmihalyi 1993; Dawkins 1976)—the units of useful information—that our forebears have discovered and that are then packaged into myths, histories, philosophies, technology, and science.

Societies that can use past information efficiently tend to provide more comfortable environments and longer life spans for their inhabitants. Such societies presumably encourage continued learning and creativity not only in childhood, but later and later into adulthood. And as more innovative individuals live longer in such societies, this mutual synergy may place in motion a benign spiral of individual and social improvement.

Creativity and Physical Aging

In terms of the relationship between creativity and adult development, it is useful to distinguish between the effects of physical and social aging. However, it is quite difficult to untangle the purely physical effects of aging from those due to social aging. Clear physiological effects include declines in memory functions in old age, impairment of fluid intelligence, and loss of energy. These changes, however, are of relatively little consequence to many forms of creativity. In many ways, social aging is more consequential. This involves passing through social roles that require different behaviors from the person, either enhancing or jeopardizing his or her creativity. Social aging will be discussed in the following section; here we review the scant information available on the purely physiological impact of aging on creativity.

Contrary to popular belief, age—even considerable old age—need not be an impediment to creativity, Michelangelo was 79 years old when he painted the strikingly original frescoes in the Pauline Chapel of the Vatican. Benjamin Franklin was 78 when he developed the bifocal lens for eyeglasses, Giuseppe Verdi composed the opera *Falstaff* at 80, and he never wrote anything as joyfully playful as that composition in the 60 years of his musical career. Frank Lloyd Wright broke new architectural ground at age 91 with the building of the Guggenheim Museum in Manhattan. One could go on and on with examples that show how originality and perseverance need not decrease until the very end of life.

It is true that beginning with the 7th decade of life, it is usual to report a waning of energy and troubles with memory and sustained effort, especially in tasks requiring what has been called "fluid intelligence" (Cattell 1963). However, age decrements in intellectual functioning appear to be less severe than they were once held to be (Schaie 1996), and they may be more than compensated for by increased knowledge that accrues with life experience (Baltes and Staudinger 2000).

It is likely that age presents more obstacles to scientific than to artistic creativity (e.g., Chandrasekhar quoted in Wali 1991; Lehman 1953). In our study of creativity in later life (Csikszentmihalyi 1996; Nakamura and Csikszentmihalyi 2003), some of the scientists complained that memory decrements were constraining the assimilation of new knowledge, or learning, needed for creative work. For example, a scientist in his 90s observed that he can no longer store and retrieve effortlessly the information he reads. Another complains, "At my age it's a lot harder to learn all these techniques.... You think how lucky children are..., I get discouraged... mathematics comes easily to me. And physics... [But] all the experimental side... running the programs, does not come easily." (All excerpts quoted in this chapter refer to interview transcripts collected during the Creativity in Later Life Study; see Csikszentmihalyi (1996), Nakamura and Cskiszentmihalyi (2003).)

At 75, one social scientist whose research plate is overflowing, cast an interested eye toward a neighboring specialty, but noted, "that is not anything that I am ever going to get into... I would not even have the memory." A busy physicist's reasoning was somewhat different: The demands of learning a controversial new paradigm would have required putting aside his ongoing, engaging work; besides, the new area did not promise to lead to the kind of "final" or "complete" answers that this scientist finds satisfying.

Faced with demands to assimilate new ideas and particularly new technologies to do creative work, many scientists are clearly aided by the resources accruing from earlier achievements. Some rely on collaborators' knowledge of new technologies, others on support staff's ability to use computers. In other words, above and beyond their continuing impact on productivity, the external resources at the disposal of eminent individuals can substitute for having to engage in new learning.

Social interaction is a major means of staying current in certain domains, such as physics. Some scientists even return to the role of student, violating expectations concerning the conduct of distinguished older scholars. Vibrant examples of late-life learning were provided by two eminent physicists, both still active in their eighties. In recent years, each has sought younger experts at other universities in a specialty that they wished to learn. One explained: "I realized that there is a development in general relativity that I ought to learn about and I did not know.... So I got up on my hind feet and phoned and made an appointment and spent 2 days there talking with people, both this fall and the previous fall."

At the age of 80, this scientist flew from the East Coast to the Midwest to consult with a former college student who had just entered the University of Chicago. Thus, relying on networks of informants can compensate to a large extent for not being able to keep up personally with the progress of disciplinary knowledge.

Investigations of creativity based on the historiometric method pioneered by Lehman (1953), Dennis (1956), and recently expanded by Simonton (1999) and Martindale (1990), have attempted to establish the optimal ages at which creative contributions are typically made. These approaches involve arranging the achievements of a scientist or artist in chronological order and plotting them along the life span axis of the creator. In a recent review, Simonton (1999, p. 120) claimed: "Illustrious creators can be examined from the moment of conception to the very instant of death, plus everything that takes place within this long interval." However, a problem historiographers encounter is that one cannot determine from the published record when the creative ideas actually occurred. A revolutionary idea hatched in early life may not be fully developed until maturity or later; thus the attribution of a specific date for the creative accomplishment is often inaccurate.

Nevertheless, the application of this method makes it possible to come up with some generalizations about the life histories of creative people. Dennis (1966) and Lehman (1960) concluded that the peak of "superior output" for creative people occurs at age 30—the age at which Mozart composed the *Marriage of Figaro* and Edison invented the phonograph. In all, 40 % of all major contributions to the culture were made in that decade of life. Half as many (20 % each) occurred at ages 20 and 40; and the remaining 20 % were spread over the rest of life. One possible contaminant of such results is the inclination to project a more inflated evaluation of the early work of well-known creators based on their lifetime output. In any case, it is impossible to ascertain the extent to which the decline after 40 years of age is due to physical causes or to the social changes associated with age that will be discussed in the next section.

Simonton (1999, p. 122) summarizes six age-linked findings about creativity: Creative individuals tend not to be firstborn; they are intellectually precocious; they suffer childhood trauma; their families tend to be economically and/or socially marginal; they receive special training early in life; and they benefit from role models and mentors. Most of these conclusions relate to the earlier years of life, indicating the lack of systematic knowledge about creativity in the second half of life.

The relation of age to creativity is likely to depend on the particular domain in which the person is operating: "The overall age functions, including the placement of the first, best, and last creative contribution, are contingent upon the specific domain of creative activity" (Simonton 1999, p. 122). To determine answers to questions such as "Why do mathematicians and lyric poets do their most original work earlier in life than, say, architects or philosophers?" one cannot simply consider changes in the maturation of the creative person's brain. One must also explore the interaction between the mind and the symbolic system of the domain and the social constraints and opportunities of the field. For example, in symbolic domains that are very well integrated, like mathematics, chess, or musical performance, it is relatively easy for a talented person to move quickly to the cutting edge of the domain and thus be well positioned to innovate in it. In domains that are less logically ordered, such as musical composition, literature, and philosophy, there is less agreement as to what the most urgent issues are. Specialized knowledge is not enough; one needs to reflect on a great amount of experience before being able to say something new. Therefore one would expect important new contributions in these domains to be made later in life.

Social Aging: The Effects of the Field on Creativity

Although there is not much that can be said about the purely physiological effects of age on creativity, it is clear that as a person matures into adulthood and then old age, there will be many changes that affect his or her productivity, in both positive and negative ways. These changes are the consequence of different roles that the creative person is likely to play in the field, beginning as an apprentice, and then becoming an expert practitioner, and finally a gatekeeper. Each of these roles provides different opportunities and demands different responsibilities.

Careers in science or the arts—or for that matter, in any other domain as well— are rarely a matter of smooth sailing. As Thomas Kuhn, historian of science, noted, new ideas are rarely adopted by the leading figures in the field whose fame rests on an older paradigm. Instead, it is the younger scientists who wish to prove their mettle who adopt new ideas and try to change the domain (Kuhn 1962). Or as Pierre Bourdieu, French sociologist, wrote:

> The history of the field arises from the struggle between the established figures and the young challengers. The ageing of authors, schools, and works is far from being the product of a mechanical, chronological slide into the past; it results from the struggle between those who have made their mark... and who are fighting to persist, and those who cannot make their own mark without pushing into the past those who have an interest in stopping the clock (Bourdieu 1993, p. 60).

Sooner or later, a promising scientist usually becomes head of a lab, takes on duties in scientific societies, edits journals, writes textbooks, and serves on innumerable committees. Similar changes await successful artists who become public property of agents, collectors, and foundations. In this way, cutting-edge work can become restricted with advancing age; Older scientists may stop doing bench work in the lab to take on administrative positions, and older artists may become distracted from the voice of the muse by their lionizing audience.

The observation that over the course of a career one's training ages was made by Zuckerman and Merlon (1972). They noted both the possibility of career obsolescence that aging scientists may encounter and the disadvantages that neophytes in a discipline may face. Attention is finite at any age, and during the late career it may be further limited by accumulated obligations and by the slowing that accompanies physiological aging. Most original scientists and artists are primarily concerned with their own creative work. Staying abreast of developments in the wider domain or in other disciplines thus competes for attention with their own evolving work agenda. On the other hand, this agenda itself impels learning. Scientists described "trying to audit" the literature and attending seminars to hear colleagues present "hot new findings." Artists need to stay in touch with new developments on the art scene as well as new techniques. A social scientist in his fifties said:

I learn something new every year. I mean, a major area, like I'll learn a new mathematics.... Last year I studied anthropology a lot and learned about primate behavior...

So that's the other philosophy I have, which is to learn something about everything and have a wide variety of experiences because you never know, and over the years, those experiences come in handy, I think. It's a well-known statement about inventions that what you really need is some luck and a prepared mind. So I've worked hard to have a prepared mind.

The eminent older scientist plays roles other than that of an innovator; these, too, may occasion exposure to new knowledge. Gatekeeping roles, such as editing professional journals, may have this impact. A social scientist in his sixties who had recently founded a new journal, noted that it would "force me to read some kinds of things that I wanted to read, because as the editor I really need to"; "I've never paid as much attention to work by other people as I should pay." Teaching can be a way either of staying current within a domain ("students in a sense are telling us what's going on at the frontier") or of broadening one's knowledge ("the heterogeneity of inquiry and interest that come with teaching give you more back-burners to opportunistically develop"). Informal discussions with junior collaborators and other colleagues and attending conferences may have the same effect.

How extraneous demands impinge on the time and attention of renowned artists was conveyed by Canadian writer Robertson Davies, who at age 80 commented:

> One of the problems about being a writer today is that you are expected to be a kind of public show and public figure and people want your opinions about politics and world affairs and so forth, about which you don't know any more than anybody else, but you have to go along or you'll get a reputation of being an impossible person, and spiteful things would be said about you, (Csikszentmihalyi 1996, p. 206).

A similar situation is described by physicist Eugene Wigner, who recalled the sudden change in status of physical scientists after the harnessing of nuclear power at the end of World War II:

> By 1946, scientists routinely acted as public servants… addressing social and human problems from a scientific viewpoint. Most of us enjoyed that, vanity is a very human property…. We had the right and even perhaps the duty to speak out on vital political issues. But on most political questions, physicists had little more information than the man on the street (Wigner 1992, p. 254).

As the original contributions of a person are beginning to be recognized by the field, the power of the creative person as gatekeeper and leader grows apace. Ironically, but as might be expected, this rarely translates into greater creative output. Fields may restrict opportunities for creative work by escalating expectations for administrative and statesmanlike activities. And finally, the social system in which the fields are embedded may distract successful creative individuals by diluting their focus of attention from the tasks they are best qualified to perform. For instance, scientists often complain that policy makers mistake their specialized expertise for a more general wisdom and ask them to sit on committees and boards where their expertise is no better than that of the average person on the street.

In line with these considerations, the literature has focused from the start on the related questions of whether older scientists resist new paradigms or indeed actively obstruct a field's embrace of new ideas or conversely, whether they become significant contributors to the new areas themselves. In other words, literature has been concerned about the actions of the older scientist in the role of gatekeeper as much as innovator (Zuckerman and Merlon 1972, p. 309). A variety of mechanisms that could account for age-associated resistance have come to be recognized, such as the force of accrued social and intellectual investments. In addition, counter findings have also emerged, for which possible mechanisms have been suggested. In particular, older eminent scientists may be better equipped than the young to endorse revolutionary ideas when these are first publicized, because they have already achieved their professional goals and are less concerned with defending orthodox positions.

As stated earlier, the systems model suggests that the distinction between the contribution of new ideas and their adoption is not as crucial as it seems from an individualistic perspective on creativity. If the adoption of novelty is as important as its discovery, then even those scientists and artists who have abandoned active work but still exercise leadership in the field are indispensable to creativity. Thus, perhaps a better question to ask is, what does a gatekeeper have to do to contribute to creativity?

Obviously, remaining open to novelty and staying abreast of new developments are prerequisites. If gate-keepers are too rigid, the domain becomes starved for new ideas and eventually declines. But a domain can be destroyed just as well by gatekeepers who are too open to novelty and who, by admitting every fad, destroy the integrity of the domain. Thus "conservatism in science is not all bad" (Hull 1988, p. 383). Perhaps it is better to speak of skepticism rather than conservatism, in which resisting the new and clinging to the old are coupled. The shift would be consistent with Hull's basic insight ("No one complains that scientists, young or old, resisted novel theories that we now take to be mistaken").

Our data suggest an additional way in which the appearance of aged conservatism might be created. One 79-year-old Nobel laureate in economics expressed the kind of spirited rejection of a current fad in his discipline that might seem to be a typical example of resistance to new ideas with old age:

I'm about to give a speech next week... at a conference, in which I'm going to denounce the work that's been going on for 10 years... which I think has been relatively format and sterile, but it's been done by all the smart people. They've, lots of them, gotten their professorships very young.... I'm predicting that it's reaching the end of it's period of joy and happiness. Very, very clever people working on very special problems... and I think it's become a very scholastic enterprise. In the way we use that language to denounce the medieval church teachings and so forth, and that it will fail, although you can have a run with it in the market. We have fads in science.

However, from a life span perspective, a different possibility merits attention: that this scientist has challenged new ideas throughout his career, so that the upcoming speech represents a form of continuity rather than a swing toward conservatism. And, indeed, this scientist observes:

One characteristic I have, and you'd get that if you asked other people about me, is that I always have a non-faddish view of things. If a theory sweeps the profession, I'll be the last guy that accepts it, in general. I've been a critic, for example, of... the rage of the '30s, and wrote on it... I wrote what was maybe the standard refutation of [another theory], after it became very widespread. So I don't have any instincts to say that since everybody's doing it, that's right. I've more the instinct: "Well, hey, are they looking at it hard enough and from enough different attitudes?"

As this scientist readily notes, the maverick stance means that he has also been slow to accept ideas that later become "the universal truth." Nevertheless, skepticism was mentioned by a number of respondents as a valuable attribute in those who aspire to make original contributions to a domain. In this light, it is conceivable that skeptical scientists do important work, attain eminence, and go on to become eminent—and still skeptical—older scientists. A question for future investigators is: Does a characteristic skepticism come to be viewed differently by other members of the community when a scientist is old? The structure of the domain and the field are important in determining whether someone will continue to produce useful new ideas or things, but it is even more important to preserve the personal drive for playfulness and discovery.

Preserving the Passion

If there is one trait that a person must possess to continue on a creative trajectory, it is curiosity. Without a strong dose of curiosity a promising artist or scientist will be tempted to settle for a comfortable career that does not require the risk of striving for novelty. In our studies of creativity in later life, we found this trait mentioned over and over by creative respondents. "I am incredibly curious," said a neuropsychologist; "I am relentlessly curious," said a well-known composer; "I am enormously curious," said an astronomer. Joshua Lederberg, a leading geneticist, admitted to a "voracious curiosity." Cognitive scientist Donald Norman claimed that the "one thing I try to do, is always be curious and inquiring."

This curiosity does not concern just the work at hand, but often extends to the broadest issues imaginable. Nadine Gordimer, the Nobel Prize—winning novelist, explained when she was interviewed in our study of creativity in later life:

Writing is a form of exploration of life.... Of course, some people have a ready-made structure of explanation. People who have a strong religion, no matter what it is. Whether you're a Christian or a Muslim or a Jew or whatever. You have got an explanation of why you're here... what the purpose is and what the future is. That you're going to go to Heaven or whatever it is, or you're going to become part of the universal spirit; there's an explanation for your life. What if you haven't got that?

John Wheeler, one of the most distinguished theoretical physicists in the world, said that past 80 years of age he is still driven by "a desperate curiosity. I like that Danish poem... 'I'd like to know what this show is all about before it's out.' To me that is the number one thing—to find out how the world works."

In most cases, this curiosity was present in early life. There is no question that if one wished to increase the frequency of creative ideas through life, the place to start would be in trying to enhance the curiosity of children. A distinguished astronomer recalls:

When I think about my childhood, I was enormously curious. I mean, I can actually think of questions that... I don't know how old I was, I certainly wasn't ten, I might have been six....I mean really in my childhood... things that puzzled me about the physical universe. I mean, I can even remember asking questions like "why, when we drove down the road the moon was following us?" I mean I could give you five questions that bothered me as a child.... I just had an enormous curiosity from the very beginning and just wanted to do these things.... I was just curious about how things work and I was trying to—and after a while I learned that the questions that I was most curious about no one knew the answer to. So, if I wanted to get the answer I had to go out and observe and do these things myself. But in a sense it was to learn the answer to these very curious questions that drove me.

John Wheeler again: "I can remember I must have been 3 or 4 years old in the bathtub and my mother bathing me, and I was asking her how far does the universe go, and the world go, and beyond that"

A neuropsychologist recalls:

The thing that has driven me my whole life—and I have always said this and I know is true. It is curiosity. I am incredibly curious about things, little things I see around me.... My mother used to think that I was just very inquisitive about other people's business. But it was not just people it is... it is things around me. I am a noticer. I am sure much less now than when I was young. But it is noticing quirks, the things that patients do or that people do. And then I wonder why and I want to investigate it.

Oscar Peterson, renowned jazz pianist, grew up in an African American family in Montreal, and he recalls the curiosity that drove him as a child and still drives him approaching 70 years of age:

I was mischievous. I admit it I was always seeking projects to do, you know. Finding out what made things work, things that I shouldn't be fooling with.... I remember destroying a phonograph once, under the guise of repairing it And things like that. I wasn't a bad child, in the sense that I'd go out and start fires or beat up neighborhood kids or anything like that. But I was always into little nooks and crannies, getting my nose into things it shouldn't have been into. I was a very curious child.

For most creative individuals, this early curiosity is preserved through the years, and becomes a lifelong project. Gunther Schuller, one of the most original composers of our time, stated: "I'm the eternal student. I always want to learn more and study more, because... the longer I live, the more I realize that as much as I know, it's very little in the overall scheme of things. And the more I learn, the more I learn how much more there is to learn....it's an endless process."

Astronomer Vera Rubin repeats the same theme:

But, yes, just the curiosity of how the universe works.... I still have this feeling. When I am out observing at a very dark site on a clear night and I look at the stars, I stilt really wonder how you could do anything but be an astronomer, and that's the truth. How could you live looking up at those stars and just not spend your life learning about what's going on. I think when I was young I had no concept that the things that were puzzling me no one knew the answer to. I thought it was just like learning math. You just went to a book and you would learn all about these things. And I think that is the way that children's books and elementary books are written. I think the understanding of how little we know came much, much later.

This intrinsically motivated desire to learn is an organic part of the process of answering a question for oneself; it accompanies and feeds creativity. It differs from learning obliged by membership in the field (the need to maintain mastery, expertise), which can actually displace or discourage curiosity if it becomes too absorbing an obligation.

The neuropsychologist comments on the danger of being caught up in the concerns of the field, rather than following one's own interests and intuition:

So I like to see people curious and interested in things around them, including the patients and the atmosphere.... Where people are really having to do so much course work and... they are so busy doing that that the curiosity, or the adventure, the spirit of the adventure goes, and I think that, that is bad.

Creative persons take steps to make sure that the pressures placed on them by the expectations of the field do not stifle their passion for discovery. Natalie Davis, one of the most original and respected historians of her generation, said.

It's hard to be creative when you are just doing something doggedly.... If I felt my curiosity was limited, I think that the novelty part of it would be gone. Because it is the curiosity that has often pushed me to think of ways of finding out about something that people... previously thought you could never find out about or ways of looking at a subject that have never been looked at before. That's what keeps me running back and forth to the library, and just thinking and thinking and thinking and thinking.

Many other variables enter the equation that preserves creativity throughout life —from dogged perseverance to sheer luck. In fact, when asked to explain their lifelong success, creative individuals most often mentioned luck. Being at the right place at the right time was seen by many of them as the main difference that separated them from less successful peers. But curiosity, the desire to learn, seems to be one characteristic that is absolutely necessary. Without it, the temptation to abandon the quest for novelty becomes too strong; it is so much easier to rest on one's laurels and reap the benefits of one's early accomplishments.

The satisfaction of curiosity is the intrinsic reward that keeps a person struggling against high odds in an effort to come up with a new and more accurate perception of reality.

Personal Creativity

Whereas cultural creativity depends on many extraneous factors over which a person has no control—access to the domain, to the field, and sheer good fortune—personal creativity with a small c is something everyone can learn to develop. The one trait necessary for both kinds of creativity is curiosity. Individuals who are not interested in new knowledge and new experiences, who do not enjoy the thrill of discovery, are handicapped in both their professional and personal lives. The study of personal creativity, however, is still in its infancy and very little can be said about it with any authority.

Some persons, like the big C individuals quoted, are lucky in having had families that encouraged their curiosity from early on. We do not know to what extent it is possible to compensate for the lack of a stimulating early environment in later life. It is not easy to reverse habits of bored acceptance of the status quo, but perhaps it is not impossible.

At the end of our study of creativity (Csikszentmihalyi 1996, Chap. 14), a few steps for reawakening curiosity and interest were suggested. For instance, one should endeavor to be surprised each day by some experience. Even the simplest sight, sound, person, or conversation can reveal unexpected aspects if we take the trouble to attend to them with full attention. As Dewey (1934) pointed out long ago, the essence of an aesthetic experience lies in perception, which he differentiated from recognition, or the routine noticing of things that does not reveal anything new about them. Learning to perceive means being able to temporarily suspend the generic characteristics of experience and focus instead on their uniqueness. With time, the habit of perception is likely to grow into the kind of curiosity that fuels personal creativity.

Another way to break long-established routines is to surprise yourself, or others, by something you do, Instead of acting out the predictable scenario of one's personality, it helps occasionally (and appropriately) to say something unexpected, to express an opinion that one had not dared express before, to ask a question one would not ordinarily ask. It helps to take up new activities, try new clothes and new restaurants, and go to shows and museums.

As a result of breaking routine ways of experiencing and living, one might stumble on activities or interests that are enjoyable and meaningful. At that point, it makes sense to take one's experience seriously and devote more attention and time to those experiences that provide the greatest rewards. We spend far too much time doing things that are neither fun nor productive. Passive entertainment, for example, is often actually quite boring. Television viewing—which is the single most time-consuming activity people do in their free time—has many of the characteristics of addiction (Kubey and Csikszentmihalyi 2002). The more one watches the less enjoyable it is, yet the harder it is to break the habit.

What we are suggesting here about making one's life more interesting is not the same as in the Chinese curse; "May you lead an interesting life." The curse's meaning of *interesting* has the same sense as the word has in literature and the movies: The interest comes from outside in the form of danger, drama, risk, and tragedy. What makes life interesting for creative persons does not depend on external factors. It is the ability to endow even the most common experience with wonder and curiosity that makes their lives interesting. Leonardo da Vinci, who shaped our culture as deeply as any other person, led a life that to a superficial observer would have appeared miserly and drab (see Reti 1974). When he walked through the slums of Milan, looking at the peeling plaster on walls that would suggest to him new ways of representing the wonderful landscapes that formed the backgrounds for his paintings, few recognized the depth and reach of the thoughts soaring through his mind.

Many other suggestions could be reviewed, but it can all be summarized in a short principle: To increase personal creativity in one's life, one must take charge of how one perceives the world and of what one does in it. Creativity in any form does not come cheap; it requires commitment and perseverance. With some effort one can develop those habits of allocating attention that will result in realizing the awesome complexity of existence. After that, increasing joy at discovering more of its facets should sustain a life that thrives on growth and novelty rather than uniform routine.

Conclusions

Creative involvement with the world is an essential component of cultural evolution (big C creativity), and a source of enrichment in an individual's life (small c). Comparative psychology suggests that the playful, exploratory behavior underlying creativity diminishes rapidly with age and hardly exists after the reproductive age. With humans, however, whether there is decline depends on a variety of factors. First, creativity depends on the domain in which a person works; second, it depends on the opportunities and obstacles that the field offers the person; and finally, it depends on whether the person is able to sustain curiosity, interest, and passion. In many branches of the arts and some of the sciences, creative accomplishment continues until the end of life. Although the structure of the domain and the field are important in determining whether someone will continue to produce useful new ideas or things, it is even more important to preserve the personal drive for discovery.

What is true of big C creativity also applies to the ordinary, everyday kind that fails to be noticed and adopted by the culture. Here, however, the passion itself suffices; a person who can find novelty and excitement in the beauty of life in all its manifestations need not accomplish anything of note. Just experiencing life with full involvement will be a reward more important than fame and success.

References

Altmann, J. (1980). *Baboon mothers and infants*. Cambridge: Harvard University Press.
Anderson, S. R., & Ray, P. H. (2001). *The cultural creatives*. New York: Three Rivers Press.
Baltes, P. B., & Staudinger, U. (2000). Wisdom: A meta-heuristic (pragmatic) to orchestrate mind and virtue toward excellence. *American Psychologist, 55*, 122–136.
Blackmore, S. (1999). *The meme machine*. Oxford: Oxford University Press.
Brannigan, A. (1981). *The social basis of scientific discoveries*. New York: Cambridge University Press.
Bourdieu, P. (1993). *The field of cultural production*. New York: Columbia University Press.
Cattell, R. B. (1963) Theory of fluid and crystallized intelligence: A critical experiment. *Journal of Educational Psychology, 54*, 1–22.
Csikszentmihalyi, M. (1988). Society, culture, and person: A systems view of creativity. In R. J. Sternberg (Ed.), *The nature of creativity: Contemporary psychological perspectives* (pp. 325–339). New York: Cambridge University Press.
Csikszentmihalyi, M. (1993). *The evolving self: A psychology for the third millennium*. New York: HarperCollins.
Csikszentmihalyi, M. (1996). *Creativity: Flow and the psychology of discovery and invention*. New York: HarperCollins.
Csikszentmihalyi, M. (1998). Creativity and genius: A systems perspective. In A. Steptoe (Ed.), *Genius and the mind* (pp. 39–66). Oxford: Oxford University Press.
Csikszentmihalyi, M. (1999). Implications of a systems perspective for the study of creativity. In R. J. Sternberg (Ed.), *Handbook of creativity* (pp. 313–335). Cambridge: Cambridge University Press.
Csikszentmihalyi, M., & Wolfe, R. (2000). New conceptions and research approaches to creativity: Implications of a systems perspective for creativity in education. In K. A. Heller, F. J. Monks, R. J. Sternberg, R. Subornik (Eds.), *International handbook of giftedness and talent* (pp 81–93). Nailsea: Elsevier Science.
Dawkins, R. (1976). *The selfish gene*. New York: Oxford University Press.
Dennis, W. (1956). Age and achievement: A critique. *Journal of Gerontology, 11*, 331–333.
Dennis, W. (1966). Creative productivity between the ages of 20 and 80 years. *Journal of Gerontology, 21*, 1–18.
Dewey, J. (1934). *Art as experience*. New York: Minton, Balch.
Drucker, P. F. (1985). *Innovation and entrepreneurship*. New York: Harper Business.
Drucker, P. F. (1999). *Management challenges for the 21st century*. New York: Harper Business.
Estes, R. D. (1976). The significance of breeding synchrony in the wildebeest. *East African Wildlife Journal, 14*, 135–152.
Fagan, R. (1981). *Animal play behavior*. New York: Oxford University Press.
Florida, R. (2002). *The rise of the creative class*. New York: Basic Books.
Hull, D. L. (1988). *Science as a process*. Chicago: University of Chicago Press.
Kasof, J. (1995). Explaining creativity: The attributional perspective. *Creativity Research Journal, 8*(4), 311–366.
Kawai, M. (1965). Newly-acquired pre-cultural behavior of the natural troop of Japanese monkeys on Koshima Islet. *Primates, 6*(1), 1–30.
Kubey, R., & Csikszentmihalyi, M. (2002). Television addiction. *Scientific American, 286*(2), 74–81.
Kuhn, T. S. (1962). *The structure of scientific revolutions*. Chicago: University of Chicago Press.
Lehman, H. C. (1953). *Age and achievement*. Princeton: Princeton University Press.
Lehman, H. C. (1960). The age decrement in outstanding scientific creativity. *American Psychologist, 15*, 128–134.
MacKinnon, D. W. (1963). Creativity and images of the self. In R. W. White (Ed.), *The study of lives*. New York: Atherton.

Martindale, C. (1990). *The clockwork muse: The predictability of artistic change*. New York: Basic Books.

Miller, G. (2000). *The mating mind: How sexual choices shaped the evolution of human nature*. New York: Random House.

Nakamura, J., & Csikszentmihalyi, M. (2003). The motivational sources of creativity as viewed from the paradigm of positive psychology. In L. G. Aspinwall & U. M. Staudinger (Eds.), *A psychology of human strengths* (pp. 257–270). Washington, DC: American Psychological Association.

Reti, L. (Ed.). (1974). *The unknown Leonardo*. New York: McGraw Hill.

Schaie, K. W. (1996). Intellectual development in adulthood. In J. E. Birren & K. W. Schaie (Eds.), *Handbook of the psychology of aging* (4th ed., pp. 266–286). San Diego: Academic Press.

Simonton, D. K. (1999). Creativity from a historiometric perspective. In R. J. Sternberg (Ed.), *Handbook of creativity* (pp. 116–136). New York: Cambridge University Press.

Wali, K. C. (1991). *Chandra*. Chicago: University of Chicago Press.

White, J. P. (1968). Creativity and education: A philosophical analysis. *British Journal of Educational Studies, 16*, 123–137.

Wigner, E. (1992). *The recollections of Eugene P*. Wigner: Plenum Press.

Zuckerman, H., & Merton, R. K. (1972). Age, aging, and age structure in science. In M. W. Riley, M. Johnson, & A. Foner (Eds.), *Aging and society* (Vol. 3, pp. 292–356). New York: Russell Sage Foundation.

Chapter 16
Cortical Regions Involved in the Generation of Musical Structures During Improvisation in Pianists

Sara L. Bengtsson, Mihaly Csikszentmihalyi and Fredrik Ullén

Introduction

Creative behaviors and creative individuals fascinate scientists and laymen alike, and studies of creativity have a long history in psychology (see, e.g., Simonton 1999; Sternberg 1999; Csikszentmihalyi 1997; Eysenck 1995). A precise, generally agreed-upon definition of what constitutes a creative behavior has been difficult to arrive at, however, although two characteristics seem central: Creative acts are novel or original and, qualified judges will agree that they constitute valuable contributions to the field (Sternberg 1999). The novelty aspect is critical, and tests designed to measure creative ability typically require *divergent* thinking, as opposed to the *convergent* problem-solving abilities measured by traditional intelligence tests. Convergent problems have a single answer. Divergent tasks have a large number of possible solutions, and the free generation and selection of alternatives among these possibilities are fundamental processes in creative behavior (Campbell 1960).

Although psychological research has provided valuable Information on both creativity as a trait and the characteristics of divergent thinking, little is still known about the brain mechanisms underlying creative behaviors. A few neuroimaging

S. L. Bengtsson · F. Ullén
Karolinska Institutet, Stockholm, Sweden

M. Csikszentmihalyi (✉)
Claremont Graduate University, Claremont, CA, USA
e-mail: Mihaly.Csikszentmihalyi@cgu.edu

M. Csikszentmihalyi, *The Systems Model of Creativity*,
DOI: 10.1007/978-94-017-9085-7_16,
© Springer Science+Business Media Dordrecht 2014

257

studies have Investigated of motor output and sensory feedback. However, the Improvise condition required storage in memory of the Improvisation, We therefore also included a condition FreeImp, where the pianist improvised but was instructed not to memorize his performance, To locate brain regions involved in musical creation, we investigated the activations in the Improvise–Reproduce contrast that were also present in FreeImp contrasted with a baseline rest condition. Activated brain regions included the right dorsolateral prefrontal cortex, the presupplementary motor area, the rostral portion of the dorsal premotor cortex, and the left posterior part of the superior temporal gyrus, We suggest that these regions are part of a network involved in musical creation, and discuss their possible functional roles. B more complex verbal tasks involving divergent thinking, such as story generation (Howard-Jones et al. 2005), sentence completion (Nathaniel-James and Frith 2002), generation of unusual verbs in response to nouns (Seger et al. 2000), and the Brick test of unusual uses of objects (Carlsson et al. 2000). These studies generally show an activation of cortical association areas, in particular, the prefrontal cortex, during divergent thinking. Interestingly, there appears to be a tendency for the right prefrontal cortex to be particularly involved (Howard-Jones et al. 2005; Carlsson et al. 2000; Seger et al. 2000; Abdullaev and Posner 1997). A major difficulty in the Investigation of more complex actions, however, is obviously to isolate the neurocognitive components responsible for controlling different aspects of the behavior.

A systematic investigation of neural processes underlying free selection has been performed using simpler model behaviors, as a part of studies of *willed action.* Willed actions involve "free" choice as well as attention, conscious awareness, and intentionality (Jahanshahi and Frith 1998). By studying tasks such as finger or hand movements (Lau et al. 2004; Frith 2000; Playford et al. 1992; Deiber et al. 1991) or number generation (Jahanshahl et al. 2000), and by comparing pseudorandom generation of responses with stereotyped actions, a number of cortical regions involved in free selection have been characterized. These include the dorsolateral prefrontal cortex (DLPFC), medial and lateral premotor areas, and the anterior cingulate cortex. This approach has enabled an elegant analysis of the various processes involved in free selection, such as attention to action, working memory, suppression of stereotype responses, and selection per se (Lau et al. 2004; Nathaniel-James and Frith 2002; Desmond et al. 1998).

However, an interesting question is whether the brain regions involved in free selection in simple willed actions are also utilized in more complex behaviors that could qualify as ecologically valid examples of creativity. In the present study, we investigated this issue using musical improvisation in professional pianists as a model. Improvisation arguably satisfies the demands of a prototypical creative behavior. It involves freely generated choices, but these must be adapted to ongoing performance, and monitored through auditory and somatosensory feedback, as well as to an overall aesthetic goal (Pressing 1988). It is simple enough, however, to allow an experimental design where the neural processes involved in the free generation of musical structures can be separated from those involved in the sequential organization and programming of the movements (i.e., piano playing), and the processing of movement feedback, To achieve this, we used one condition, *Improvise,* where the planist improvised on the basis of a visually displayed melody. In the control condition, *Reproduce,* the participant reproduced his previous improvisation from memory. The critical contrast, Improvise-Reproduce, was thus matched in terms of motor output and sensory feedback. Because the Improvise condition required storage of the improvisation in memory, we also included a third condition, *FreeImp,* where the pianist improvised but was instructed not to memorize his performance. To find brain regions involved in music generation, but not in memorization or motor programming, we examined which activations in the Improvise-Reproduce contrast were also present in a conjunction analysis between Improvise-Reproduce and FreeImp-Rest. Activity in the Improvise-Reproduce contrast was regressed on a measure of improvisation complexity in order to localize brain regions with a higher level of activity during the generation of more complex musical structures. Finally, differences in brain activity between FreeImp and Improvise were evaluated by contrasting these two conditions in brain regions that were active in Improvise–Reproduce.

Methods

Participants

Eleven professional Swedish concert pianists took part in the study. All participants were men, healthy, right-handed (Oldfield 1971), and had a Master's degree in the performing arts (piano) from the Royal Academy of Music in Stockholm. They were between 23 and 41 years old, with a mean age of 32.0 ± 6.0 years, and had started playing the piano between 4 and 8 years old (mean 5.7 ± 1.4 years). The experimental procedures were ethically approved by the Karolinska Hospital Ethical Committee (Dn 02.194) and were undertaken with the understanding and written consent of the participants.

Experimental Setup

Magnetic resonance (MR) imaging recordings were conducted on a 1,5-T scanner (Signa Horizon Echospeed, General Electric Medical Systems), During the functional magnetic resonance imaging (fMRI) scans, the participants played with their right hand on a small piano keyboard, especially designed for usage in an MR environment (LUMItouch, Inc.). The keyboard had one octave of 12 authentic keys (from F to E), and was connected to a PC computer through a fiber-optic cable. During scanning, the participant's performance on the keyboard was recorded on the PC, using the E-Prime software (Psychological Software Tools, Inc.). Auditory feedback from the piano was provided to the participant through headphones. The pianists were lying in a supine position, with the arm supported so that the keyboard could be played by moving the fingers and the wrist without arm movements. A plastic bite bar was used to restrict head movements.

A projector located outside the scanner room was used to project task instructions and musical scores onto a semitransparent screen, positioned approximately 3 m from the participants' eyes. The participants viewed the screen through a custom-made binocular/mirror system (Lorentzen Instrument AB) mounted directly on top of the head coil.

Conditions

All participants performed three conditions: Improvise, Reproduce, and Rest. These were performed in trials lasting 40 s, During the first 4 s of a trial, the name of the condition was projected onto the screen. For the Rest condition, the screen after this went blank for the remaining 36 s of the trial. For the other conditions, a musical score consisting of a simple eight-bar melody was displayed (Fig. 16.1a),

Fig. 16.1 Examples of a musical template and ornamentations used during improvisation. **a** One of the musical templates presented to the participants. **b** The five most common types of modification of templates used in improvise and FreeImp. Two bars of the original melody are shown to the *left* of the *double bar line*, and the improvised modification to the *right*

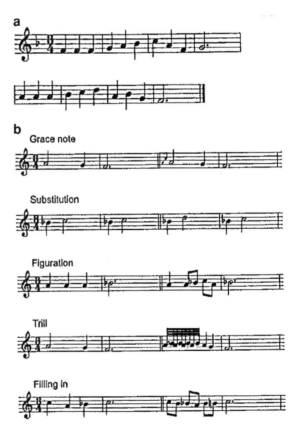

For a preparatory period of 8 s, the score was surrounded by a red, rectangular frame. This frame was then removed, signaling to the participant to start playing. These final 28 s of the trial, when the task was performed on the keyboard, were later used in the data analysis. A total of 12 musical scores of similar complexity were used in the study, six in F major, six in F minor. The main reason to use improvisation based on melodic templates, rather than completely free improvisation, was to make the improvisations more constrained, and thus, easier to remember. The scores were especially written for the present study, and thus, were unfamiliar to the participants. They were notated using the Finale music notation software (MakeMusic, Inc.).

In Improvise, the displayed melody was used as a basis for an improvisation. The Instructions to the participants were to employ any kind of modifications of the presented melodic template they wished, and when the improvisation was finished, to rest without any active movements until the next condition began (for examples of the employed modifications, see Figs. 16.1b and 16.3a, b). They were also instructed to memorize the performance for subsequent reproduction. In Reproduce, the task was to reproduce, as faithfully as possible, the improvisation previously made upon the same melody. In Rest, the participants relaxed, viewing the screen without any movements. Five of the participants performed an additional condition, FreeImp, where the instruction was to improvise on the melody, as in Improvise, but without trying to memorize the performance.

Experimental Procedure

Before the experiment, the participants were familiarized with the tasks and were given one practice trial of each condition outside the scanner room. When the participant was lying in the MR-scanner in a supine position, the conditions were practiced a second time. The pianists found the tasks enjoyable and interesting. The musical examples used during the practicing sessions were not used again during the experiment.

We started the experiment by collecting a high-resolution Tl-weighted anatomical image volume of the whole brain. Thereafter, fMRI data were recorded while the participants performed three sessions, each containing three trials of the different tasks. Musical scores were selected randomly from the database of 24 scores. For the same participant, a particular melody was only used once in each of the four conditions. Four such trials, where the same score was used, were always performed consecutively. To minimize task order effects, four different task orders were used in different sessions. A necessary constraint on the task order was obviously that Improvise had to be performed before Reproduce.

MRI Scanning Parameters

The imaging parameters for the three-dimensional Tl-weighted image were as follows: field of view, 22 cm; echo time, 6 ms; repetition time, 24 ms; flip angle, 35°; and voxel size, 0.86 × 0.86 × 2 mm. Functional imaging data were recorded as gradient-echo, echo-planar (EPI) T2*-weighted images with blood oxygenation level dependent (BOLD) contrast, Image volumes of the whole brain were built up from 30 continuous axial slices. The following parameter values were used: field of view, 22 cm; echo time, 60 ms; repetition time, 4 s; flip angle, 90°; pixel size, 3.4 × 3.4 mm; slice thickness, 5.0 mm; matrix size, 64 × 64. During one session, 122 image volumes were collected continuously. At the beginning of the session, four "dummy" image volumes were scanned, but not saved, to allow for Tl equilibration effects.

Analysis of Behavioral Data

The onset time and identity of all keys played during scanning were recorded on the PC. The main purpose of the behavioral analysis was to determine how accurately participants reproduced a previous Improvise trial in the Reproduce condition. For this purpose, we performed three types of analysis.

First, the total number of keys played in each trial were calculated. Paired t tests were employed to analyze differences in this parameter for corresponding trials of Improvise and Reproduce (i.e., trials where the same musical score was presented). This analysis was performed on all the trials pooled together, as well as separately for the individual participants. Secondly, the same analyses were performed on the total duration of the performance in each trial. For descriptive purposes, number of played keys and duration were calculated also for the FreeImp trials.

Finally, we evaluated the structural similarity of the performances in corresponding trials of Improvise and Reproduce. The Levenshtein edit distance (LED) is a measure of the degree of similarity between two arbitrary sequences (Levenshtein 1966). It is defined as the minimum number of single element deletions, insertions, or substitutions required to transform one of the sequences into the other. For example, the LED between the two sequences F–A–C and F–G is 2 (F–A– C → F–G–C → F–G). It can easily be seen that the LED is at least as large as the difference in length between the two sequences, and 0 only in the case of identical sequences. The LED between different melodic structures, that is, the sequences of played keys, was calculated using a standard algorithm (Knuth 1981) implemented in Matlab 6 (The MathWorks, Inc.). The LED between corresponding Improvise-Reproduce trials was investigated as a measure of the accuracy of the improvisations. The LED between each improvisation and its original template melody was used as a measure of the complexity of the improvisation. All statistical analyses were performed in Statistica (StatSoft, Inc.).

Processing and Statistical Analysis of the fMRI Data

The fMRI data were analyzed using the SPM99 software package (Wellcome Department of Imaging Neuroscience, London, UK). The scanned brain volumes were realigned to correct for head movements. Subsequently, they were coregistered to each individual's Tl-weighted image (Ashburner and Friston 1997) and normalized to the standard space (Talairach and Tournoux 1988). Proportional scaling was applied to eliminate the effects of global changes in the signal. The time series were smoothed spatially with an isotropic Gaussian fitter of 10 mm full width at half-maximum, and temporally with a Gaussian kernel of width 4 s.

The fMRI data were modeled with the general linear model, where we defined four conditions of interest corresponding to the periods in each epoch when the participants performed the task (the last 28 s of the 40 s epochs). We modeled the first 12 s of each epoch (i.e., the presentation of the task instruction and the preparatory period) as conditions of no interests. The significance of the effects was assessed using one-tailed t statistics for every voxel from the brain image, to create statistical parametric maps, which were transformed into Z statistics. Analyses were performed for contrast subtractions of Interest within participants, followed by a between-participants random-effects analysis based on summary-statistics of the subtraction images created for each participant. In this way, the interparticipant variance was accounted for, and inferences can be extended to the population from which the participants are drawn,

To localize brain regions involved in real-time improvisation and recall of a previous improvisation from memory, respectively, the contrasts Improvise–Reproduce and Reproduce–Improvise were investigated. To exclude the possibility that differences in these conditions reflected a deactivation, the contrasts Improvise–Rest and Reproduce–Rest, respectively, were used as inclusive masks. For both masks, an uncorrected p value of 0.05 was used. To investigate whether the brain activity seen in Improvise–Reproduce could reflect reproduction errors, a regression analysis was performed across participants, to test if the parameter estimates for the Improvise–Reproduce contrast correlated with the mean LED between Improvisations and reproductions for all trials performed by each participant. In a second between-subject regression analysis, Improvise–Reproduce activity was regressed on the mean LED between the original melodic template and improvisation, in order to localize brain activity related to the generation of more complex improvisations.

Brain activity in the Improvise–Reproduce contrast could reflect storage in memory, as participants were required to reproduce the Improvise trials during Reproduce. We therefore investigated which of the activations in Improvise–Reproduce were also seen in the contrast FreeImp–Rest, using a conjunction analysis between these two contrasts, We utilized a "minimum statistic compared to the conjunction null" analysis, as described in Nichols et al. (2005), which can be interpreted as a logical AND-operation between the two contrasts. Because only five participants performed the FreeImp condition, the conjunction was analyzed using a fixed-effects model to increase statistical sensitivity. Finally, to Investigate differences in activity between FreeImp and Improvise in regions that were involved in improvisation, the contrasts FreeImp–Improvise and Improvise–FreeImp were examined. Small volume corrections for multiple comparisons were employed, with spherical regions of interest (radius 10 mm) centered around the peak coordinates of the activations in Improvise–Reproduce,

We report activations that were significant at $p < 0.05$ according to a False Discovery Rate (FDR) analysis (Genovese et al. 2002). In this analysis, the results are corrected for multiple comparisons and a threshold is set to control the rate of false positives. The threshold of $p < 0.05$ thus means that, on average, less than 5 % of the suprathreshold voxels are not truly active. For the contrast Improvise–Reproduce, no activity was found at this threshold in the presupplementary motor area (pre-SMA), However, a recent study by Lau et al. (2004) found the pre-SMA to be the one region where a parametrical relation between brain activity and performance in a free selection task was found, We therefore used a small volume correction within a spherical region of Interest (radius 10 mm) in the pre-SMA, using the coordinate of the peak of activity *(x, y, z* = 8, 16, 64) in Lau et al. as the center of the sphere. Anatomical localizations of the activated regions were determined from an average image of normalized and intensity standardized Tl-weighted images from all 11 participants. We used the anatomical terminology of Duvernoy (2000), To localize cerebellar activations, we used the atlas of Schmahmann et al. (2000).

Results

Descriptive Characteristics of the Improvisations in Improvise and FreeImp

The identity and onset time of all piano keys played during scanning were recorded. Each condition was performed nine times, each time with a different melodic template, by each of the 11 participants, giving a total of 99 trials each of Improvise and Reproduce. During three of these trials (each in a different participant), a temporary mechanical error in the keyboard prevented proper recording of the behavioral data. Ninety-six trials of Improvise and Reproduce are thus included in the analysis below. FreeImp was performed by five subjects. Here, two trials in two different subjects had to be discarded for technical reasons, giving a total of 43 trials included in the analysis. The displayed melodic templates had, on average, 17.0 ± 2.6 (mean ± SD) notes.

For Improvise trials, the total number of played keys was 29.1 ± 9.4, and the mean duration of the improvisations was 17.8 ± 3.2 s. The mean LED between the melodic template and Improvisation was 20.7 ± 10.6, The improvisations in FreeImp were slightly more elaborate than in Improvise, They contained a larger number of notes (mean number of played keys 36.4 ± 9.2) than the corresponding performances in Improvise [paired *t* test; $t(42) = 6.02; p = 0.000$). The total duration

Table 16.1 Modifications of the melodic templates used in improvise and FreeImp

Modification	Improvise		FreeImp	
	η	% of Total	η	% of Total
Grace note	247	40.1	157	46.4
Substitution	112	18.2	76	22.5
Figuration	74	12.0	31	9.2
Trill	73	11.9	35	10.4
Filling in	38	6.2	9	2.7
Repetition	23	3.7	13	3.8
Elimination	23	3.7	9	2.7
Two part	12	1.9	3	0.9
Rhythmization	10	1.6	3	0.9
Tremolo	3	0.5	1	0.3
Minor/major shift	1	0.2	1	0.3
Total	616	100	338	100

For each condition, the total number of modifications of a particular type (η), as well its relative frequency (% of total), is shown

of the FreeImp Improvisations was also longer (18.4 ± 3.6 s) than in Improvise, although this trend did not reach significance [paired t test; $t(42) = 1.84$; $p = 0.07$]. The LED between FreeImp improvisations and their templates was higher (27.8 ± 9.6) than for Improvise [paired t test: $t(42) = 4.12$; $p = 0.000$].

During both Improvise and FreeImp, participants always played **a** modified version of the entire original melodic template, as written, that is, in no cases were only a part of the template or transformed (e.g., retrograde, mirrored) versions of template utilized as a basis for the improvisation. A qualitative analysis of all Improvisations revealed that all modifications could be classified Into 11 categories (Table 16.1): (i) Insertion of a fast group of one or more grace notes before a template note; (ii) substitution of a template note for another note; (iii) figuration, that is, expansion of the original template Into melodic figures; (iv) insertion of 1 trill on a template note; (v) filling in, that is, insertion of chromatic or diatonic scales between template notes; (vi) repetitions of template notes; (vii) elimination of template notes; (viii) insertion of figures giving, a broken two-part polyphony; (ix) rhythmization of the template; (x) insertion of a tremolo, that is, a trill-like figure between two notes with a larger interval than a second; and finally, (xi) switching of tonality from major to minor, Examples of the five most common types of modification (1–v), which together constitute more than 88 % of the modifications in both Improvise and FreeImp, are shown in Fig. 16.1b.

The larger number of notes in the FreeImp improvisations was due to a larger mean number of modifications per improvisation [t test: $t(137) = 3.40$; $p = 0.001$) in FreeImp (7.9 ± 2.5) than in Improvise (6.4 ± 2.2). No differences in the relative frequencies of the 11 different modifications (Table 16.1) were found between the two conditions [paired t test: $t(10) = 0.000$; $p = 1.0$], nor was the mean number of notes per modification different [t test: $t(134) = 0.30$; $p = 0.77$]. In Improvise (5.3 ± 3.0) and FreeImp (5.5 ± 4.2).

Accuracy of the Reproductions

Pooling data from all participants, no significant difference [paired t test: $t(95) = 158; p = 0.12$] was found between the total number of keys played in Improvise and Reproduce trials (29.6 ± 9.8). Similarly, no difference [paired/test: $t(95) = 1.51; p = 0.131$ was found in the total mean duration of Improvise and Reproduce (17.6 ± 3.4 s) trials, Nor could any significant differences in these variables be found within single participants. The mean number of played keys per trial in Improvise and Reproduce is shown for each participant in Fig. 16.2a. When analyzing all participants individually with repeated paired/tests, no significant differences were found (all Bonferroni·corrected p values >0.20). Individual data for trial durations are shown in Fig. 16.2b. No significant differences were found in the durations using paired /tests within each participant (corrected p values >0.52).

In terms of overall motor output—number of key strokes and duration of the performances—participants were thus highly consistent in improvise and Reproduce. To further investigate how well each Improvisation was reproduced structurally, we calculated the LED) between the key sequences played in corresponding trials of Improvise and Reproduce (see Methods). The mean LED for all trial pairs was 7.5 ± 4.9. Many of these single key edits were due to minor, and musically irrelevant, differences for instance, in the number of notes included in a trill or other ornament. An example of an Improvise–Reproduce trial pair where the reproduction was of average accuracy (LED 8) is illustrated in Fig. 16.3.

Fig. 16.2 Behavioral data recorded during the scanning **a** The mean number of played keys per trial in improvise and reproduce for each individual participant. **b** The mean duration of improvise and reproduce trials for each participant. In both (**a**) and (**b**), *error bars* indicate standard deviations

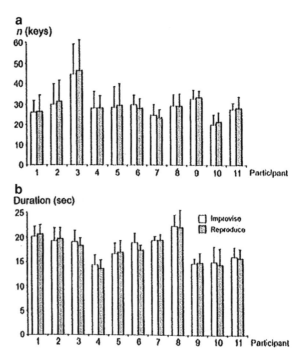

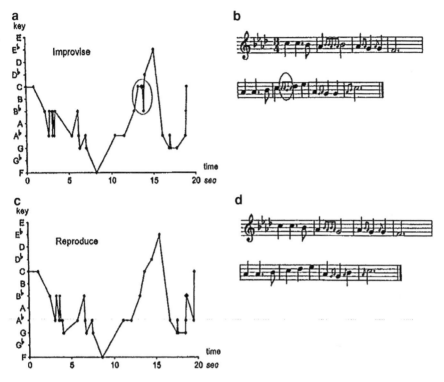

Fig. 16.3 An example of a typical improvise–reproduce trial pair. The diagrams **a**, **c** show the onset time of each key stroke of the performance. The same trials are illustrated in musical notation in panels (**b**) and (**d**). One ornament, which was not properly reproduced, is encircled in (**a**) and (**b**)

The diagrams (Fig. 16.3a, c) show the onset time of each key stroke. The same trials are illustrated in musical notation in panels b and d. The two trials are practically identical in overall conception, and highly similar also in the individual details. In this case, four single edits were due to that fact that one single ornament (encircled) was forgotten in the Reproduce trial, The remaining single key edits are due to minor differences in the execution of the details of other ornaments. In summary, the participants were able to reproduce their performances in Improvise with remarkable accuracy in the Reproduce condition. To further investigate whether differences in reproduction accuracy influenced the observed brain activity, a participant level regression analysis was performed between mean LED and activity in the Improvise–Reproduce contrast (see below).

fMRI Data

Brain areas with significantly higher BOLD response during Improvise than during Reproduce are summarized in Table 16.2 and illustrated in Fig. 16.4. The histograms in Fig. 16.1 show, for those subjects who performed ail four conditions, the mean percent signal change in BOLD signal for each condition in peak voxels of the active regions, with the Rest condition as zero. In the frontal lobe, activations were found in the right DLPFC and pre-SMA, and bilaterally in the rostral portion of the dorsal premotor cortex (PMD). Temporal lobe activations were found in the left posterior superior temporal gyrus (STG), close to the temporoparietal junction, and in the fusiform gyrus. Bilateral occipital activity was found in the middle occipital gyrus. For each peak of activity found in this contrast, we have indicated (Table 16.2, right-most column) whether the same region was also activated In a conjunction between Improvise–Reproduce and FreeImp–Rest. This was the case for all activations, except for the peak in the left STG and one of the peaks in the left PMD. However, peaks were found in the close vicinity of these regions (Table 16.2, footnotes). The durations of the improvisations were variable, and shorter than the 28-s epoch length (mean duration 17.8 s; see above). To verify that

Table 16.2 Brain regions with significantly increased BOLD contrast signal in improvise–reproduce

Brain region	Side	x	y	z	t value	Conj[a]
Frontal lobe						
Middle frontal g (DLPFC)	R	33	39	27	5.24	+
Superior frontal sulcus (PMD)	L	−24	12	48	4.41	−[b]
		−27	9	60	8.73	+
		−33	−3	60	5.06	+
	R	27	12	48	6.60	+
Superior frontal g (pre-SMA)	R	9	12	54	2.88[c]	+
Middle frontal g (PMD)	L	−33	3	42	6.14	+
		−36	−3	45	6.58	+
Temporal lobe						
Posterior STG	L	−60	−39	15	7.42	−[d]
Fusiform g	R	45	−51	−12	4.70	+
Occipital lobe						
Middle occipital g	L	−36	−78	18	4.20	+
		−27	−87	−3	4.21	+
	R	39	−78	6	4.57	+
		39	−81	0	4.77	+

[a] A (+) sign in this column indicates that activity (FDR < 0.05). In this region was also found in *a* conjunction between improvise–reproduce) and (FreeImp–rest)
[b] The nearest active voxel in the conjunction was found in the L PMD at −33, 6, 45 (*x, y, z*)
[c] Significant at FDR < 0.05 after a small volume correction based on an a priori hypothesis, but not In a whole-brain analysis
[d] The nearest active voxel in the conjunction was found In the Inferior parietal cortex immediately above the temporo-parietal junction, at −51, −39, 30 (*x, y, z*)

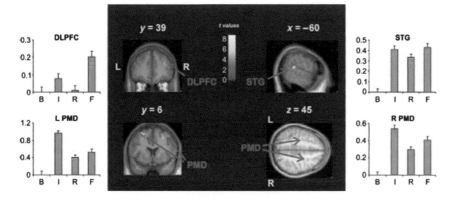

Fig. 16.4 Brain regions active in the Improvise–Reproduce contrast. Activity maps of brain regions with significantly increased BOLD contrast signal are shown for the right dorsolateral prefrontal cortex (DLPFC; slice y = 39), the left superior temporal gyrus (STG; slice x = −60), and the bilateral dorsal premotor cortices (PMD; slices y = 6 and z = 45). The color scale shows *t* values. R and L denote the *left* and *right* sides, respectively. The histograms show mean percent signal change in BOLD, signal for each condition in peak voxels of the active regions, with the rest condition as zero. Error bars show standard error of the mean (*SEM*). Names of conditions are abbreviated as follows: B = Rest (baseline); I = Improvise; R = Reproduce; F = and FreeImp

the observed activations were not confounded with brain activity occurring after the improvisations, we therefore also performed a separate analysis where only the first 16 s of the improvisations were included. All activations in Table 16.2 were found also in this analysis.

To test whether the activations in Improvise–Reproduce correlated with the accuracy of the reproductions, we regressed single-participant activations in this contrast on the mean LED between improvisations and reproductions in all trials performed by each participant. No significant positive or negative correlations were found. Neither were significant correlations found in the Reproduce–Improvise contrast at the current threshold (FDR < 0.05), or when using *a* more liberal threshold of FDR < 0.2. To localize brain activity related to the complexity of the improvisations, brain activity in Improvise–Reproduce was regressed onto the mean LED between improvisations and the original melody template for each participant. A significant positive relation was found in the pre-SMA (Fig. 16.5). The diagram shows the correlation (r = 0.71; p = 0.01; Pearson Product-Moment Correlation) between BOLD activity in the peak coordinate of the cluster (x, y, z = 12, 15, 54) and improvisation complexity. As can be seen, one of the participants produced much more complex improvisations than the rest of the group. When removing this outlier, a positive trend remained (r = 0.28), but did not reach significance (p = 0.43).

No activations were significant at $p < 0.05$ (FDR) in the contrasts FreeImp–Improvise and Improvise–FreeImp. In FreeImp–Improvise, nonsignificant trends were found in the DLPFC (p = 0.27; t = 2.24; x, y, z = 30, 45, 21) and the middle

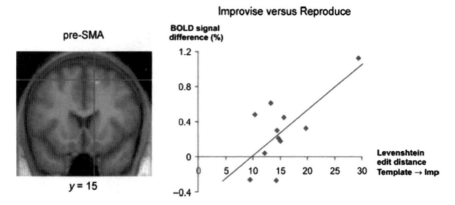

Fig. 16.5 The pre-SMA and improvisation complexity. In the pre-SMA, a positive relation was found between brain activity in the Improvise–Reproduce contrast, and the degree of complexity of the improvisations, operationalized as the LED between improvisation and template. Adjusted fMRI data from the peak voxel of the cluster (the red cross in the activity map; $x, y, z = 12, 15, 54$) are plotted against mean improvisation complexity for each participant in the graph, each *dot* in the plot represents an individual participant

occipital gyrus (p = 0.12; $t = 2.41$; $x, y, z = -42, -81, 2$). In Improvise–FreeImp, nonsignificant trends were seen in the PMD (p = 0.15; $t = 2.48$; $x, y, z = 24, 9, 60$) and the middle occipital gyrus (p = 0.07; $t = 2.65$; $x, y, z = -33, -78, 27$). In no other regions were voxels found above a threshold of $p = 0.05$, uncorrected.

Discussion

We compared brain activity during on-line improvisation (Improvise) and the reproduction of a previously created improvisation from memory (Reproduce), Three Important questions have to be considered when interpreting the Improvise–Reproduce contrast.

First, the pianists did not reproduce their improvisations with perfect accuracy. Does the brain activity in Improvise–Reproduce reflect these minor differences In motor output? Several observations speak against this. The number of played keys did not differ between the two tasks. In fact, a nonsignificant trend was found for a *larger* total motor output in Reproduce than in Improvise. One could therefore expect brain activity related to differences in motor output to appear in the Reproduce–Improvise contrast, but no significant activations were seen in that comparison. Furthermore the duration (i.e., time on task) of improvisations and corresponding reproductions did not differ. Finally corresponding trials were highly similar in terms of sequential structure, and no correlations were found between an index of structural similarity (LED) and brain activity at the single-participant level. Had the activations reflected motor output differences, one would have expected a higher level of activity in participants with a higher mean LED value, as this implies larger discrepancies between the improvisations and the reproductions. For the same reasons, we consider Improvise and Reproduce to be essentially equivalent in terms of sensory input (I.e., auditory and somatosensory feedback).

Secondly, the improvisations were of variable duration. Could activations In the Improvise–Reproduce contrast be confounded with non-task-related brain activity occurring after the performance? Two facts speak against this. First, the same set of activations were seen in the Improvise–Reproduce contrast when analyzing only the first 16 s of the improvisations. Secondly, participants were instructed to rest passively after finishing the performance,

Thirdly, because the improvisations had to be reproduced, the Improvise condition required both improvisation and storage of the performance in working and long-term memory. To what extent does the neural activity in Improvise–Reproduce reflect the latter processes? To evaluate this question, we investigated which of the activated brain areas were also seen in the contrast FreeImp-Rest. For the FreeImp condition, the participants had been instructed to improvise without memorizing their performance. The fact that the same types of modifications of the template were used with the same relative frequencies in FreeImp and Improvise suggests that no major differences in improvisatory strategies were used in these two conditions. All major regions active in Improvise–Reproduce—the DLPFC, the rostral PMD, the left temporo-parietal region, and the middle occipital gyri— were also active In the conjunction analysis. In summary, we therefore argue that the activity in these brain regions reflects neural processes involved in the generation of new musical material during improvisation.

Dorsolateral Prefrontal Cortex

A key finding in the present study is that the DLPFC Is involved in the generation of musical structures during improvisation. This is of interest because it demonstrates that the DLPFC is involved in the creative aspects of a complex and ecologically relevant behavior, where the free selection of responses is adapted to an overall goal of producing an aesthetically satisfactory end-result.

The finding is in line with the many earlier studies that have used simpler model behaviors to investigate the involvement of the DLPFC in free response selection. The DLPFC is consistently more active during motor tasks when movement parameters such as effector (Frith et al. 1991), movement direction or target (Rowe et al. 2005; Playford et al. 1992; Deiber et al. 1991), and movement timing (Jahanshahi et al. 1995a, b) are freely chosen, as opposed to repetitive or externally determined by a stimulus. Similarly, DLPFC activity is related to free selection in cognitive tasks. This has been shown, for instance, for word generation (Frith et al. 1991; Petersen et al. 1988), number generation (Jahanshahi et al. 2000), word-stem completion (Desmond et al. 1998), and sentence completion (Nathaniel-James and Frith 2002). It can also be noted that there was a trend for higher DLPFC activity during Free-Imp than during Improvise, which could be related to the slightly higher level of complexity (larger number of modifications) of the improvisations in FreeImp.

What are the specific functional roles of the DLPFC in this type of tasks? Part of the activity may relate to attention to the selection of action, rather than free choice per se (Lau et al. 2004; Jueptner et al. 1997). Lau et al. (2004) found that the DLPFC was activated during selection between several possible responses, whether these were externally specified or free. However, other studies have reported a positive relation between the number of available alternatives in a free choice situation and the level of DLPFC activity (Nathaniel-James and Frith 2002; Desmond et al. 1998), suggesting that the DLPFC is also involved in the selection process,

It should be noted that "free" in free-selection tasks typically means pseudo-random. The apparent simplicity of such a task is obviously deceptive (Jahanshahi et al. 1998). To emulate randomness, participants must rely on some strategy to produce an irregular output. One task for the DLPFC is thus presumably to maintain earlier responses in working memory. In this way, different response alternatives can be compared to previous output to avoid regularities. The DLPFC Is strongly implicated in working memory for action-relevant information (for a review, see Fuster 2001), and is important for the continuous comparison of consecutive stimuli (Petrides 1995). Transcranial magnetic stimulation experiments show that disruption of DLPFC activity during pseudorandom generation of numbers (Jahanshahi et al. 1998) or letters (Jahanshahi and Dirnberger 1999) tends to make the responses more stereotyped. One role of the DLPFC in free selection may thus be to inhibit unwanted, habitual responses.

All these subfunctions of the DLPFC—attention to action, monitoring in working memory, response selection, and suppression of stereotype responses—may be of importance during improvisation. In addition, it appears likely that improvisation, perhaps to a larger degree than attempts at random behavior, relies on the higher, Integrative mechanisms of the DLPFC. During Improvise, a whole set of freely selected modifications of the original melody must be temporally organized according to a musically meaningful overall plan. A central role for the DLPFC in planning and performance of novel or complex behavioral sequences, including language and thought, Is demonstrated by a vast body of neurological and experimental data (for reviews, see Fuster 2001; Cummings 1993; Baddeley 1986; Luria 1966). Our data are in line with that one central function of the DLPFC during improvisation is supervisory, to maintain and execute an overall plan for the Improvisation through top-down influences on the activity, for instance, In subordinate premotor areas. One aspect of this may be "sculpting of the response space" (Frith 2000), that is, the selection of a set of responses suitable for a particular Improvisation. These influences can be mediated by the extensive connections from the DLPFC to the motor system, including the rostral premotor areas (Fuster 2001; Picard and Strick 2001). Notably, the DLPFC activation was In the right hemisphere. This is consistent with a number of earlier studies which also found predominantly right-sided activity during divergent tasks Howard-Jones et al. 2005; Carlsson et al. 2000; Seger et al. 2000; Abdullaev and Posner 1997).

Rostral Premotor Cortices

Activity in Improvise–Reproduce was also found In rostral premotor areas, mesially in the pre-SMA as well as laterally in the PMD. Our findings fit the general view that the rostral portion of the premotor cortex is Involved In cognitive aspects of action (Picard and Strick 2001). Both the pre-SMA (Johansen-Berg et al. 2004; Lu et al. 1994; Bates and Goldman-Rakic 1993) and the rostral PMD (Lu et al. 1994; Barbas and Pandya 1987) are, unlike caudal premotor areas, interconnected with the DLPFC.

The pre-SMA has been implicated in free choice, in particular, when the *timing* of a response is selected (Jahanshahi et al. 1995a, b). Interestingly, Lau et al. (2004) recently found that not only was the pre-SMA active in free selection but the level of pre-SMA activity also correlated with response time between participants. The finding of a positive relation between pre-SMA activity and the complexity of the Improvisations is in line with a role of the pre-SMA in the selection process. This correlation did not remain significant when removing one outlier participant that produced highly complex Improvisations. However, because a positive trend was still seen, it seems likely that this reflects a restriction of range in terms of improvisational complexity among the other participants. Our data thus indicate that the pre-SMA is involved In response selection also In more complex divergent tasks such as musical improvisation. The Involvement of the pre-SMA in temporal selection Is of interest in relation to the consistent finding that this region is active during rhythmic sequence performance (Bengtsson et al. 2004, 2005; Lewis et al. 2004; Schubotz and von Cramon 2001; Lutz et al. 2000; Larsson et al. 1996) as well as during perceptual timing tasks (Macar et al. 2002). One could therefore suggest that the pre-SMA activity during improvisation may be particularly related to decisions about timing and rhythmic patterning. In addition, it seems plausible that demands on temporal processing are higher during Improvisation, when generated ornaments have to be fitted into a given metric structure, than during reproduction.

The PMD receives a large input from the superior parietal lobule, and plays important roles for visuo-motor control, sequencing, and spatially targeted movements (Andersen et al. 1997; Wise et al. 1997). As for the medial wall motor areas, more rostral activations are associated with higher-order, non-movement-related processing (Picard and Strick 2001). Two findings on the rostral PMD can be mentioned, in particular, in relation to our results. First, the rostral PMD Is implied in response selection in visual choice reaction time tasks (Grafton et al. 1998). Secondly, neurons in this region have been shown to be Involved in transforming a series of positional cues kept In working memory, into a sequential motor program of targeted movements (Ohbayashi et al. 2003). The rostral PMD could be Involved in similar operations—response selection based on visual cues, that is, musical notation, and transformation of information held in working memory by the DLPFC and the pre-SMA into movement sequences—during improvisation. The trend for higher PMD activity during Improvise than during FreeImp could reflect a higher load on working memory in Improvise, where the participants had to memorize their performance.

Earlier work on movement sequence production has Indicated that medial premotor areas are more important for timing, whereas lateral premotor cortex activity is more related to sequencing of the movements in the correct order (Bengtsson et al. 2004; Schubotz and von Cramon 2001). An Interesting possibility is that a similar division of labor holds also during improvisation so that the rostral PMD and the pre-SMA are more involved in the shaping of melodic and rhythmic structures, respectively.

Temporal and Occipital Areas

We found activity specifically related to Improvise in a portion of the posterior STG, close to the temporo-parietal junction. This region, area Spt (Hickok et al. 2003), has consistently been found active in studies that require auditory-motor integration, such as rhythmic sequence performance (Bengtsson et al. 2004, 2005; Lewis et al. 2004; Jäncke et al. 2000; Lutz et al. 2000) and vocal rehearsal of words or music (Hickok et al. 2003). It can affect the motor system through connections with inferior frontal regions, via the arcuate fasciculus (Hickok and Poeppel 2000). We suggest that the area Spt activation in the present study may reflect a larger load on auditory—motor feedback loops during Improvise, for example, to adapt the improvisation to ongoing performance. In addition, the posterior superior temporal cortex is involved in auditory working memory of melodic structures (Gaab et al. 2003; Patterson et al. 2002; Griffiths et al. 1998), and may thus be of Importance for auditory monitoring of the ongoing performance. Finally, the different modifications of the original template employed in the improvisations are obviously part of a common "vocabulary" of ornaments used In Western art music (see Palmer 2001). One possibility is that the area Spt is involved in retrieval of such musical structures from long-term memory, in analogy with its role in lexical retrieval in linguistic tasks (Hickok and Poeppel 2000).

A number of small clusters of activity were found In higher-order visual areas in the fusiform and middle occipital gyri. These activations may be due to a more intense visual processing of the musical score when this was used as a basis for improvisations, rather than as a template to recall a previous performance. Notably, two of these regions (right fusiform and left middle occipital gyri) were found to be involved in music reading in another study on the same group of participants (Bengtsson and Ullén 2006).

Conclusion

We have provided evidence that a set of frontal and temporal association areas are specifically involved in the free creation of musical structures during Improvisation. We suggest that the DLPFC interacts with the rostral PMD and the pre-SMA in processes of free selection, selective attention, as well as the sequential and temporal organization of the behavior, and with area Spt in the superior temporal cortex for auditory working memory, retrieval of musical standard ornaments from long-term memory, and auditory—motor integration. For the pre-SMA, increased activity related to the generation of more complex improvisations could be demonstrated.

We believe this study demonstrates that musical improvisation may be a useful behavior for studies of the neurocognitive processes underlying all ecologically relevant creative behavior. An important next step will be to analyze the neural underpinnings of the cognitive components of improvisation, such as production of melodic and rhythmic structures, and the interaction between systems for planning, motor attention, response generation, and selection. The brain regions shown to be involved In musical improvisation in the present study are part of a larger set of neural regions active during piano performance (Bengtsson and Ullén 2006; Parsons et al. 2005). It would be of interest to examine to what extent these are specifically involved in creative behaviors in other domains.

Acknowledgments We thank Lea Foreman, Hans Forssberg, Guy Madison, and Jeanne Nakamura for comments on the manuscript. This work was funded by the Swedish Research Council; the Freemasons in Stockholm Foundation for Children's Welfare, Sweden the Medici II symposia on positive psychology; the Templeton Foundation; and Linnea och Josef Carlssons Stiftelse, Sweden. The present address of S. L. B. is Wellcome Department of Imaging Neuroscience, Institute of Neurology, London, UK.

Reprint requests should be sent to Dr. Fredrik Ullén, Stockholm Brain Institute, Neuropediatric Research Unit Q2; 07, Department of Women and Child Health, Karolinska Institutet, SE-171 76 Stockholm, Sweden, or via e-mail: Fredrik.Ullen@kl.se.

References

Abdullaev, Y., & Posner, M. I. (1997). Time course of activating brain areas in generating verbal associations. *Psychological Science, 8*, 56–59.

Andersen, R. A., Snyder, L. H., Bradley, D. C., & Xing, J. (1997). Multimodal representation of space in the posterior parietal cortex and its use in planning movements. *Annual Review of Neuroscience, 20*, 303–330.

Ashburner, J., & Friston, K. J. (1997). Multimodal image coregistration and partitioning: A unified framework. *Neuroimage, 6*, 209–217.

Baddeley, A. (1986). *Working memory*. Oxford: Clarendon Press.

Barbas, H., & Pandya, D. N. (1987). Architecture and frontal cortical connections of the premotor cortex (area 6) in the rhesus monkey. *Journal of Comparative Neurology, 256*, 211–228.

Bates, J. P., & Goldman·Rakic, P. S. (1993). Prefrontal connections of medial motor areas in the rhesus monkey. *Journal of Comparative Neurology, 336*, 211–228.

Bengtsson, S., Ehrsson, H. H., Forssberg, H., & Ullén, F. (2004). Dissociating brain regions controlling the temporal and ordinal structure of learned movement sequences. *European Journal of Neuroscience, 19*, 2591–2602.

Bengtsson, S. L., Ehrsson, H. H., Forssberg, H., & Ullén, F. (2005). Effector-independent voluntary timing: Behavioural and neuroimaging evidence. *European Journal of Neuroscience, 22*, 3255–3265.

Bengtsson, S. L., & Ullén, F. (2006). Different neural correlates for melody and rhythm processing during piano performance from musical scores. *Neuroimage, 30*, 272–284.

Campbell, D. T. (1960). Blind variation and selective retention in creative thought as in other knowledge processes. *Psychological Review, 67*, 380–400.

Carlsson, I., Wendt, P. E., & Risberg, J. (2000). On the neurobiology of creativity. Differences in frontal activity between high and low creative subjects. *Neuropsychologia, 38*, 873–885.

Csikszentmihalyi, M. (1997). *Creativity: Flow and the psychology of discovery and invention.* New York: Perennial.

Cummings, J. L. (1993). Frontal-subcortical circuits and human behavior. *Archives of Neurology, 50*, 873–880.

Deiber, M. P., Passingham, R. E., Colebatch, J. G., Friston, K. J., Nixon, P. D., & Frackowlak, R. S. J. (1991). Cortical areas and the selection of movement: A study with positron emission tomography. *Experimental Brain Research, 84*, 393–402.

Desmond, J. E., Gabrieli, J. D. E., & Glover, G. H. (1998). Dissociation of frontal and cerebellar activity in a cognitive task: Evidence for a distinction between selection and search. *Neuroimage, 7*, 368–376.

Duvernoy, H. M. (2000). *The human brain: Surface, blood supply and three-dimensional sectional anatomy.* Wien: Springer.

Eyscnck, H. (1995). *Genius. The natural history of creativity.* Cambridge: Cambridge University Press.

Frith, C. D. (2000). The role of dorsolateral prefrontal cortex in the selection of action. In S. Monsell & J. Driver (Eds.), *Control of cognitive processes: Attention and performance* (Vol. 18, pp. 429–565). Cambridge: MIT Press.

Frith, C. D., Friston, K. J., Liddle, P. F., & Frackowiak, R. S. J. (1991). Willed action and the prefrontal cortex in man: A study with PET. *Proceedings of the Royal Society of London, Series B, 2.14*, 241–246.

Fuster, J. (2001). The prefrontal cortex: An update time is of the essence. *Neuron, 30*, 319–333.

Gaab, N., Gaser, C., Zaehic, T., Jancke, L., & Schlaug, G. (2003). Functional anatomy of pitch memory: An fMRI study with sparse temporal sampling. *Neuroimage, 19*, 1417–1426.

Genovese, C. R., Lazar, N. A., & Nichols, T. (2002). Thresholding of statistical maps in functional neuroimaging using the false discovery rate. *Neuroimage, 15*, 870–878.

Grafton, S. T., Fagg, A, I. I., & Arbib, M. A. (1998). Dorsal premotor cortex and conditional movement selection: A PET functional mapping study. *J Neurophys, 70*, 1092–1097.

Griffiths, T. D., Buchel, C., Frackowiak, R. S., & Patterson, R. D. (1998). Analysis of temporal structure in sound by the human brain. *Nature Neuroscience, 1*, 422–427.

Hickok, G., Buchsbaum, B., Humphries, C., & Muftuler, T. (2003). Auditory-motor interaction revealed by fMRI: Speech, music, and working memory in area Spt. *Journal of Cognitive Neuroscience, 15*, 673–682.

Hickok, G., & Poeppel, D. (2000). Towards a functional neuroanatomy of speech perception. *Trends Cogn Sci, 4*, 131–138.

Howard-Jones, P.A., Blakemore, S. J., Samuel, E. A., Summers, I. R., & Claxton, G. (2005). Semantic divergence and creative story generation: An fMRI investigation. *Cognitive Brain Research, 25*, 240–250.

Jahamhahi, M., & Dirnberger, G. (1999). The left dorsolateral prefrontal cortex and random generation of responses: Studies with transcranial magnetic stimulation. *Neuropsychologia, 37*, 181–190.

Jahanshahi, M., Dirnberger, G., Fuller, R., & Frith, C. D. (2000). The role of the dorsolateral prefrontal cortex in random number generation: A study with positron emission tomography. *Neuroimage, 12*, 713–725.

Jahanshahi, M., & Frith, C. D. (1998). Willed action and its impairments. *Cognitive Neuropsychology, 15*, 483–533.

Jahanshahi, M., Jenkins, I. H., Brown, R. G., Marsden, C. D., Brooks, D. J., & Passingham, R. E. (1995a). Self-initiated versus externally-triggered movements: Effects of stimulus predictability assessed with positron emission tomography. *Journal of Psychophysiology, 9,* 177–178.

Jahanshahi, M., Jenkins, I, H., Brown, R. G., Marsden, C. D., Passingham, R, E., & Brooks, D. J., (1995b). Self-initiated versus externally triggered movements: I. An investigation using measurement of regional cerebral blood flow with PET and movement-related potentials in normal and Parkinson's disease subjects. *Brain, 118,* 913–933.

Jahanshahi, M., Profice, P., Brown, R. G., Ridding, M. C., Dirnberger, G., & Rothwell, J. C. (1998). The effects of transcranial magnetic stimulation over the dorsolateral prefrontal cortex on suppression of habitual counting during random number generation. *Brain, 121,* 1533–1544.

Jäncke, L., Loose, R., Lutz, K., Specht, K., & Shah, N. J. (2000). Conical activations during paced finger-tapping applying visual and auditory pacing stimuli. *Cognitive Brain Research, 10,* 51–66.

Johansen-Berg, H., Behrens, T. E., Robson, M. D., Drobnjak, I., Rushworth, M. F., Brady, J. M., et al. (2004). Changes in connectivity profiles define functionally distinct regions in human medial frontal cortex. *Proceedings of the National Academy of Sciences USA, 101,* 13335–13340.

Jueptner, M., Stephan, K. M., Frith, C. D., Brooks, D. J., Frackowiak, R. S., & Passingham, R. E. (1997). Anatomy of motor learning: I. Frontal cortex and attention to action. *Journal of Neurophysiology, 77,* 1313–1324.

Knuth, D. E. (1981). Supernatural numbers. In D. A. Klarner (Ed.), *The mathematical gardener* (pp. 310–325). Belmont: Wadsworth.

Larsson, J., Gulyás, B., & Roland, P. E. (1996). Cortical representation of self-paced finger movement. *NeuroReport, 7,* 463–468.

Lau, C, I. I., Rogers, R. D., Ramnani, N., & Passingham, R. E. (2004). Willed action and attention to the selection of action. *Neuroimage, 21,* 1407–1415.

Levenshtein, V. I. (1966). Binary codes capable of correcting deletions, Insertions and reversals. *Soviet Physics Doklady, 6,* 707–710.

Lewis, P. A., Wing, A. M., Pope, P. A., Praamstra, P., & Mlall, R. C. (2004). Brain activity correlates differentially with increasing temporal complexity of rhythms during initialisation, synchronisation, and continuation phases of paced finger tapping. *Neuropsychologia, 42,* 1301–1312.

Lu MT, Preston JB, Strick PL (1994) Interconnections between the prefrontal cortex and the premotor areas in the frontal lobe. J Comp Neurol 341:375–392

Luria, A. R. (1966). *Higher cortical functions in man.* New York: Basic Books.

Lutz, K., Specht, K., Shah, N. J., & Jäncke, L. (2000). Tapping movements according to regular and irregular visual timing signals Investigated with fMRI. *NeuroReport, 11,* 1301–1306.

Macar, F., Lejeune, H., Bonnet, M., Ferrara, A., Pouthas, V., Vidal, F., et al. (2002). Activation of the supplementary motor area and of attentional networks during temporal processing. *Experimental Brain Research, 142,* 475–485.

Nathaniel-James, D. A., & Frith, C. D. (2002). The role of the dorsolateral prefrontal cortex: Evidence from the effects of contextual constraint in a sentence completion task. *Neuroimage, 16,* 1094–1102.

Nichols, T., Brett, M., Andersson, J., Wager, T., & Poline, J. -B. (2005). Valid conjunction inference with the minimum statistic. *Neuroimage, 25,* 653–660.

Ohbayashl, M., Ohki, K., & Miyashita, Y. (2003). Conversion of working memory to motor sequence in the monkey premotor cortex. *Science, 301,* 233–236.

Oldfield, R. C. (1971). The assessment and analysis of handedness: The Edinburgh inventory. *Neuropsychologia, 9,* 97–113.

Palmer, K. (2001). *Ornamentation according to C. P. B. Bach and J. J. Quantz.* Bloomington, IN: Authorhouse.

Parsons, L. M., Sergent, J., Hodges, D. A., & Fox, P. T. (2005). The brain basis of piano performance. *Neuropsychologia, 43,* 199–215.

Patterson, R. D., Uppenkamp, S., Johnsrude, I. S., & Griffiths, T. D. (2002). The processing of temporal pitch and melody information in auditory cortex. *Neuron, 36,* 767–776.

Petersen, S, E., Fox, P. T., Posner, M. I., Nintus, M., & Raichle, M. E. (1988). Positron emission tomographic studies of the cortical anatomy of single word processing. *Nature, 331,* 585–589.

Petrides, M. (1995). Impairments on nonspatial self-ordered and externally ordered working memory tasks after lesions of the mid-dorsal part of the lateral frontal cortex in the monkey. *Journal of Neuroscience, 15,* 359–375.

Picard, N., & Strick, P. I. (2001). Imaging the premotor areas. *Current Opinion on Neurobiology, 11,* 663–672

Playford, E. D., Jenkins, I. H., Passingham, R. E., Nutt, J., Frackowiak, R. S., & Brooks, D. J. (1992). Impaired mesial frontal and putamen activation in Parkinson's disease: A positron emission tomography study. *Annals of Neurology, 32,* 151–161.

Pressing, J. (1988). Improvisation: Methods and models. In J. A. Sloboda (Ed.), *Generative processes in music* (pp. 129–178). New York: Oxford University Press.

Rowe, J. B., Stephan, K. E., Friston, K., Frackowlak, R. S., & Passingham, R. E. (2005). The prefrontal cortex shows context-specific changes in effective connectivity to motor or visual cortex during the selection of action or colour. *Cerebral Cortex, 15,* 85–95.

Schmahmann, J. D., Doyon, J., Toga, A. W., Petrides, M., & Evans, A. C. (2000). *MRI atlas of the human cerebellum.* San Diego: Academic Press.

Schubotz, R. I., & von Cramon, D. Y. (2001). Interval and ordinal properties of sequences are associated with distinct premotor areas. *Cerebral Cortex, 11,* 210–222.

Seger, C. A., Desmond, J. E., Glover, G, H., & Gabrieli, J. D. (2000). Functional magnetic resonance Imaging evidence for right-hemisphere Involvement in processing unusual semantic relationships. *Neuropsychology, 14,* 361–369.

Simonton, D. K. (1999). *Origins of genius. Darwinian perspectives on creativity.* New York: Oxford University Press.

Sternberg, R. J. (1999). *Handbook of creativity.* Cambridge: Cambridge University Press.

Talairach, J., & Tournoux, P. (1988). *Co-planar stereotaxic atlas of the human brain.* Stuttgart: Thleme.

Wise, S. P., Boussaoud, D., Johnson, P. B., & Caminiti, R. (1997). Premotor and parietal cortex: Corticocortical connectivity and combinatorial computations. *Annual Review of Neuroscience, 20,* 25–42.

Chapter 17
Creativity and Responsibility

Mihaly Csikszentmihalyi and Jeanne Nakamura

> *Fatti non foste a viver come bruti ma*
> *per seguir virtute e conoscenza.*
> —Dante, *The Divine Comedy, Inferno*, Canto 26, 118–120

In the popular imagination, creative individuals are often seen as oblivious to the ties of responsibility that hobble lesser mortals. They tend to be depicted as arrogant and insensitive, disdaining social values and obligations. In part this image has been the unintended result of Europe's emancipation from the weight of tradition that followed the humanistic turn of the Renaissance. The still largely conformist masses, on the one hand, were gradually estranged from the few individuals who, on the other hand, were ready to break away from tradition. Those who rejected the constricting ethos of the Middle Ages and developed new maps of the heavens or dissected cadavers to see how the body was put together were often suspected of breaking the boundaries not only of knowledge but of morality as well.

Even artists who explored subjects beyond traditional religious themes and adopted new styles were suspect. When Vasari wrote the first biographies of Western artists in 1550, he complained bitterly about their lack of polish and morality: they "had received from nature a certain element of savagery and madness, which, besides making them strange and eccentric... revealed in them rather the obscure darkness of vice than the brightness and splendor of those virtues that make men immortal" (Vasari 1959, p. 232).

Centuries later the ideology of Romanticism emphasized the chasm between the creative individual and the conforming masses. In Goethe's masterpiece, Faust rejects traditional morality in order to gain knowledge and experience novelty— even at the price of selling his soul to the devil. The perception that to be creative

Reference: "Creativity and Responsibility" by Mihaly Csikszentmihalyi and Jeanne Nakamura, in H. Gardner (Ed.) Responsibility at Work. San Francisco: Jossey-Bass, 2007, pp 64–80.

This chapter focuses on the cultivation of responsibility for others. It does not explore—despite their prominence as aims of undergraduate education—the cultivation of responsibility for self or the nurturing of responsibility for a particular domain or discipline.

You were not born to live like brutes do, but to pursue virtue and knowledge. (Ulysses, trying to convince his shipmates to be the first to sail out into the open Atlantic Ocean.)

M. Csikszentmihalyi, *The Systems Model of Creativity*,
DOI: 10.1007/978-94-017-9085-7_17,
© Springer Science+Business Media Dordrecht 2014

one must reject social mores led to a vicious circle: Young people who sought recognition found it easier to attract attention by acting extravagantly rather than by actually producing valuable novelty, thus reinforcing the stereotype (Kasof 1995).

It is therefore not surprising that when Lombroso, in 1889, wrote the first modern treatise on creativity and mental health, *The Man of Genius,* he argued that artistic creativity was a form of inherited insanity. Creative scientists had an equally dubious reputation. Frankenstein's monster and *Dr. Strangelove* of Stanley Kubrick's film are prototypes of what happens when a person's *hubris* lets him trespass the limits that keep most mortals in line.

But is it actually true, as popular wisdom suggests, that men and women at the cutting edge of culture operate without a moral compass? Our claim in this chapter is that, to the contrary, the culture has much to learn from the distinctive ethical sense that directs most creative individuals. An extremely intransigent sense of responsibility is a distinctive trait of creative persons. They feel an almost religious respect for human accomplishments of the *past,* at least within the domain of their interest and activity. Musicians revere the classics of the past, and scientists revere the laws of nature and those who uncovered them. So a sense of responsibility for staying true to the best practices of one's domain is a constant aspect of creativity. Conversely, creative individuals also respect the possibilities of the *future.* They are open to novelty and curious about how to make things better. Whenever they can, they try to combine the achievements of the past with the possibilities of the future and express them in the *present.* Thus, responsibility for good work in the present that combines the best of what was and the best of what is to be is the hallmark of creativity.

What binds the behavior of creative persons is a response to a call that is neither less urgent nor less essential to the well-being of humankind than the dictates of conventional morality. The responsibility felt by creative persons involves integrity, honesty, and excellence in the performance of their tasks—qualities that are not always foremost among conventionally moral people. Thus, understanding the creative ethos might help expand our notions of what constitutes responsible behavior and provide a broader basis for moral education.

In what follows, we examine interviews conducted with approximately one hundred creative individuals in an attempt to extract what these persons consider the most important guiding principles in their lives and work. The participants in the study included artists, scientists, inventors, businesspersons, and politicians who had in some ways transformed their domain and the broader culture. Eleven of them had been recognized with the Nobel Prize (Csikszentmihalyi 1996).

In an analysis of a subset of 47 interviews from the study, Choe and Nakamura (1996) found that these creative individuals mentioned at least three values that reflected concern for responsibility: *responsibility* (the tenth most often mentioned value), *doing good work* (the seventh most frequently mentioned value), and *social concerns* (the fourth most often mentioned value out of 81 cited altogether). These three coded values overlapped substantially, and hereafter we shall refer to them collectively as *responsibility.*

What did *responsibility* mean to these creative individuals? Most of our interviewees employed a language that stressed notions of calling, duty, loyalty, obligation, and responsiveness. In the most circumscribed instances, these notions applied to the conscientious performance of professional roles. Doing careful, sound, original work was a value essential to their self-image. One scientist defined it as "dealing with information rigorously," another as "getting things right and formulating things perfectly"; an astronomer aimed to "collect very good data" and a poet said "one wants really to write very good poems."

But in at least one third of the cases, the sense of responsibility extended much further. Some felt they owed a duty to mentors, colleagues, and students, to be available, supportive, critical, or responsive, as needed. Others felt they had to enhance the visibility and status of the discipline in which they worked. On a more idiosyncratic note, a novelist expressed "concern that what I write is not destructive [to readers]," and a leading journalist embraced his mission of being "the eyes and ears for the little guy."

Finally, several of these eminent scientists and artists extended the scope of their concern far beyond the boundaries of their discipline. For instance, nuclear physicist Victor Weisskopf became a vocal opponent of the Cold War arms race "to see that the negative influences of science are mitigated"; so did Benjamin Spock, the pioneering pediatrician. Linus Pauling, who earned a Nobel Prize in chemistry in 1954 and 8 years later the Nobel Peace Prize for his courageous stand against the irresponsible use of nuclear energy, was detained by the police for his efforts. In fact, at least a dozen of the 91 creative individuals studied were jailed or attacked for their beliefs—for supporting union strikers in the United States, for standing up to Stalin or Hitler in Europe, or for expressing candid views about cultural and religious changes in Egypt, as happened to Nobel Prize novelist Naguib Mahfouz, who just months after our interview was critically wounded by a Muslim fundamentalist assassin.

Responsibility as a Call to Excellence

Of all the forms of responsibility that these creative persons mentioned and demonstrated in their lives, perhaps the most important is their duty to do excellent work as defined by the traditions and current standards of the particular activity in which they are engaged. To know how a person learns to heed this call is enormously important for society, because the excellence of the whole depends disproportionately on the energy and commitment of those few who, in all walks of life, want to change society for the better. Yet the link between creativity and responsibility is little understood.

It is easy to assume that by *responsibility* we mean only a contractual obligation that develops between a person and a community that imposes certain moral expectations. According to this limited view, each of us internalizes, consciously or not, a set of rules and demands that we then feel obliged to follow.

But responsibility is often also manifested in a broader form. The term itself derives from the noun *response* and connotes a feeling that one must answer a call, a summons, that comes from somewhere outside the person. Thus the notion of responsibility overlaps with what in Christian religious thought, and later in the sociology of Max Weber, has been referred to as a calling or vocation—the sense a person has that he or she must answer a call and take on a task that a higher power expects him or her to fulfill. When a person is immersed in a religious worldview, the call is interpreted as coming from God. This is how billionaire investor Sir John Templeton, for instance, recalls his response to the call: "When I was very small, maybe as young as 8 years old, I wondered why humans were created... and coming from a religious town, I thought God must have made people for some purpose.... I wanted to find out what God wanted me to do." After reflecting on his strengths and weaknesses, when he reached college Templeton decided that investing in tech-nologically less advanced countries would help him "accelerate God's creativity," and this is the call he has followed ever since (Csikszentmihalyi 2003, p. 159). Creative individuals—and most people to a greater or lesser extent—seem to hear intimations of such a vocation, even though the personal call from a divinity is often missing. But if not from God, from whence does the call to excellence come?

The Call of the Past

The interviews suggest that in most cases creative individuals recognize a specific talent or strength they possess, and if they take this advantage seriously, they react to it in a way that is not unlike the acceptance of vocation or calling that people with a religious background describe. In other words, they feel they have a responsibility to do their best to use the special tools that genes, family, or sheer luck has given them. The bottom line is, they feel responsible to do work of such high quality that it would stand up to the best of what one's predecessors were able to accomplish.

To do so means internalizing the highest standards of the past. When asked what he felt responsible to at the time of the interview, Canadian novelist Rob-ertson Davies, who was 80 years old then and spending much time giving public talks about his latest book, answered, "I feel that I must be very careful about what I say and not just talk off the cuff, you know, because that is so shallow and stupid, and it's not fair to the people who've asked you to speak."

Care in avoiding shallowness and stupidity was a constant theme in all of the interviews. Whatever one's craft is—art or science, medicine or engineering—one can aim either to do well or to just get by. It is difficult to achieve eminence in any field if one is not committed to the first of these two choices.

It is clear that the network of loyalties to which Davies felt responsible was wide and complex. Above all else, he felt responsible to his own experiences; even though he knew they were subjective and probably unique to him, he defended their reality and importance. It is out of these personal memories that Davies constructed his dense narratives. He had no doubt that all novels are essentially autobiographical—their value depends on the author's faithfulness to what he or she actually feels.

("You remember that story about Gustave Flaubert when someone said to him, 'Where did you achieve this extraordinary knowledge of feminine psychology that appears in Madame Bovary?' and he said, 'Madame Bovary, *c'est moi.'* And he was right, where else would he get it from? Not out of a book, certainly").

Extending beyond his own experience, Davies felt a sense of responsibility for his ancestry and ethnic roots—his Welsh paternal lineage ("because of my father, I always had one eye turned toward the past, almost looking back toward the days of King Arthur.... The Welsh have very long memories"), and the British loyalists on his maternal side who were exiled from New England to Canada after the United States gained its independence ("and so I had both the old land and the new land constantly before me in my childhood and in the things that influenced me, and I was always turning from one to the other, and feeling the pull of one against the other").

Davies illustrates two common sources of responsibility reaching out from the past. Although accessible to everyone, these sources are rarely noticed by most people. One is the call of excellence in one's task, the second is responsibility to one's experience and to one's roots. These are among the most insistent voices to which creative individuals respond.

Although this pattern is most evident among artists and humanists, it is also present in a less obvious form among scientists. For them, responsibility to the demands of the craft is so taken for granted that it seldom even comes up. Thorough knowledge of the best work in one's field is a given. Excellence that demands hard work is well illustrated by Freeman Dyson, the mathematical physicist who has laid down the formal theory of quantum electrodynamics:

I have always to force myself to write.... You have to put blood, tears, and sweat into it first. It's awfully hard to get started.... You have to force yourself and push and push and push with the hope that something good will come out. You have got to go through that process before it really starts to flow easily, and without that preliminary forcing and pushing, probably nothing would ever happen.

Like all other creative scientists, Dyson believes that one cannot do anything new without first becoming thoroughly immersed in the past. Respect for the insights of previous scientists is essential; they know, as did Isaac Newton, that if they are able to see farther than others, it is because they are standing on the shoulders of giants. Similarly, scientists are committed—almost by definition—to take seriously their responsibility to evidence, to their own experience.

Less clear in the case of scientists is the link to their personal past or ethnic origin. Yet in most cases those interviewed remembered a parent or teacher they admired and whose strengths they wished to emulate. For instance, Dyson spoke with respect of his father, an orchestra conductor who sat down at his desk at home every day to compose music: "I remember very well when we were children, he would compose quite systematically for three hours every morning.... He had a very strong self-discipline. His hero was Haydn. He also, like Haydn, put on his best suit when he was composing... and I think that is very largely true of me as well." Respect for past excellence is not restricted to one's own craft, but can emanate from any form of outstanding accomplishment.

But how does a person learn to respect and emulate the accomplishments of others? While there are almost as many ways to do so as there are creative persons, some qualitative similarities emerged in the interviews. Creative persons tend to become interested, intrigued, almost obsessed with an aspect of life for which they have a special knack—a small advantage over their peers. When the interest becomes established, the budding creator tries to find our as much about it as she or he can, approaching with wonder the skills and knowledge that previous generations achieved in that domain. E. O. Wilson, the great naturalist, described how this process occurred in his childhood, when in grade school he and a friend became deeply interested in fire ants:

> We would go over to the zoo in Washington and to the National Museum... I was enthralled by the grandeur, by federal grandeur, the idea that the citizenry of this great country could make magnificent institutions, full of animals and insects and scientists who studied them and so on. This was grand stuff, and I just wanted to be part of it. And Ellis and I soon got a copy of an advanced textbook in entomology, which I now realize is one of the most... densely technical books ever written. Quite unnecessarily so. But we were awestruck by this. You know, there was the mystique that goes with terminology and complex drawings and so on. Well, we started studying it together. And this gave us new impetus, something to shoot for, that we would be competent enough to do that kind of work some day. Oh, I was, I was committed from then on.

One note of caution about perhaps overestimating the importance of respect for the past is the fact that all creative individuals studied, whether by us or by others, tend to be adults at the time they are interviewed. So it could be that a sense of responsibility to the best work of the past is more the result of maturity than of creativity. Perhaps when they were young the Dysons and Davies had no interest in or respect for their predecessors; perhaps all their energies were focused on leaving their mark on the domain by rejecting traditions. This is certainly a popular view in the social sciences; for instance, Bourdieu (1993) attributes the historical change in science and art to the struggle between older cohorts intent on preserving the past and younger cohorts bent on dethroning them.

Certainly many older creative persons recalled that by their teens they felt a sense of awe for the best work of their predecessors. As Wilson's recollection suggests, wanting to continue in their forerunners' footsteps was something they felt early; it does not seem to be a later reconstruction from an adult perspective. It is difficult to resolve this issue without following cohorts of young people in a longitudinal study and determining whether respect for tradition differentiates creative individuals early in life as well as late. In any case, our present uncertainty suggests an interesting topic for future research: The hypothesis is that, other things being equal, young people who feel a sense of responsibility for the past are more likely than those who do not to become creative as adults—provided, of course, that they also feel responsible for improving on what their predecessors accomplished. While *deference* to the past can be paralyzing, *responsibility* for it can be liberating and constructive.

The Call of the Future

Respect for the past is not sufficient to provide an ethos conducive to creativity. In fact, by itself an excessive concern for past accomplishments might breed excellent performance, but it is unlikely to lead to novelty, let alone striking originality. As one might expect, creative individuals are also extremely interested in future possibilities. For them the old adage *rerum novarum cupidus*—lusting for new things—is an apt description.

Robertson Davies, the writer who described himself as being constantly pulled back and forth between the "old land" of his ancestors and the "new land" where he grew up, expressed this dynamic in his works. In his last book, he traced the trajectory of how his city, Toronto, emerged from provincialism into a dynamic metropolis: "One of the principal themes in it is the growth of a city, and the city is this city, Toronto. I have seen it in my lifetime emerge from a place which was still gripped in the form of a British colony into an independent place.... What the book is about is [this growth] as seen by a single character who observes it... without, by any means, taking the line that progress has always been positive."

At age 69, Freeman Dyson was also still "lusting for new things." Having ridden the crest of quantum physics 50 or so years earlier, he now found physics too specialized, too congested: "When I first came into physics, I would go to meetings of the American Physical Society, and essentially all the physicists of the United States would be there in one room, you know? I mean it was still a small community.... Now, of course, the Physical Society has 25,000 members, and meetings are completely different... specialized." As a result, Dyson has become more interested in astrophysics and is searching-out colleagues in that still manageable field, learning from them and contributing to their thinking. There are about 12 young astronomers in this building who are doing fantastic things. I mean, astronomy is now in a golden age, much as physics was 40 years ago.... In astronomy there are new things being discovered every week.... Those people are really enjoying themselves." In fact, one could say of any of the individuals interviewed what has been said of Paul Cezanne: "He was obsessed with tradition and obsessed with overturning it" (Trachtman 2006, p. 82).

Of course an excessive focus on what is to come presents its own dangers. It can breed impatience with what is at hand. Lusting for new things may lead to risky shortcuts, to a disregard for process in favor of the desired outcome. Without roots in the best practices of the past, a commitment to the future can easily become out of touch with lived experience and result in chaos instead of creativity. The emphasis on novelty for the sake of novelty that has become so prevalent in the contemporary visual arts is just one of many examples.

Past and Future Folded into the Present

How past and future excellence can be combined in a fulfilling quest for creativity in the here and now is shown by the life of ceramicist Eva Zeisel. She was born to a prominent intellectual family in Budapest in the early part of the twentieth century. Two of her relations eventually obtained Nobel Prizes in science. She was a very independent young girl, in part because she believed she lacked her mother's social graces and her brother's intellectual ambition and training. In her late 70s she still remembered that as a teenager she overheard some people sitting a couple of rows back in a theater talking about her: "Her grandmother is such a clever, bright, intellectual person. Her mother is such a beauty. And now, look at her."

Zeisel turned out to have one talent that was missing from the rest of the family: drawing. She meant to become a painter, but in the meantime she also dabbled in making ceramic ware—vases, plates, pitchers, and bowls. Eventually she took it upon herself to become a "professional" ceramicist, which involved the unheard-of step, for a girl from a good family (or any girl for that matter), of apprenticing to a master potter so she could get an official guild certificate at the end of the training.

In this decision she was inspired, in large part, by her belief that well-designed objects of folk art were being replaced by cheap, mass-produced tableware and that poor people were being deprived of one of the last opportunities to be surrounded by things of beauty. At the same time she understood how quixotic it would be to try to provide handmade plates and glasses to those living close to poverty. So she decided next to study the mass production of china; toward this end, she went to work for a large factory in Germany.

When she felt ready to combine her appreciation of beautiful ceramics inspired by tradition with the new manufacturing opportunities, Zeisel asked herself, Where could I apply this knowledge? In the early 1930s, one obvious answer presented itself: in the Soviet Union, the paradise of the proletariat. So Zeisel went to Russia and offered to set up a factory to manufacture beautiful chinaware cheaply. The Soviet regime appreciated the public relations opportunity—daughter of wealthy Western family comes to work for Russia—and accepted her offer, putting her in charge of an existing factory.

To make a long story short, Zeisel soon came into conflict with the Soviet authorities, who wanted her to make things cheap but did not care about how they looked. The conflict ended with her being imprisoned, m solitary confinement, waiting any moment to be executed. The Soviets finally relented because of international pressures and allowed her to leave for Turkey. From there Zeisel moved to New York, where her inexpensive but elegant lines of chinaware became best sellers all over the world and are now exhibited at the Museum of Modern Art and other museums.

Although in no way a moralistic person by conventional standards, Zeisel responded to the calls for excellence that issued from many directions. She felt responsible for continuing what was best in traditional folk art, and she felt responsible for sharing beauty with those who could not otherwise afford it. These senses of responsibility led her to learn modem ceramic technology so she could satisfy these two calls. At every step she was directed by the enjoyment she derived from making the most beautiful objects she could at the least expense.

Although she was always playful in her work, the responsibilities Zeisel shouldered were no trifling matters. While in solitary confinement in Moscow she was tempted to commit suicide several times. In her loyalty to beauty, she showed the steely determination that one usually associates with religious martyrs determined to follow their vocation to the bitter end.

Another example of how respect for the past and a vision of the future come together in a creative present is provided by Ravi Shankar, Indian composer and musician. Shankar trained since childhood as a *sitar* player and composer, and reached great fame in doing so. He felt enormous commitment to the traditional roots of this music and to its preservation. But by the middle of the twentieth century he realized that these traditions were endangered by a variety of economic and cultural changes: "[In] the olden days, when the maharajas and all these aristocrats were sponsoring famous musicians, it was no problem keeping 15 or 20 students, you know.... And for all these years they would really concentrate [on] learning and practicing—that's all they did." Now, however, with the maharajas gone, young people had to earn money to support themselves and could no longer focus on learning the traditional skills.

Shankar saw the possibility of combining the traditional music of India with the avant-garde music of the West. In the 1960s he became the guru of George Harrison and performed with Harrison and the other members of the Beatles—thus revitalizing both the content of the music and the economy that supported it. Respect for the past and respect for the unfolding reality of the future together allowed Shankar to keep doing good work in the present.

The notion of responsibility shown by these people is not the usual kind based on ethical values and conformity to community pressures. It is based instead on a desire to do good work for its own sake—to achieve excellence in a domain at any cost. While the desire for excellence may actually lead to questionable outcomes— as with Robert Oppenheimer's fascination with the "sweet problem" of how to build a nuclear bomb—it is also a necessary component of the evolution of culture. Without reverence for the achievements of the past and a clear-eyed respect for the unfolding reality of the future, one can expect only chaos or rigidity.

The Sources of Calling

Table 17.1 summarizes the responsibilities that attract the allegiance of creative individuals. The 18 cells of the figure are not intended to be exhaustive; they are provided only to suggest how a full classification might be developed. Basically, the taxonomy refers to the direction from which the call for action is perceived to be coming, and thus the direction toward which the person is likely to commit his or her energy. It contains three prime dimensions of concern for excellence: the

Table 17.1 Major sources of the call for responsibility mentioned by creative individuals

		Past	Present	Future
Domain	Chosen discipline	Learn	Act	Expand
(culture)	Relation to the discipline	Learn	Integrate	Expand
Field (society)	Coworkers	Be trained	Collaborate	Train
	Broader social milieu	Respect traditions	Support community	Innovate
Person (self)	Personal growth	Find meaning	Act with integrity	Reshape goals
	Relation to others	Filial	Partnering	Generative

past, the present, and the future; and three major areas of investment: the culture, society, and the self. Each of the nine cells and the intersection of these dimensions can in turn be subdivided into at least two subsets.

For example, the first row refers to the responsibility a creative person is likely to feel toward the content of his or her discipline—for a doctor, the knowledge of medicine; for a mechanic, the craft of making a car run. Practitioners of any domain would be remiss if they did not master the knowledge of the past, did not apply it in their own work, and did not try to expand the existing knowledge so that their domain would contain more of it in the future.

The second row in Table 17.1 refers to the fact that many creative achievements take place at the boundaries of domains. When the quantum theory that had been developed at the subatomic level was applied to chemistry, the latter domain was able to expand exponentially. Sometimes ideas from music, art, and literature influence neighboring forms at art, and even science. Thus creative individuals are often patrolling the borders of their domain to see if they can learn something from outside them that can be integrated into their own work and thereby expand the domain.

The third row of Table 17.1 indicates that creative individuals feel three sense of responsibility toward the people who trained them—such as the master craftsman, the guru, or the lab head who shaped their approach to the craft. They also learn continually from peers and often collaborate with them, or are involved in the organization of the field of practitioners as reviewers, editors, department chairpersons. They are also involved in training the next generation of practitioners and may take responsibility for how the discipline will be practiced in the future.

The fourth row suggests that eventually many creative persons feel the call of the larger human context in which they live and get involved in causes beyond the borders of their discipline, first by becoming involved in the community as it is, and then by working to change it in line with their values—as did Benjamin Spock, Eva Zeisel, and Linus Pauling, among others.

The fifth and sixth rows of the table deal with the personal development that creative individuals tend to pursue throughout their lives, not only in their professional role but also in their full humanity. Starting from a firm foundation of curiosity, interest, and meaning, they try to act in the present in conformity with the self-image they have created. But this image does not become static: even in the late decades of their lives they often find new knowledge to learn, new activities to engage in, and new goals to pursue. The relationships that define them also reflect this threefold attachment—to their origins, ancestors, and family; to their partner, and colleagues; and to the generations that will follow.

The Implications of Creativity for an Expanded View of Responsibility

The most important message that creative individuals have to convey on this matter is a simple but vital one: there is no responsibility without care. Persons who do not care enough for *something* are unlikely to extend themselves except for reasons of self-interest. But if they care enough for something, then they feel responsible for the well-being of the object of their care. If they do not care, they do not even hear the call; or if they hear it, they do not bother to respond.

The most obvious and universal objects of care are other people we love: our parents, siblings, friends, spouses, and children; the members of our sport team or army platoon; our coworkers, fellow parishioners, and compatriots. When they call, we hear and heed the summons. Then we feel responsible to the institutions that order our lives—the laws, the church, or the workplace. We also feel responsible to legal, professional, religious, and civic virtues that we have learned make a good person and a good citizen.

All of these reasons for caring are necessary for civilized human existence. But creative individuals show us yet another way of caring. Their concern is for all aspects of life—for galaxies and molecules, for towering buildings and subtle human feelings. They care for the excellence of human artifacts such as music or mathematics, life sciences or poetry. They care not only for the best examples of the past, but also for how best to perform in their chosen medium right now—and how to improve and enrich the tradition.

The call to excellence is a joyful calling: Creative people may at times be lonely, depressed, and even suicidal; but when they respond to a call, they feel connected to the dynamic trajectory of human evolution. It is an ecstatic experience that benefits everyone—the creator who is lifted out of limited-individual existence, and the community that is enriched by the quest for excellence.

Is this kind of care something only geniuses feel, or can the rest of us benefit from their expanded view of responsibility through education? It seems quite obvious that we not only can, but we also desperately need to apply the lessons of creativity to the rearing of children in all walks of life. Alas, formal education is not overly concerned with teaching passion, which is the prerequisite for caring, and hence for beginning to feel responsible for something beyond self and the closest circle of one's social network. Some teachers understand the importance of getting students to care about some aspect of life, whether the fire ants that so fascinated naturalist E. O. Wilson or the pottery that Eva Zeisel so loved. But it is very difficult for teachers to do so under the current conditions of schooling, where numbing tests take top priority and even sullen obedience is difficult to achieve, let alone burning passion.

In fact, one of the most distressing changes in the context of child rearing is a widespread reduction of opportunities for children to care and to feel responsible. In the prevailing environment of a century ago, on the farms and in the small towns of America, children learned that cows had to be milked each morning, chickens needed to be fed, the garden plot needed to be watered, the firewood had to be split, and so on and so forth—and if the tasks were not completed competently and on time, the consequences were felt by all, and the responsibilities could be clearly-assigned. This kind of experience is now very rare. Many children grow into adulthood with hazy notions of how cause and effect work in the real world— notions made even more confusing by the steady diet of virtual reality absorbed from the media.

Visionaries and some educational pioneers have pointed at possible solutions that might serve as stimuli for planning what we should do next. In his novel *Island,* Aldous Huxley described a Utopian community where the first formal training of children was to learn rock climbing.

This way, the author argued, they would learn to take responsibility for their own lives as well as those of their partners on the rope. Moreover, they would learn to trust their peers by placing the responsibility for their own life in the hands of their partners, Huxley's educational program has never been implemented, to our knowledge, but less extreme versions have entered child-rearing practices quite successfully. For instance, one of the major goals of Montessori teachers is to get children to learn to care for their clothes, their food, and the well-being of their peers; as well as to care for the orderliness of the classrooms and the learning tools they contain. Children who learn to care for such simple things will be able to care for increasingly more complex objects, ideas, and forms of order.

Creative lives bear witness to the fact that one can learn to care and be responsible for practically any aspect of the world and of human activity. How to implement their experience into a viable pedagogy, however, is a challenge that still needs to be confronted. Some initial suggestions include the following:

Help the child find his or her interest. The passion of creative persons often arises serendipitously, by chance. It is aroused by an exceptional event or experience. But just as often it seems to be prepared for by the intervention of parents and teachers. We know only a little at this point about how to ignite a child's passion.

One obvious way is to expose the young person to as many forms of experience as possible, without pressure or coercion. Role models who love what they are doing help, and so do exemplars of excellence. Taking traditional accomplishments seriously is also useful. So is considering future possibilities in the child's life, in connection with possible careers in various fields.

Basically, the issue is to communicate to the child a love for life in its myriad forms, in the hope that the child will find a connection between his or her interests and some aspect of the world. Once the connection is established, the child is likely to begin caring for that aspect in its past, present, and future forms.

Trust the child while helping to develop the child's interest. If the child learns, to care for an object or activity, a dialectic spiral of autonomous learning tends to develop. Care implies a desire for excellence, which leads to more skilled activity—a desire to play the piano better or to solve more advanced calculus problems, for example. In turn, this cycle leads to deeper caring for the medium, and hence a greater sense of responsibility. When this commitment coalesces, the adult needs only to stand on the sidelines, ready to lend a hand when needed or to point to the next level of challenge.

The love for learning that develops in a child needs to be sustained into maturity if it is to lead to responsible adult behavior. A physician or business-person who sees his or her work exclusively as a means to wealth or prestige is likely to take the easy way out when hard choices are called for. A plumber who does not care for excellence is going to be more prone to take shortcuts in his work than one who does care for excellence. A civil society depends on institutions that support in people a feeling of responsibility to their callings. As John W. Gardner so aptly wrote, "An excellent plumber is infinitely more admirable than an incompetent philosopher. The society which scorns excellence in plumbing because plumbing is a humble activity and tolerates shoddiness in philosophy because it is an exalted activity will have neither good plumbing nor good phi-losophy. Neither its pipes nor its theories will hold water" (Gardner 1961, p. 86).

Unfortunately, training in the occupations, and even in the professions, is ignoring the fact that good work depends on whether workers come to love and respect what they are meant to do. The notion that one's work is a calling, a vocation, is not a fashionable one to hold these days. The close mentoring, the teaching by example, that used to be a safeguard that young workers would rec-ognize the beauty and value of a job well done, is getting harder to find. Yet if a young person fails to learn this and sees instead that success and promotion in the workplace depend on cleverness and compromise rather than on responsibility to the craft, the temptation to be irresponsible becomes more attractive. Of course the responsibility that a budding poet learns for his craft or that a young biologist learns for hers might not transfer to other aspects of life outside their respective domains of interest. The extremely punctilious business-person and the uncom-promising plumber could be lax and remiss as citizens. But considering the alternative—cohorts of children growing up without any interest in or concern for the past or the future, without any motivation to do their best—it is hard to argue that life in the next generation would not improve if children learned to care for at least one aspect of the world, and thus be led to appreciate excellence in it and to feel responsible for preserving and improving it.

References

Bourdieu, P. (1993). *The field of cultural production*. New York: Columbia University Press.

Choe, I., & Nakamura, J. (1996). Values of creative individuals (Unpublished manuscript).

Csikszentmihalyi, M. (1996). *Creativity: Flow and the psychology of discovery and invention*. New York: HarperCollins.

Csikszentmihalyi, M. (2003). *Good business: Leadership, flow, and the making of meaning*. New York: Viking.

Gardner, J. W. (1961). *Excellence: Can we be equal and excellent too?*. New York: Harper & Row.

Kasof, J. (1995). Explaining creativity: The attributional perspective. *Creativity Research Journal, 8*, 311–366.

Lombroso, C. (1889/1891). The man of genius. London: Walter Scott.

Trachtman, P. (2006). Cézanne, the man who changed the landscape of art. *Smithsonian, 36*(10), 80–89.

Vasari, G. (1959). Lives of the most eminent painters, sculptors, and architects. New York: Modern Library (Original work published 1550).

Chapter 18
The Early Lives of Highly Creative Persons: The Influence of the Complex Family

R. Routledge, Gary Gute, Deanne S. Gute, Jeanne Nakamura and Mihaly Csikszentmihalyi

Introduction

Over the last 50 years, theoretical, speculative, and empirical scholarship has examined the influence of early family context on subsequent accomplishments in children of high ability. Building upon 40 years of creativity literature focusing on optimal experience, this exploratory study applied the Complex Family Framework in a systematic analysis of creative adults' recollections of their early family lives. The study identifies evidence of the interplay of integration and Differentiation, a catalyst for individual optimal experience, in the families of nine creative exemplars who have made significant contributions to contemporary culture. Five participants represented the Arts and Humanities, three the Social Sciences, and one the Physical Sciences. The study demonstrates the utility of the Complex Family Framework in understanding families' contributions to children's later creative achievement.

Over the last 50 years, much theoretical, speculative, and empirical scholarship has described the influence of early family context on subsequent accomplishments in children of high ability (e.g., Albert 1971, 1980, 1994; Albert and Runco

R. Routledge (✉)
Taylor & Francis Group, Boca Raton, USA

G. Gute · D. S. Gute
University of Northern Iowa, Cedar Falls, USA

J. Nakamura · M. Csikszentmihalyi
Claremont Graduate University, Claremont, USA

M. Csikszentmihalyi, *The Systems Model of Creativity*,
DOI: 10.1007/978-94-017-9085-7_18,
© Springer Science+Business Media Dordrecht 2014

1986; Amabile 1989, 1996; Bloom 1985; Colangelo 1988; Goertzel et al. 1978; Helson 1968; McCurdy 1960; Milgram and Hong 1999; Runco and Albert 2005; Simonton 1984; Walberg 1981; Walberg et al. 1996).

Although several studies have investigated the relationship between family context and significant achievement in adulthood, few have drawn upon existing models to provide a conceptual framework for understanding how families can contribute to children's later creative achievement. The present study explores the utility of the Complex Family Framework (Csikszentmihalyi et al. 1993) in illuminating that relationship. The framework is particularly promising because it has helped researchers empirically identify a specific pathway toward the development of talent during adolescence (Csikszentmihalyi et al. 1993; Rathunde and Csikszentmihalyi 1991).

This study builds upon 40 years of creativity literature focusing on optimal experience. Seminal studies include Getzels and Csikszentmihalyi's (1976) longitudinal study of 290 artists; a 4-year longitudinal study of talented teenagers (Csikszentmihalyi and Larson 1984, 1987; Csikszentmihalyi et al. 1993); a study of 91 persons whose creative achievements continued throughout later life (Csikszentmihalyi 1996); and studies of vital engagement in adulthood (Nakamura 2001, 2002). A recurring finding in these publications was that complexity is central to the lives of creative persons.

Complexity, Complex Families, and Flow

Since the 1970s, terms such as *complexity* and *complexity theory* have been widely used with differing perspectives and emphases in the social sciences, engineering, computer science, and the study of chaos. It is important to distinguish *complex* from *complicated,* which commonly implies a dysfunctional lack of organization. As it has developed over several decades of optimal experience research, Csikszentmihalyi's theory of complexity shares chaos theory's premise that an order underlies the apparent disorder of all enduring systems. This order is characterized by two complementary, but often seemingly oppositional, processes: differentiation and integration. It is the ongoing processes of differentiation and integration that account for the ontogenesis of all living things, "from the simplest amoeba to the most sophisticated human creature" (Csikszentmihalyi 1996, p. 362). All complex systems, whether biological, cognitive, familial, or societal (Rathunde and Csikszentmihalyi 1991), seek differentiation: movement toward uniqueness, seeking change by taking on new parts and functions. Within a family, individuals differentiate by constructing a unique identity and working toward personal goals (Csikszentmihalyi and Rochberg-Halton 1981; Damon 1983), Complex systems, also seek integration: working to maintain continuity and stability. Within an integrated family, members provide emotional support, working to maintain relationships by investing in common goals, traditions, and values

(Rathunde and Csikszentmihalyi 1991). In such a family, clear rules, limits, and expectations provide structures that minimize chaos.

Within an optimized complex system, these ongoing processes of differentiation and integration keep the system healthy and growing. The complexity dialectic, similar to Baldwin's (1911) developmental theory, suggests that a system's growth results from the ongoing syntheses of these two opposing, but complementary, processes.

When a person within the complex family feels anxiety, "creating order through a higher level of integration becomes a conscious goal; when faced with boredom, seeking change through differentiation becomes the aim" (Rathunde and Csikszentmihalyi 2008, p. 470), It is in the space between anxiety and boredom that the person is poised to experience flow, a state of complete engagement in an activity. Within a complex family, the integration force provides a consistently cohesive, supportive family context, an optimal backdrop for flow experiences in the daily lives of family members. The complex family's ongoing encouragement of differentiation results in family members experiencing flow as a result of their investing attention in activities that, over time, demand increasing skill and challenge.

The simultaneous forces of order and novelty result in a coordinated stabilizing and broadening of attention (Fredrickson 1998). From early childhood on, creative persons find deep enjoyment in an area of talent or skill. These rewarding experiences motivate them to replicate the enjoyment and fulfillment that the activity brings, which leads to the development of vital engagement with the endeavor: "Artists become fascinated by painting, musicians by music, and scientists by the pursuit of elusive relationships in Nature" (Csikszentmihalyi and Csikszentmihalyi 1993, p. 188). Sustained over long periods of time, the person's talent, skill, knowledge, and expertise, if channeled and accepted by established gatekeepers, might result in "breakthroughs", significant creative contributions to the culture or a specific domain (Csikszentmihalyi 1999).

Several theorists and researchers have proposed frameworks in which optimal functioning within family and individual systems is explained by the presence of opposing attributes and processes. A few examples include demandingness and responsiveness (Baumrind 1977, 1989), ego control and ego resiliency (Block and Block 1980), love and discipline (Damon 1983; Irwin 1987; Maccoby and Martin 1983), agency and communion (Bakan 1966), psychological safety and psychological freedom (Rogers 1954), connection and individuality (Grotevant and Cooper 1983), and affect enabling and cognitive enabling (Hauser 1991). Complexity theory's processes of integration and differentiation, however, form the only dialectical framework that has been empirically demonstrated to foster creativity in families and to facilitate the development of creativity across the lifespan (Csikszentmihalyi and Rathunde 1998; Rathunde and Csikszentmihalyi 2008).

Empirical Research on Complex Families

Drawing data from a 4-year longitudinal study of 200 adolescents with superior intellectual, physical, and/or artistic talent (for a detailed discussion, see Csikszentmihalyi et al. 1993), Rathunde (1988) sought to better understand the role of flow in the family context by investigating participants' subjective interpretations of family situations. For the study of 200 adolescents, Rathunde developed the 24-item Complex Family Questionnaire. That instrument, in addition to interviews, the Experience Sampling Method (ESM) (Csikszentmihalyi and Larson 1984, 1987), and systematic matching of children's perceptions with their parents' independently measured perceptions, was used to explore the families' role in the teenagers' development of their abilities.

Factor analysis of the Complex Family Questionnaire data identified two factors, each comprising two lower-order factors: support (comprised of harmony and help) and stimulation comprised of involvement and freedom; (Rathunde and Csikszentmihalyi 1991). Complex families were high on both stimulation and support; differentiated families were high on stimulation and low on support; integrated families were low on stimulation, but high on support; simple families were low on both dimensions. Of the four family types, teens from complex families reported the greatest number of positive home experiences; greater numbers of optimal experiences while spending time with their families than in other contexts; and the highest level of positive feelings when working in the area of their talent (e.g., mathematics, science, music, athletics, or art) or on schoolwork, regardless of location. Specific positive subjective rewards these teens reported included feeling happy, cheerful, alert, excited, sociable, and open, as well as experiencing greater cognitive efficiency, motivation, and self-esteem. Compared to participants in the other groups, the teens from the complex families more often reported living up to their own and others' expectations and doing projects important to themselves and the fulfillment of their goals. Moreover, parents in complex families were frequently viewed as helpful teachers; children from differentiated families saw their parents as pressuring them to achieve (Rathunde and Csikszentmihalyi 1991).

Rathunde's findings demonstrated that family context facilitates flow experiences in adolescents by consistently providing experiences that balance choice, clarity, centering, commitment, and challenge. As Rathunde and Csikszentmihalyi (1993) described the process, within complex families, many small, experiential "building blocks" over time "accumulate toward positive subjective rewards" (pp. 158–159).

Method

With respect to the development of creativity (Sawyer et al. 2003), few attempts have been made to understand the family as an early flow-producing context for highly accomplished, creative persons. This exploratory study applies the

Complex Family Framework in the systematic analysis of creative adults' recollections of their early family lives and experiences with flow.

Data for the present study were gathered from verbatim transcripts of semi-structured interviews conducted for the Creativity in Later Life Study (Csikszentmihalyi 1996). Although not originally generated solely for the purpose of examining family influence on later creativity, the transcripts provide rich and powerful descriptions and interpretations of the participants' families of origin. Complexity theory contributed the two concepts—integration and differentiation—that served as broad initial categories for coding all portions of the transcripts related to early family life. First, all portions of the transcripts describing participants' early lives within their families of origin were identified. Second, Rathunde's (1989) descriptors were used to guide review and annotation of transcripts: examples of family harmony and help, as well as descriptions involving the concepts of belongingness, security, rules, values, and synonymous ideas, were marked as evidence of integration. Evidence of differentiation included stimulating and challenging children to develop existing skills (or to take on new ones), and modeling perseverance and achievement-producing work habits. All excerpts illustrating participants demonstrating autonomy from specific family values or expectations were also included.

Excerpts were organized in a word processing program and reviewed multiple times for best fit as new, more refined categories were generated in answer to the question, "What specific markers of integration and differentiation are present in the life stories of the participants?" This framework permitted us to identify four specific markers of integration within the families described; (a) supporting children's existing aptitudes and interests; (b) spending time together; (c) teaching core values and behavioral boundaries; and (d) demonstrating tolerance for failure. The analysis also yielded four markers of differentiation: (a) coping with difficult circumstances; (b) stimulating new interests and challenges; (c) modeling habits of creativity; (d) and building a demographically and psychologically diverse family unit. Table 1 illustrates the distribution of markers in the transcripts. Absence of a marker indicates only that no reference was made in the transcript to that concept, not that the trait was absent within the participant's family.

We do not claim to know definitively that the present study measures the degree of complexity in the families described or that all nine of these families are, in fact, complex. Our study is limited to descriptions of subjective experience generated voluntarily while the participants reflected on a range of topics, including direct questions about early family life. However, based upon the theoretical premise that all complex systems are highly integrated and differentiated, and upon the studies of optimal experience demonstrating that complexity is central to the lives of creative persons, we did anticipate that the Complex Family Framework would provide a useful tool for plumbing these interviews for markers of complexity.

Table 18.1 Markers of integration and differentiation: references to traits in the interview transcripts

Participant	Integration	Marker I–1	Marker I–2	Marker I–3	Marker I–4
1 Booth	X	X		X	
2 Franklin	X	X		X	
3 Peterson	X	X	X	X X X X	- X
4 Lanyon	X	X X			
5 Holton	X	X		X X	
6 Henderson	X			X	
7 Dyson	X		X X		
8 Davies	X	X X		X	X
9 Anonymous	X	X		X	
Participant	Differentiation	Marker D–1	Marker D–2	Marker D–3	Marker D–4
1 Booth	X	X	X	X X	
2 Franklin	X	X		X	
3 Peterson	X	X X	X X		
4 Lanyon	X	X		X X	
5 Holton	X	X X			
6 Henderson	X		X X	X	X
7 Dyson	X	X	X X	X X	
8 Davies	X			X	X
9 Anonymous	X		X X		

Note 1–1 = supporting existing interests and aptitudes; 1–2 = spending time together; 1–3 = teaching core values/setting rules; 1–4 = tolerating failure; D–1 = dealing with difficult circumstances; D–2 = stimulating new interests and challenges; D–3 = modeling habits of creativity; D–4 = building a demographically diverse family

Participants

The sample consisted of 9 of the 91 participants in the Creativity in Later Life Study (Csikszentmihalyi 1996), All 91 participants made a significant impact upon a major cultural domain, and continued active" involvement in that or a different domain in later life. The present sample was chosen because it provided a varied range of backgrounds. Given the exploratory nature of the study, we considered the sample size adequate because during the coding process, the same markers recurred across the corpus of nine interview transcripts, indicating that we had sampled until redundancy.

Participants included one male social scientist, an author and developer of social programs who chose to maintain anonymity, along with eight additional participants (five male and three female) who granted consent for identification by name when quoted. The sample, although small, represents a balance of nationalities (five American-born, four immigrants to the United States) and domains (five from the Arts and Humanities, three from the Social Sciences, one from the Physical Sciences). The S we can identify include (1) Wayne Booth, literary critic and author of such seminal works as *The Rhetoric of Fiction* and *The Company We Keep*; (2) John Hope Franklin, African American historian best known for his scholarship about slavery and the Civil War; (3) Oscar Peterson, world-renowned jazz pianist and composer; (4) Ellen Lanyon, painter and art educator; (5) Nina Holton, Austrian-born sculptor, whose work has been widely exhibited at international galleries; (6) Hazel Henderson, economist and scholar well known for her contributions to the study of sustainable economies; (7) Freeman Dyson, physicist and author of books and essays about the future of the universe; and (8) Robertson Davies, Canadian novelist and playwright.

The Interviews

In spite of the many ways in which the interview participants in the present study differ on particulars, all provide evidence of early family contexts that are both integrated and differentiated. Through the qualitative analysis of transcripts, we constructed a depiction of what these apparent opposites look and feel like when experienced simultaneously in a family context.

Integration

Rathunde's analysis (Rathunde 1989) suggested that integration can be best understood as the coexistence of harmony and help, qualities that participant's families maintained in environments where each individual felt a strong sense of belongingness, value, and security. Two themes emerged in almost every interview. Participants described warm, caring parents who maintained family harmony by enforcing consistent values, reasonably stable routines, and active rule-setting. These rules, they say, saved them confusion and facilitated good decision-making. As important as these behavioral boundaries, however, was families' unconditional emotional support for their children's personal interests and aptitudes, The four specific themes that emerged as markers of integration in participants' lived experience are described in the following.

Supporting children's existing aptitudes and interests The transcripts provided ample illustrations of how, once parents recognized an interest or talent in their children, they cultivated integration by providing material, verbal, and emotional support and encouragement. In answer to a question about what makes a fulfilling and effective teaching career, Wayne Booth named authentic vitality, optimism, and strength of ego sufficient to "get people really to express what they think". Booth directly attributed his development of these qualities to the enthusiastic confidence his mother and other family members conveyed to him throughout his childhood and adolescence:

I have thought a lot about this question. And I really think the answer is quite conventional: a very powerful introduction to life, with a mother who thought I was the… the King of the Beasts. And grandparents who thought I was terrific, and expected me to become President of the United States or something, you know. Just absolute, total faith.

The interviews' themes of confidence and faith were sometimes accompanied by examples of investments of material help. Artist Ellen Lanyon's maternal grandfather was a muralist. When Lanyon demonstrated an early interest in art, her family passed on her grandfather's painting tools to her, confident in their belief that she "must have inherited" his talent:

There was this confidence from the family that it would happen. You know, everybody believed it, it had to be. And when I was about 12 years old, my grandfather died and my father and mother had put together his equipment that was left plus tubes of paint, et cetera, and it was presented to me on my twelfth birthday as a sort of a, you know, a gesture. This is passing the torch or something.

Some families' belief in the intergenerational continuity of creativity extends the idea of the integrated family beyond the present, linking members through an awareness of their ancestry.

Robertson Davies, similarly, described his parents as "very, very kind and generous to me", a recollection that prompted him to express that he had "great cause to be grateful to them… though often we had strong differences of opinion", Davies' reminiscence of more concrete forms of help primarily consisted of his parents' providing opportunities to go places that fed his interests. Trying to describe his parents, he said

It's very hard to describe what they all were, but one of the things they were, which I very, very greatly appreciate: They were very generous to me because I showed an aptitude for education, and so they helped me get a lot of education. And also, they helped me to get a kind of grounding in music and literature, and so on and so forth, by their example and their advice, and just by sending me where that was to be found.

Asked if his parents helped facilitate his development because he showed aptitude, or if they attempted to impose their view of what he should be, Davies emphasized that he demonstrated aptitude first, and his parents responded by actively seeking ways to help: "No. No, they weren't (imposing their view). They did recognize what was—well, what I was and what my brothers were and what we could do and wondering in what directions we could be helped".

Oscar Peterson's experiences provide another example of parents offering more help than parental control, He was asked if his parents introduced him to jazz:

Peterson: No, I was busy pursuing that for myself (Both laugh)
Interviewer: Was that something they tried to keep you away from because...
Peterson: No, they didn't, not in any way. They tried to keep me in bed at night, but (both laugh) they never prevented me or inhibited me listening to jazz in any way.

John Hope Franklin's narrative provided a reminder that for many of the participants, most of whom grew up during the Depression, material resources were scarce. He suggested that affective forms of support can compensate for lack of material ones: "I got all the encouragement that I needed from them. What they didn't have in the way of money they made up in the way of encouragement". Ellen Lanyon's family illustrates other ways creative interests could be fed without adequate financial resources, and demonstrates that help can come from extended family, not only from parents:

> I grew up when, you know, every weekend the Metropolitan Opera was on the radio. It was a standard thing that the family would listen to. So, everything that we could have we had, even though funding was not there. Now, ah, but my father's sister was a business woman, and she had the means to send my sister and I to Saturday school at the Art Institute when we were kids, you know, maybe eight years old or something. So, that my training and my familiarity with the museum and the school was very early.

Lanyon expressed an opinion that synthesized what all these examples suggest about the relationship between family support and creativity:

> I just think that when family is supportive of someone who, you know, a child, who shows that they want to do something no matter what it might be, it helps that child to become more convinced that this is something they can do, and it gives you confidence. And I think that is so important in the making of a… especially making a creative person…If that kind of support comes gently and is not a force that one rebels against, then it's a very positive thing, I think.

Even though these selections indicate the support and faith that the family extended to these participants, and were therefore coded as examples of the underlying concept of integration, they also clearly indicate that confidence and harmony did not constitute passive support, but active efforts to identify and build upon the child's budding interest.

Spending time together Families build integration as a result of something quite uncomplicated: time spent together. Lanyon's recollection of her family listening to opera together on the radio is an illustration. It is easy to infer how some of these activities shaped professional choices. Davies, the novelist, "Grew up in a talking family where there was endless conversation, endless talk about politics and about the theater. My parents were both mad for the theater and music, and all that sort of thing and that was very lucky for me". Freeman Dyson singled out his sister as someone with whom he most enjoyed spending time: "She is completely unscientific… but she is intelligent and enjoys most of the things that I enjoy". This companionship eventually served a professional purpose, his sister figuring into his creative achievement. He noted that except for his more technical works in physics, he would begin projects by imagining he was composing a letter to her.

Other narratives compellingly demonstrate that time spent together shaped positive recollections of childhood and helped create an atmosphere of warmth and harmony. Dyson recalled several activities that built a sense of closeness with his mother:

> My mother and I were very close. We used to go every month to Kew Gardens and look at the latest flowers. They would always have fresh displays of flowers and bushes and the

gardens all year round, and we would go to art museums… and generally she was the stronger cultural influence on me…It is no question that I was very fortunate.

Reflecting on time spent with his own family, Oscar Peterson observed a trend toward less integration in today's families compared to those in the era in which he grew up:

It was much—families were much more closely knit then. And most of my time was spent with the family. I had the odd friends outside in the very young years, later on in high school of course I had friends. But I still made a big thing about my home life. It was always my family that was important. I don't see that as much today, as you well realize. Perhaps one of the problems today.

Parents cultivate family integration in another way: by holding their children responsible for their actions. These families—provide a core set of values—ethical, moral, religious, intellectual, aesthetic, or some combination—that define the boundaries of individual family members' behavior. These stable conditions minimize chaos. Research has suggested that the message "be responsible, independent, and mature… filtered through a context that is also supportive and reliable" (Rathunde and Csikszentmihalyi 1991, p. 155) makes everyday routines more enjoyable and frees children to invest psychic energy in creative activity rather than feelings of insecurity, regret for bad choices, poor self-image, or other negative emotions.

Religious faith is one manifestation of a core value. Franklin described the home where he grew up as "moderately religious". Along with familial religious traditions came lessons about "certain elements of honesty and integrity", Davies felt a more specific religious guidance:

I was brought up—I would not say strictly, because there was nothing harsh about it—but my parents brought me up in a kind of religious atmosphere so that I had a very profound respect for truth, and I was perpetually being reminded, because my parents were very great Bible-quoters, that God is not mocked.

Some of the families centered their values around political and social ideas. The social scientist in our sample provided an illustration:

My father died early. My mother was a very strong, independent-minded person. She had ideas which, for her time, were very advanced, about women's rights and about race relations. She had very strong standards of conduct but they didn't fit some of the conventional hypocrisies of the time. For example, she simply would not allow us to look down on any other race or any other group. It just wasn't permitted in our family. We weren't even conscious of it. Years and years later my brother and I would talk about it and realize that we both had exactly the same attitudes. She had instilled those attitudes early.

A content area or skill can also be inculcated as a family value, through modeling (as in the case of Lanyon and Davies), or through direct persuasion. Franklin offered an example: "And so I said in the *Life of Learning,* in that essay, my parents had an enormous influence on my intellectual as well as my social development. I learned from them the value of studying and reading and that sort of thing".

When asked "In what way do you think your family background was special in helping you to become the person you are?" Oscar Peterson offered examples that shaped him musically, as well as personally.

> Well, I think my family gave me—first of all, the love of music. They helped me appreciate some of the music that I was hearing, and that of course catapulted me into the medium. But they also gave me a—a set of personal rules to live by, that kept me from getting into some of the troubles that musicians were getting into at that time.

The interviewer pursued a line of questioning about musicians' "troubles", noting that "Especially several decades ago, jazz music was associated to some degree with drugs…" Peterson pointed out that his parents' teachings prevented him from making certain choices. Peterson's remark illustrates how the thought of disappointing or hurting family members by acting contrary to their values guided a decision. His description suggested that he rejected what he perceived as unnecessary risk-taking by considering two consequences: (a) loss of family harmony and acceptance and (b) potential harm to his father's well-being.

> They let me know they would never tolerate or accept that. And I knew that all—I remember telling a, I won't call any names, but a very famous musician once who offered me cocaine—I guess it was cocaine—no heroin, excuse me. As he called it, "a hit with heroin". And I told him quite frankly, I said, I would never be able to go home if I did this. And that's the thing that terrified me, more than anything else. I didn't, I couldn't figure out what I would tell my mother, far less my father, if I came home with a habit. There would be no reason for it. It wasn't a fear of what he would do to me, it was a fear of— maybe destroying him altogether. I didn't know how I could ever explain this to him.

This value system helped Peterson navigate peer pressure in his profession, and he interpreted his father's expectations as protecting his creativity.

John Hope Franklin also interpreted his family's guidance and rule-setting as a help, not a hindrance. He recalled, "I didn't have to wonder later whether I should or should not do certain things. It was part of my being because of their influence".

Learning to tolerate failure The parents of these interviewees set high expectations for their children, but they balanced their expectations with support. We see this in how the parents reacted to their children's crises of confidence or outright failure. Oscar Peterson described such a situation as he was developing his musical ability.

Peterson: The first time I heard Art Tatum it almost crippled me! Mentally and physically (Both chuckle).
Interviewer: How old were you then?
Peterson: Oh God. I'm not sure exactly what age I was. I know I was in high school and my dad brought this friend, who happened to be a musician, home with him. And he had, they had this record of Art Tatum's "Tiger Rag". And played it for me. And that sort of stopped my career for a month or two.
Interviewer: It really did? You didn't—

Peterson: Yes, it did. I just decided to give it up. I said, "If someone can play that well, and that inventively, there isn't room for me". And you know, you get into that self-pity area, which I had to fight my way out of, with the help of my father, who encouraged me.

Interviewer: Wow. So he said—what did your father say to you? What did he say?

Peterson: Well, his logic was, "He did it, why can't you?" You know, "You're both human beings, if he found an avenue, you can find one.

Davies' parents provided support by accepting the possibility that their children might *not* succeed in one domain, and reminding them that they could succeed in others. Davies said,

> They were understanding about failures. You see, as a young man, that is, a boy, I was an absolute fool at mathematics and was perpetually failing my examinations in school, and I remember-one time, I was very downcast because I had done dreadfully badly on that examination, and my father gave me some advice which was terribly immoral but very comforting. He said, "Don't worry too much about mathematics. As you grow older, you will find that there are always people who'll do it for you, for money. And because they're interested in getting the right answer they're usually honest" (both laugh). And that was it because he was a terrible mathematician himself, but was very successful in business because he was awfully good at people, and he chose very good helpers, and assistants, and associates.

Franklin's mother used to tell him regularly, "Now, you just do your best, and understand this, the angels cannot do any better than their best!"

Differentiation

Within a differentiated family, members are encouraged to "be themselves" by seeking out new challenges and opportunities. They are encouraged to develop an identity independent of others in the family. The participant narratives demonstrate that both the principle of integration, with its emphasis on harmony and shared values, and differentiation, with it emphasis on autonomy, can be active within a family system. One need not preclude the other: They can work together as a complex mechanism, one part counterbalancing the other. The following section explores, in detail, the four specific markers of differentiation exhibited by families in the present sample, with attention to the ways they coexisted with the integrative aspects of family life already described. They are (a) coping with difficult circumstances; (b) stimulating new interests and challenges; (c) modeling habits of creativity; and (d) building a demographically and psychologically diverse family unit.

Coping with difficult circumstances A concept central to differentiation is the pursuit of challenge. Research describes parents in differentiated families as people who not only permit or facilitate opportunity, but also exercise a degree of *demandingness* (Baumrind 1989; Rathunde 1996) that encourages children to strive beyond present levels of challenge and skill. This was a persistent theme in the transcripts. Challenge is sometimes a function of history-graded influences (Baltes et al. 1998), such as social and macro-economic forces. Throughout John Hope Franklin's childhood, during the Great Depression, his father was unemployed. During the same period, Oscar Peterson's father worked as a porter for the railroad; artist Ellen Lanyon's father worked in a foundry. After Nina Holton and her family immigrated to the United States from Europe, and she subsequently moved alone to New York City to pursue her interest in the arts, she did so without financial support. How the participants responded to the challenges created within their historical milieu can help illuminate ways difficult circumstances contributed to their differentiation and creative achievement.

Freeman Dyson, recalling the era in which he grew up, looked farther into the past, describing pretechnological, less affluent conditions as positive stimuli for cognitive challenge:

> When you look at the way people used to be 100 years ago, they were forced to develop their spirit, sort of their spiritual resources because essentially there was nothing else. They had these long winter evenings with nothing else to do except read or write or do something creative. That is what kids lack these days. They are never given the chance to be bored because there is so much entertainment all the time.

Although powerless to change the macroeconomic environment, participants' parents did actively steer the family's response to Depression-era conditions. Most of these participants experienced no lack of harmony or emotional support as a result of material deprivation. Franklin described his family's tenuous income as supplemented by ample affective support:

> What you have to understand is that a black lawyer in Oklahoma in the Depression years is as unemployed as an unemployed street sweeper. I mean all of his clients were not employed; therefore, he did not get any money. We lost our home and all of that sort of thing during the Depression. I had to work in college. I couldn't have stayed there without working. They did what they could but that was not all that much and I understood that. As a matter of fact, I was 16 when I went to college and I understood the limits. And I got all the encouragement that I needed from them. What they didn't have in the way of money they made up in the way of encouragement. You know? And I was stimulated to do my best.

Similarly, Lanyon's family of "working class people" had abundant appreciation for music and art, even though they "weren't a family that had the means to have leisure to travel or go to museums or go to the opera or ballet.... There simply wasn't the money. But there was encouragement in that direction, I knew that it existed".

A question asked of Oscar Peterson illustrates Differentiation-seeking through exploration and openness to new experience, even within a Depression-era context. He suggested that his parents encouraged differentiation amid scarce material resources by being both tolerant of childhood curiosity and aware of their roles as rule-makers.

Interviewer:	How did you spend most of your free time as a child?
Peterson:	Getting into mischief. (Both laugh). I was mischievous. I admit it. I was always seeking projects to do, you know finding out what made things work, things I shouldn't be fooling with. You know. I remember destroying a phonograph once, under the guise of repairing it. And things like that, I…I wasn't a bad child, in the sense that I'd go out and start fires or beat up neighborhood kids or anything like that. But I was always into little nooks and crannies, you know, getting my nose into things it shouldn't have been into. I was a very curious child.
Interviewer:	How did your parents respond? Let's say you've taken apart their phonograph. Was it—were they angry or were they like—what would they do?
Peterson:	Well, they didn't think I was another Ben Franklin. I'll tell you that (Both chuckle). They didn't react too well to it. They—they were most upset. Because don't forget those were the poverty years. And that was a tremendous luxury just having a phonograph. So you can figure the rest of that out.

The family's financial circumstances necessitated certain rules about preserving scarce resources and making material objects last, but lack of money also opened opportunities for Peterson to explore his surroundings and amuse himself.

Holton's family illustrates a possible exception to the rule that the participants' parents encouraged their children to strive beyond their financial or social limitations:

> They were a very warm family. But. My family, you know, left during the Hitler regime…. I was very young and therefore I had the possibility to enter this new country, this new life, while they could not, and therefore they were very frightened by it… And I think also, refugee families, I believe by and large, want their children to succeed in a material way, so that they will not have wants. And maybe to support them a little bit in the old age, quite rightly, you know, but above all that their children are secure somewhere. The idea of having a girl who would go off to some uncertain future, seemed to them utterly loony and terrifying, you see? And I think most refugee families who have a background like that would feel that way, perhaps.

Holton's story may exemplify a case of family warmth and protectiveness inhibiting openness to new experience, the unique physical and financial risks of the time outweighing their desire to see their daughter maximize her creative opportunities. Desire for economic security and, at that time, perhaps Holton's gender, also would have restricted the family's receptiveness to her desire to move to New York City to attend a theatrical school; it was a decision that would differentiate their daughter from the family in ways that the family could perceive as intolerable. Yet, although her family refused to offer financial support, they did not forbid her to act on her decision.

Stimulating new interests and challenges In our analysis, we distinguish between providing emotional support for existing interests and aptitudes, a marker of integration, and encouraging children to try new challenges or aspire to a higher level of skill or achievement, a marker of differentiation. Our participants' families overtly encouraged each other to grow. Peterson's father told him to "find a way" in reaction to his son's crisis of self-doubt. Many of the families insisted that the children read, write, and work hard. Dyson pointed out that understanding children's interests, even those most incompatible with the parents' own, can be a less direct, but still an effective, motivator: "They were both of them such strong characters. And yet still they left me complete freedom to do my stuff which was science. And neither of them was a scientist but they understood what it was about". Wayne Booth's grandmother encouraged a technique whereby Booth could record achievements and aspirations: keeping a diary at the age of 14, "Just a regular journal... not a small diary but a discursive diary. My grandmother gave it to me. 'You should keep a journal, because what you do is important.' And I did... As if that were, you know—I gotta have achievements".

For Booth, a particularly strong motivation to rise to a challenge resulted from a difficult family circumstance. Booth's father died when he was six, a loss provoking what Booth interpreted as an inevitable move toward autonomy and questioning. The family's Mormon faith was his first target: "Though initially, all my family rationalized the death of my father as in God's plan, I am sure that it set up a context of inquiry and doubt". The directed challenge-provocation on the part of Booth's mother manifested in his "mother always saying, 'You've got to be the man of the house now.' Which is another pressure to... achieve. 'You've got to be... your sister's father now.' I had... a sister 5 years younger than I".

Apparently, by then, Booth already had an intrinsic drive to complete his father's goal. He recalled "a kind of sense that I had to live my father's life. He died at the age of 35 just, without having—he had just finished his BA and had taught one year, when he died. So my father's life had to be lived by me". He recalled his father's death as devastating, leaving his mother "working as a first grade teacher. And with not enough money in the house, just barely able to make ends meet... emotionally I suffered terrific—I wept for—for years I was a crybaby about my father's having died". Yet, harmony and help did not become Booth's dominant needs, a refuge from accepting challenge. Instead, his loss changed his perspective of himself in relation to the world in a motivating way: "I think it really taught me, you just are not the center. And it's important for you to live your life knowing that you are not the center. And to find forms of meaning that don't have to make you the center..." As a result, what took priority became "a sense of needing to achieve, and needing to achieve not just externally, but you've got to have a life; (to) make up for that loss".

Stimulating children to take up new interests and challenges is important for the ultimate development of creativity. A developmental irony, from parents' perspective, is that new interests, and the autonomy that follows during adolescence and young adulthood, can lead children to rebel against earlier influences. Differentiated individuals might not choose precisely the path their parents would have hoped. However, in the narratives described in this study, the counterbalance of integration apparently kept the family's emotional bond and its core teachings intact, albeit, perhaps, in different forms, Wayne Booth serves as an illustration. The diary his grandmother suggested he keep served as an outlet for questioning his childhood mentors and teachers. He recounted that by the age of 17 or 18, he not only believed he was no longer the center of the universe, he decided that "I would no longer believe the Mormon theology". Furthermore, Booth rebelled against his mother's expectations for his success after he finished his PhD:

> You know, I went on a mission; came out and spent 2 years in the Army,... most of the time as a private. I deliberately eschewed all attempt to achieve; I was repudiating those norms I was telling you about. My mother wants me to be President of the United States; I'm not going to do anything other than simply read books and talk with people and, and be an intellectual.

Although he had turned away from some of his church's teaching and practices, he did not reject the idea of rigorous effort, inquiry, and belief. As he put it, "the religion of education, you might say, became my substitute; I turned from one church to the other".

Modeling habits of creativity The parents described in these interviews did not expect their children to rise to standards they themselves could not uphold. They created environments in which habits of productivity were modeled on a daily basis. Freeman Dyson, John Hope Franklin, Ellen Lanyon, Robertson Davies, and others learned important habits by imitation. Dyson, for example, described his father's intense concentration on his own creative work. Although Dyson pursued physics, not music as his father did, he interpreted the example of his father as highly significant because it demonstrated the satisfaction that can come from intense concentration on a challenging task.

Dyson: My father was a composer and so...I have perhaps more understanding of his creative process than my own, in a way.
Interviewer: Can you describe his?
Dyson: Well,... he would compose quite systematically for three hours every morning and when he was not busy with other things, he would sit down at his desk at 9 o'clock and compose until 12, He had a very strong self-discipline.

Self-discipline was the theme for Franklin as well:
My father was the most disciplined man I ever saw. And, ah, when he was not with a client... I used to go out in the office and be with him. I admired him greatly, When he was not with a client he was studying. At night he was reading or writing. And as I said in *The Life of Learning,* I thought that was what you were supposed to do in the evening. I thought that you were supposed to read or write so that is what I did and that is what I still do. People say, "Well, I will settle back and look at me some television"; well, I will settle back and do me some writing or some reading, that is just the way that I am.

Some of Lanyon's role models came from outside the immediate family and showed her some possibilities for women's achievement that were relatively uncommon at the time:

My father had these sisters who were working women, and so as a woman, I think, it was set very early in my mind that there was no reason—I mean—it never occurred to me that I couldn't do anything a man could do. So I just went ahead and did it. I didn't question it.

Davies, perhaps more than any of the other participants, learned from a family of role models working in the same field. He described how the process of writing became naturalized in his mind. Writing is a challenge, he learned, that not everyone welcomed:

Another very lucky thing for me was that I was born into a family where really everybody wrote: my father, my mother, my brothers all wrote. They were journalists and wrote newspaper things. And my father had been—he'd written fiction. I had great uncles and people like that who were journalists and commentators for newspapers and political commentators and that. And you know, I honestly say that it was—I was 12 years old before I realized that not everybody wrote all the time. I thought everybody did it, and I was astonished to find later on that some people found it dreadfully difficult. And there it was. I just grew up in a writing family, so I was very lucky in that way and in those early impressions.

In describing his interpretation of his family's tragedy, Booth raised the point that one's developmental path may not be influenced only by family members who model or insist on achievement, but also by antimodels, images of what one does not want to become:

I also had a grandfather who didn't have much of a life.... He had eight children, never had an adequate salary, we lived with him for 5 years and I saw him as a kind of dried-up, miserable, day-by-day slave to his necessary financial needs. And I think I've been kind of trying to live his life, too, to make up for his loss.

Building a demographically and psychologically diverse family unit Some interview participants grew up in families whose members represented diverse geographical backgrounds, personalities, and worldviews. Some of the families, in addition, were shaped in complex historical and cultural contexts. Some participants directly credited this diversity of family influences with opening them up to multiple ways of seeing the world and dealing with new experiences—hallmarks of differentiation. These families illustrate, in more than one way, how opposites can coexist and how children can reconcile, even capitalize on these differences.

Henderson described her mother as the nurturing counterbalance to a demanding father within a "typical patriarchal family in a typical patriarchal culture":

My mother had much less power than my father did. And my mother was really my role model. She was, you know, very loving. And always had enough time for all of her four kids. And she was the person in town, you know—I grew up in a small town of about 3,000 people. And she was the person who did the Meals on Wheels on Tuesdays and went and did the Well Baby Clinic, and everybody greeted her when we went up into the village and she knew all of the people, you know, and, and everybody sort of, you know, there was a tremendous amount of recognition and respect for her. Because she was, she is, a very good person. And so she was definitely my role model.

Yet, interpreting her family life retrospectively, Henderson came to realize that it was not exclusively her mother's influence that shaped her, but the interplay of maternal and paternal forces. She described the sometimes tense relationship between her mother and her father:

> The only thing that was really a great conflict for me was that she, she was the one who kind of got trashed in arguments with my father, of which there were quite a few. You know, he would tend to be authoritarian because that's the way… men were supposed to be. And so she never won an argument. And you know, he was always wielding power. And, I didn't want to be like him. Although I realized that power was very useful. And I did want to be like him in terms of, well, I want to be effective, and I don't want to get trashed, I don't want to be a doormat. And so that was a tremendous tension in my childhood, you know, what the hell to do with this.

Henderson was eventually able to reconcile the opposites and make them work for her. They contributed to her own creative achievement, "although I didn't particularly appreciate it or verbalize it at the time". Henderson described her insight into how psychological opposites, love and power, could be united—had to be united to effect change in the world: "Love has to be powerful. Because otherwise it's, you know, not going to be effective in the world". She reflected on people she knew who "could be very effective at doing social change, but they're afraid of power". The problem, according to Henderson, is that "They distrust themselves…There's all kinds of people doing reasonably evil things in the world that don't have any of these qualms. You know, don't you think you have a right to have your little light shine?"

Without being asked to explore the differentiated family in those terms, Davies applied the concept in his narrative, attributing his "ability to produce this enormous complex order" (the interviewer's words) to experiencing at an "impressionable age…two very sharply differentiated attitudes… apparent in my parents":

> My father had come from the United Kingdom. He came from Wales. He was very Welsh in his character. And consequently, because of him, I always had one eye turned toward the past, almost looking back toward the days of King Arthur. The Welsh have very long memories. But my mother, her family had lived in Canada since the American Revolution, and they had been the refugees from the American Revolution who had been driven north because, you know, the Americans don't like to think of it, but they were very unkind to the people who lost in the Revolutionary War, And so a lot of them had to escape north to Canada, and her family were in that group, and they were not of English descent primarily, they were mostly Dutch.

Davies, like Henderson, was able to figure out a way to reconcile polarities and use both in his decision-making throughout life:

> And so I had the old land and the new land constantly before me in my childhood and in the things that influenced me and I always was turning from one to the other, and feeling the pull of one against the other, and forming judgments about one which were related to what I had learned in the other.

Discussion

This qualitative investigation adds to the extant quantitative assessments of complexity in families by demonstrating that the Complex Family Framework can provide a useful analytical tool for the retrospective mining of family context data. It is our hope that this study, seeded in the early family lives of the participants, will encourage creativity scholars to further investigate the crucial role of a balanced interaction between integration and differentiation within the family system. Although this analysis does illuminate relationships and processes heretofore poorly understood—or presumed not to exist—it does not fully resolve issues regarding the relationship between family context and the development of creativity.

Issue 1: Is It Necessary for the Family Environment to Be Both Stimulating and Supportive?

Research on children and adolescents has suggested an important symbiosis between family stimulation and support, showing that children who feel supported by their families and challenged to develop their independence and individuality fare better than those who receive just support, just challenge, or neither (Cooper et al. 1983; Howe 1999; Irwin 1987; Rathunde 1996). Three major explanations have been offered: (a) the combination of stimulation and support helps transmit productive habits for young people, increasing the likelihood that such habits will be perceived as enjoyable, rather than as work to be avoided (Howe 1999); (b) the combination strengthens self-esteem and life satisfaction (Furstenberg et al. 1987; Wenk et al. 1994); and (c) the combination of stimulation and support creates a unique experience for young people "that makes them unusually competent" (Howe 1999, p. 433).

It is not our claim that more stimulation is necessarily better. Rather, differentiation occurs in the presence of optimal stimulation and challenge. A goodness of fit between the skill of the child and the demands of the environment is crucial. Parents who can help their children find just the right amount of challenge and stimulation are more likely to help the child negotiate an optimal person-environment fit (Rathunde and Csikszentmihalyi 2008), This position is consistent with theoretical literature such as Vygotsky's (1978) concept of scaffolding, which stresses modifying support to fit the child's skill, and by Rogoff 's (1990) research on the value of guided participation. Our position is that too much stimulation can prove counterproductive. This position is supported by Albert's (1992) caution of the risks to creative children

> when the immediate environment of family and friends organizes itself and the child too soon and loo tightly, encouraging the gifted child to foreclose on his or her identity development. When this happens—and it does—the environment prematurely shuts off or drastically reduces the range and variety of experiences and, with them, of possibilities and choices (p. 12).

Our finding is that a context of support characterized the lives of these children who later demonstrated creative achievements, a finding validated by other studies of optimal experience, as well as Milgram and Hong's (1999) longitudinal study of gifted adolescents. Our finding is also fundamentally compatible with Rogers' Theory of Creative Environments (1954), which states that constructive creativity is more likely to occur under the presence of two conditions: psychological safety and psychological freedom, the former a construct bearing similarity to Rathunde's conception of support. Rogers' theory was later validated by Harrington et al. (1987).

However, our findings about the contribution of support are at odds with a large body of literature arguing that children who will later prove creative come from families lacking harmony, Albert (1992), summarizing a long tradition in the study of eminence (e.g., Barron 1963; Brooks 1973; Dewing and Taft 1973; Getzels and Jackson 1962; Helson 1965, 1966; MacKinnon 1962, 1964, 1967; Terman 1954) characterized these families as having a *wobble* "built into many of its relationships, roles, allocation of attention and resources, and clarity of communication". That is, "the creative person-to-be comes from a family that is anything but harmonious.... Such families often generate and live through a good deal of tension if not profound disturbances most of the time" (Albert 1992, p. 175).

The present research cannot determine how the interview participants' lives would have been altered had the element of either harmony/help or stimulation/challenge been substantially altered. However, our study contributes a description of the mechanisms by which productive habits, enjoyment of one's work, self-esteem, and competence can be nurtured within families. The participants' lifetime enjoyment of a content area, resulting in domain-changing achievement, may provide some of the strongest evidence of complex, rather than one-dimensional, functioning: "The ability to enjoy work for its own sake can be... split into two seemingly opposite personality traits. Persistence, endurance, or 'driving absorption' (Roe 1952; Simonton 1988) and curiosity, openness, and intense interest" (Csikszentmihalyi and Csikszentmihalyi 1993, p. 188). No studies on the synergistic influence of family stimulation and support on optimal achievement have been published since Rathunde (1996), suggesting that the significance of these consistent findings has been missed in the field of creativity research. It is our hope that this study will help reopen the conversation.

Issue 2: What Are the Roles of Economic and Social/Cultural Capital?

Economic capital The adverse effects of poverty on cognitive development, academic achievement, and physical well-being have been well-documented (Bradley et al. 2001; Uhlenberg and Mueller 2003). A direct causal link may not be economic deprivation itself, but deprivation of support, shown in the present study to have been so important in the participants' development. Economic hardship can lead to diminished parental involvement and support, which has been associated with low self-esteem and behavior problems (Skinner et al. 1992; Whitbeck et al. 1991). Csikszentmihalyi (1999) summarized another pair of negative associations between poverty and creativity, based upon 30 years studying creativity:

> Too much deprivation does not seem to lead to innovative thinking. When survival is precarious... there is little energy left for learning and experimenting.... It is not

impossible for a talented person to emerge from a ghetto or a third-world country, but much potential is lost for lack of access to the basic tools of the domain, (p. 328)

In fact, most of the highly creative individuals considered in Csikszentmihalyi's research have represented the two socioeconomic poles, rather than the middle. Csikszentmihalyi (1999) speculated, "A person who is comfortably settled in the bosom of society has fewer incentives to change the status quo" (p. 329). As our study has shown, economic hardship can stimulate productivity.

Can family context be the great equalizer? Does it stimulate creativity that individuals can use to rise above low socioeconomic status? The present study, with a very specific and small sample, cannot make the predictive claims of studies with large samples and sophisticated statistical analyses that have demonstrated that scarcity of material resources leads to negative outcomes. In addition, regardless of methodology, cohort effects must be considered when examining the equalizing potential of complex families. The spirit of the times (Simonton 1984) and political climate, as well as the socioeconomic status of the family (Urban 1995), influence opportunities for cultivating creativity. Many of this study's participants were part of the generation that grew up during the Great Depression. Although the Depression was an experience shared by all Americans at that time, it was a transitory event. Living one's formative years during a traumatic, history-graded event, is not the same as growing up in a family that has experienced poverty across generations. However, our findings do provide a rationale for more sophisticated, quantitative investigations to explore the mitigating effects of support and stimulation on economic hardships.

Social/cultural capital Cultural capital, according to Csikszentmihalyi (1999), "consists of educational aspirations of one's parents, the nonacademic knowledge one absorbs in the home, the informal learning one picks up from home and community" (p, 328). Parental expectations, time parents spend with their children working on projects together, and transmittal of positive attitudes about hard work are influential. The literature offers much support for creativity's intergenerational effects (Albert 1980, 1996; Helson 1968; Simonton 1984), a phenomenon Albert (1996) referred to as family transfer, a process evident in the lives of many of our study's participants. Sometimes, however, unexpected deprivations of social/cultural capital such as parental favoritism (Hertig et al. 2002), parental loss (Albert 1971; Csikszentmihalyi 1996), and limited family resources (Sulloway 1996) can facilitate an individual family member's drive toward creative outcomes. Sulloway's evolutionary argument, for example, asserted that parental withholding of emotional support from some children results in their developing creative potential as they rebel in an attempt to distinguish themselves from their siblings. Simonton (1984) made a case for birth order as an additional source of differentiation within families, arguing that first-born males are more likely to excel at higher levels than their siblings.

Conclusion

One of the interview participants, reflecting on his own lifetime of creative achievement, argued that active facilitation of creativity is essential:

> It's very common to think of creativity as some very special ingredient in people's personality that leaps out like a bubbling spring, A great many people take an almost fatalistic view. You have it or you don't have it.... My own feeling is that a very substantial number of people are potentially creative but it's imprisoned. It's imprisoned by fears they develop very early, or by self-estimates they develop very early or by the constrictions of convention and so on that tell them that they can only function in certain ways.... People can... grow beyond the fears,... if they get the affirmation, sometimes on their own, sometimes with the help of mentors, that will bring out what's in them.

Forty years of optimal experience literature has demonstrated that complexity is central to the lives of creative persons. The present study's use of the Complex Family Framework contributes specific descriptions of family systems that facilitate the development of an individual's adult creativity. The participants' families were able to perform a skillful balancing act between a number of opposites: establishing ethical and material limits versus providing generous support for individual interests; spending time together versus leaving children alone; holding high expectations versus accepting experimentation and failure. Parents such as these foster integration by providing a cohesive psychological and social infrastructure and by resisting the urge to wield too much instrumental control over their children's activities, which could risk the loss of warmth and connection with children's interests and aptitudes. They foster differentiation by resisting the temptation to exercise too much emotional control, which could smother opportunities for independence and exploration. Just as the integrative principle moves parents to exercise influence by establishing support and behavioral guidelines, so the differentiating principle moves them to exercise influence by pushing children to higher levels of challenge and skill. It is our thesis that such families provide optimal conditions for cultivating creativity, environments that help children find self-fulfillment and mature into adults who can make important contributions to the culture.

References

Albert, R. S. (1971). Cognitive development and parental loss among (the gifted, the exceptionally gifted and the creative. *Psychologkai Reports, 29*, 19–26.

Albert, R. S. (1980). Family position and the attainment of eminence: A study of special family positions and special family experience. In R. S. Runco (Ed.), *Genius and eminence* (pp. 141–154). New York; Oxford University Press.

Albert, R. S. (Ed.). (1992). *Genius and eminence* (2nd ed.). New York: Pergamon.

Albert, R. S. (1994). The contribution of early family history to the achievement of eminence. In N. Colangelo & S, Assouline (Eds.), *Talent development* (pp. 311–360). Dayton: Ohio Psychology Press.

Albert, R. S. (1996). Presidential address to division 10 of the American Psychological Association: what the study of creativity can teach us. *Creativity Research Journal, 9*, 307–315.

Albert, R. S., & Runco, M. A. (1986). The achievement of eminence: A model based on a longitudinal study of exceptionally gifted boys and their families. In R. J, Sternberg & J. E. Davidson (Eds.), *Conceptions of giftedness* (pp. 332–360). Cambridge, UK: Cambridge University Press.

Amabile, T. M. (1989). *Growing up creative: Nurturing a lifetime of creativity.* New York: Crown.

Amabile, T. M. (1996). *Creativity in context.* Boulder: Westview Press.

Bakan, D. (1966). *The duality of human existence.* Chicago: Rand McNally.

Baldwin, J. M. (1911). *Thought and things: A study of the development and meaning of thought* (Vols. 3–4). New York: Macmillan.

Baltes, P., Lindenberger, U., & Staudinger, U. M. (1998). Life-span theory in developmental psychology. In R. M. Lemer (Ed.), *Handbook of child psychology: Vol. 1. Theoretical models of human development* (5th ed., pp. 1029–1143). New York: Wiley.

Barron, F. (1963). *Creativity and psychological health: Origins of personal vitality and creative freedom.* Princeton: Van Nostrand.

Baumrind, D, (1977, March). *Socialization determinants of personal agency.* Paper presented at the biennial meeting of the Society for Research in Child Development, New Orleans.

Baumrind, D. (1989). Rearing competent children. In W. Damon (Ed.), *Child development today and tomorrow* (pp. 349–378). San Francisco: Jossey-Bass.

Block, J. H., & Block, J. (1980). The role of ego-control and ego—resiliency in the organization of behavior. In W. A. Collins (Ed.), *Minnesota symposia on child psychology* (Vol. 13, pp. 39–101)., Development of cognition, affect, and social relations Hillsdale: Lawrence Erlbaum Associates.

Bloom, B. S. (Ed.). (1985). *Developing talent in young people.* New York: Ballanline Books.

Bradley, R. H., Corwyn, R. F., McAdoo, H. P., & Garcia-Coll, C. (2001). The home environments of children in the United States. Part I: Variations by age, ethnicity, and poverty status. *Child Development, 72*, 1844–1867.

Brooks, J. B. (1973). Familial antecedents and adult correlates of artistic interests in childhood. *Journal of Personality, 41*, 110–120.

Colangelo, N. (1988). Families of gifted children: The next ten years. *Roeper Review, 11*, 16–18.

Cooper, C. R., Grotevant, H. D., & Condon, S. M. (1983). Individually and connectedness in the family as a context for adolescent identity formation and role-taking skill. In H. D. Grotevant & C. R. Cooper (Eds.), *Adolescent development in the family* (pp. 43–59). San Francisco: Jossey-Bass.

Csikszentmihalyi, M. (1996). *Creativity; Flow and the psychology of discovery and invention.* New York: HarperCollins.

Csikszentmihalyi, M, (1999). Implications of a systems perspective for the study of creativity. In R. J, Sternberg (Ed.), *Handbook of creativity* (pp. 313–335). Cambridge, UK: Cambridge University Press.

Csikszentmihalyi, M., & Csikszentmihalyi, I. S. (1993). Family influences on the development of giftedness. In G. R. Block & K. Ackrill (Eds.), *Ciba Foundation Symposium. The origins and development of high ability* (Vol. 178, pp. 187–206), Chichester, England: John Wiley & Sons.

Csikszentmihalyi, M., & Larson, R. (1984). *Being adolescent: conflict and growth in the teenage years.* New York: Basic Books.

Csikszentmihalyi, M., & Larson, R. (1987). Validity and reliability of the experience sampling method. *Journal of Nervous and Mental Diseases, 175*, 526–536.

Csikszentmihalyi, M., & Rathunde, K, (1998). The development of the person: An experiential perspective on the ontogenesis of psychological complexity. In W. Damon (Series Ed.) & R. M. Lerner (Vol, Ed.), *Handbook of child psychology: Theoretical models of human development* (5th ed., Vol. 1, pp. 635–684). New York: Wiley.

Csikszentmihalyi, M., Rathunde, K., & Whalen, S. (1993). *Talented teenagers: The roots of success and failure*. Cambridge: Cambridge University Press.

Csikszentmihalyi, M., & Rochberg-Halton, E. (1981), *The meaning of things: Domestic symbols and the self* New York: Cambridge University Press.

Damon, W. (1983). *Social and personality development*. New York: Norton.

Dewing, K., & Taft, R. (1973). Some characteristics of the parents of creative twelve-year-olds. *Journal of Personality, 41*, 71–85.

Fredrickson, B. L. (1998). What good are positive emotions? *Rev Gen Psychol, 2*, 300–319.

Furstenberg, F. F, Jr, Morgan, S. P., & Allison, P. D. (1987). Parental participation and children's well-being after marital dissolution. *American Sociological Review, 52*, 695–701.

Getzels, J. W., & Csikszentmihalyi, M. (1976). *The creative vision: a longitudinal study of problem-finding in art*. New York: Wiley.

Getzels, J. W., & Jackson, P. (1962). *Creativity and intelligence: Explorations with gifted students*. New York: Wiley.

Goertzel, M. G., Goertzel, V., & Goertzel, T. G. (1978). *300 eminent personalities*. San Francisco: Jossey-Bass.

Grolevant, H. D., & Cooper, C. R. (Eds.). (1983). *Adolescent development in the family*. San Francisco: Jossey-Bass.

Harrington, D. M., Block, J. H., & Block, J. (1987). Testing aspects of Carl Rogers's theory of creative environments: Child-rearing antecedents of creative potential in young adolescents. *Journal of Personality and Social Psychology, 52*, 851–856.

Hauscr, S. T. (1991). *Adolescents and their families: Paths of ego development*. New York: Free Press.

Helson, R. (1965). Childhood interest clusters related to creativity in women. *Journal of Consulting Psychology, 29*, 352–361.

Helson, R. (1966). Personality of women with imaginative and artistic interests: the role of masculinity, originality, and other characteristics in their creativity. *Journal of Personality, 34*, 1–25.

Helson, R. (1968). Effects of sibling characteristics and parental values on creative interest and achievement. *Journal of Personality, 36*, 589–607.

Herlwig, R., Davis, J. R., & Sulloway, F. J. (2002). Parental investment: how an equity motive can produce inequity. *Psychological Bulletin, 128*, 728–745.

Howe, M. J. A. (1999). Prodigies and creativity. In R. J. Sternberg (Ed.), *Handbook of creativity* (pp. 431–446). Cambridge; Cambridge University Press.

Irwin, C. E. (Ed.). (1987). *Adolescent social behavior and health*. San Francisco: Jossey-Bass.

Maccoby, E. E., & Martin, J. Λ. (1983). Socialization in the context of the family: Parent-child interaction, In E. M. Heatherington (Ed.), *Handbook of child psychology: Socialization, personality, and social development* (Vol, 4, pp. 1–101). New York: Wiley.

MacKinnon, D. W. (1962). The nature and nurture of creative talent. *American Psychologist, 17*, 484–495.

MacKinnon, D. W. (1964). Creativity and images of the self. In: R. W. White (Ed.), *The study of lives (pp.* 250–278). New York: Atherlon.

MacKinnon, D. W. (1967). Assessing creative persons. *Journal of Creative Behavior, 1*, 291–304.

McCurdy, H. G. (1960). The childhood pattern of genius. *Horizon, 2*, 33–38.

Milgram, R. M., & Hong, E. (1999). Creative out-of-school activities in intellectually gifted adolescents as predictors of their life accomplishment in young adults: A longitudinal study. *Creativity Research Journal, 12*, 77–87.

Nakamura, J. E. (2001). The nature of vital engagement in adulthood. In M. Michaelson & J. Nakamaura (Eds.), *Supportive frameworks for youth engagement* (pp. 5–18). San Francisco: Jossey-Bass.

Nakamura, J. E. (2002). *Sustaining engagement: Continuity and change into later life (unpublished doctoral dissertation)*. Chicago: University of Chicago.

Rathunde, K. (1988). Optimal experience and the family context. In M. Csikszentmihalyi & I. S. Csikszentmihalyi (Eds.), *Optimal experience: Psychological studies of flow in consciousness* (pp. 342–363). New York: Cambridge University Press.

Rathunde, K. (1989). The context of optimal experience: An exploratory model of the family. *New Ideas in Psychology, 7,* 91–99.

Rathunde, K. (1996). Family context and talented adolescents' optimal experience in school-related activities. *Journal of Research on Adolescence, 6,* 605–628.

Rathunde, K., & Csikszentmihalyi, M. (1991). Adolescent happiness and family interaction. In K. Pillemer & K. McCartney (Eds.), *Parent—child relations throughout life* (pp. 143–162). Hillsdale: Lawrence Erlbaum Associates.

Rathunde, K., & Csikszentmihalyi, M. (2008). The developing person: An experiential perspective. In W. Damon & R. M. Lerner (Series Eds.) & R. M. Lerner (Vol. Ed.), *Handbook of Child Psychology: Theoretical models of human development* (6th ed., Vol. 1, pp. 465–515). New York: Wiley.

Roe, A. (1952). *The making of a scientist.* New York: Dodd Mead.

Rogers, C. R. (1954). Towards a theory of creativity. *ETC: A Review of General Semantics, 11,* 249–260.

Rogoff, B. (1990). *Apprenticeship in thinking: Cognitive development in social context.* New York: Oxford University Press.

Runco, M. A., & Albert, R. S. (2005). Parents' personality and the creative potential of exceptionally gifted boys. *Creativity Research Journal, 17,* 355–367.

Sawyer, R. K., John-Steiner, V., Moran, S., Sternberg, R. J., Feldman, D. H., Nakamura, J., et al. (2003). *Creativity and development.* Oxford: Oxford University Press.

Simonton, D. K. (1984). *Genius, creativity, and leadership.* Cambridge: Harvard University Press.

Simonton, D. K. (1988). Developmental antecedents of achieved eminence. *Ann Child Dev, 5,* 131–169.

Skinner, M. L., Elder, G. H, Jr, & Conger, R. D. (1992). Linking economic hardship to adolescent aggression. *Journal of Youth and Adolescence, 21,* 259–276.

Sulloway, F. J. (1996). *Born to rebel: Birth order, family dynamics, and creative lives.* New York: Pantheon.

Terman, L. M. (1954). The discovery and encouragement of exceptional talent. *American Psychologist, 9,* 221–230.

Uhlenberg, P., & Mueller, M. (2003). Family context and individual well-being: Patterns and mechanisms in life course perspective. In J. T. Mortimer & M. J. Shanahan (Eds.), *Handbook of the life course* (pp. 123–148). New York: Kluwer Academic/Plenum.

Urban, K. K. (1995). Different models in describing, exploring, explaining and nurturing creativity in society. *European Journal of High Ability, 6,* 143–159.

Vygotsky, L. (1978). *Mind in society: The development of higher psychological processes.* Cambridge: Harvard University Press.

Walberg, H. J. (1981). Childhood traits and environments of highly eminent adults. *Gifted Child Quarterly, 25,* 103–107.

Waiberg, H. J., Zhang, G., Cummings, C,, Fillipelli, L. A., Freeman, K. A., Haller, E. P., et al. (1996). Childhood traits and experiences of eminent women. *Creativity Research Journal, 9,* 97–102.

Wenk, D., Hardesly, C. L., Morgan, C. S., & Blair, S. L. (1994). The influence of parental involvement on the well-being of sons and daughters. *Journal of Marriage and the Family, 56,* 229234.

Whilbeck, L. B., Simons, R. L., Conger, R. D., Lorenz, F. 0., Huck, S., & Eider, G. H., Jr. (1991). Family economic hardship, parental support, and adolescent self-esteem. *Social Psychology Quarterly, 54,* 353–363.

Printed by Printforce, the Netherlands